Clinical Management of Voice Disorders

Clinical Management of Voice Disorders

FOURTH EDITION

James L. Case

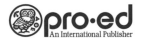

pro·ed
An International Publisher

8700 Shoal Creek Boulevard
Austin, Texas 78757-6897
800/897-3202   Fax 800/397-7633
www.proedinc.com

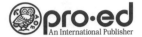
An International Publisher

© 1984, 1991, 1996, 2002 by PRO-ED, Inc.
8700 Shoal Creek Boulevard
Austin, Texas 78757-6897
800/897-3202   Fax 800/397-7633
www.proedinc.com

Library of Congress Cataloging-in-Publication Data

Case, James L.
    Clinical management of voice disorders/James L. Case.—4th ed.
        p. ; cm.
    Includes bibliographical references and indexes.
    ISBN 0-89079-883-4 (alk. paper)
    1. Voice disorders—Treatment.   2. Speech therapy.   I. Title.
    [DNLM: 1. Voice Disorders—therapy.   WV 500 C337c 2002]
    RF510.C37   2002
    616.85'5—dc21
                                                            2001048263

This book is designed in Utopia Roman and Goudy.

Printed in the United States of America

1   2   3   4   5   6   7   8   9   10   06   05   04   03   02

9/14/04

The fourth edition of this book is greeted by a new century and a new millenium. Even with all of the significant changes that have occurred leading up to these milestones, however, my dedication remains to the same individuals who have made my academic life at Arizona State University so joyful for the past 32 years.

First, I dedicate it to the many persons with voice disorders with whom I have worked and from whom I have learned so much about clinical management. Since 1996 and the third edition, I have evaluated and treated hundreds of new patients with conditions challenging even for the experienced clinician. New waves of graduate students with unique characteristics greet me each year. They seem to enjoy what and how I teach, and they challenge me intellectually and clinically to continue teaching better.

I am also profoundly appreciative of the long-term, ongoing support from my wife, Diane, and children, Jeff, Brian, Darren, and Christy, and their spouses. It is great to have happy children who marry well.

Finally, I rededicate this book to my 13 wonderful grandchildren, whose voices bring great joy to my life as I listen to them talk and sing.

Contents

Chapter 4   Clinical Management of Vocal Abuse ♦ 121

Chapter 5   Neurogenic Voice Disorders ♦ 167

Chapter 6   Psychogenic Voice Disorders   ◆   211

Chapter 7   Alaryngeal Communication   ◆   257

Chapter 8 Resonance and Miscellaneous Disorders ◆ 307

Preface

Professionals who daily manage persons with voice disorder are challenged by the many aspects of this area of communication dysfunction. Voice disorders range from a simple case of laryngitis, which usually is resolved spontaneously by time and body healing, to a life-threatening condition such as laryngeal cancer. Between these extremes the speech–language pathologist is challenged by numerous organic, psychogenic, and functional voice disorders. To manage these clients successfully requires great skill from the speech–language pathologist, along with the cooperation of many other professionals, primarily from the medical profession.

Although this book is intended primarily for speech–language pathologists, other professionals will find it helpful as a reference to voice management. It is designed to provide comprehensive coverage of the many clinical aspects of voice disorder.

I recognize that several less common voice disorders are not discussed. My focus has been on the voice disorders most often seen in clinics and discussed in the litera ture. The general principles of management, however, will likely apply to any form of voice disorder faced by the speech–language pathologist.

Chapter 1 deals with normal aspects of laryngeal and voice function, including the anatomy and physiology of laryngeal and vocal tract structures. Specific characteristics of voice, such as pitch, loudness, voice quality, and resonance, are described, as are age- and sex-related characteristics. The instrumentation that has helped clarify the inner workings of the larynx is also discussed.

In Chapter 2, I discuss some common procedures of medical management for patients with voice disorder. Medical specialties, general medical procedures generic to the evaluation and treatment of most voice disorders, information regarding common drug usage, and some common surgical techniques are covered.

Chapter 3 presents the general procedures involved in the evaluation of persons with voice disorder without respect to etiology. Principles of taking a good case history and of evaluating laryngeal parameters of pitch, loudness, and voice quality are covered. Both instrumental and perceptual evaluation procedures are discussed, along with a case example of a voice evaluation. A major focus of this chapter is the use and interpretation of video-recorded laryngeal endoscopic and stroboscopic images.

Chapter 4 studies the broad aspect of vocal abuse and phonotrauma that is common in society. The disorders of vocal nodules and contact ulcers, including details of significant etiological, symptomatic, evaluative, and treatment aspects, are covered. This chapter contains a checklist that provides a practical guide to identify most specific forms of vocal abuse as well as describe each abuse form. Case examples discuss management of vocal nodules, contact ulcers, and associated vocal abuse and misuse disorders.

In Chapter 5, on neurogenic disorders, it was difficult to determine what to include and what to omit. Entire books could have been written on many of the topics in this text, particularly neurogenic disorders. A review of general aspects of this problem lays the foundation for understanding the many neurogenic voice disorders. Several specific disorders of the nervous system that have laryngeal and voice sequelae are analyzed. Many forms of dysarthria are omitted, but the more common ones with significant voice involvement are discussed. There is considerable detail on the disorders of adductor and abductor spasmodic dysphonia, which I believe to be essentially neurogenic in etiology.

Chapter 6 covers the varied aspects of psychogenic, or nonorganic, voice disorder. One unique aspect of this chapter is the section about physiological changes in the speech system that occur under stress and other emotional states. The coverage of all mental disorders in the *Diagnostic and Statistical Manual of Mental Disorders– Fourth Edition–Text Revision* (American Psychiatric Association, 2000) provides an opportunity to discuss those mental disorders that specifically affect voice. Conversion aphonias, psychogenic dysphonias, puberphonia (mutational falsetto), and gender dysphoria voice changes are covered.

Chapter 7 includes a description of medical aspects of laryngeal cancer, with special emphasis on the speech–language pathologist's role in the rehabilitation of persons who have been laryngectomized. Details of the use of intrinsic and extrinsic forms of alaryngeal phonation are supplemented by case examples of alaryngeal management. Considerable detail on prosthetic devices for alaryngeal phonation is provided. There is a new section on recent advances in laryngeal transplant.

Chapter 8 serves two main functions: (a) to provide background for the management of persons with the resonance disorders of hypernasality and hyponasality and (b) to provide a forum for the discussion of miscellaneous disorders of voice that do not fit in previous chapters. These miscellaneous disorders include the vocal quality of persons with hearing impairment, papillomatosis, ventricular dysphonia, laryngeal webs, and other less commonly observed disorders.

I have provided a list of significant and recent references for each chapter, and these references, to both primary and secondary sources, will help readers fill gaps of information not provided directly in this text.

Anatomy and Physiology of Phonation

Any discussion of the anatomy and physiology of phonation is likely to generate in many readers as much enthusiasm as is experienced by the prisoner on death row who is about to "enjoy" a last meal. It is simply something that must be endured before the real excitement begins. One might ask whether it is necessary to know "that anatomy and physiology stuff" in such pedantic detail. Although some individuals—especially anatomy professors in university training programs—actually become excited about the details of muscle origin, insertion, course, and function or about how anatomical processes relate to each other, others might think, "Who cares?"

Nearly every book on voice disorder contains the ominous anatomy and physiology chapter, and it usually is the first one. Is this necessary? Could the author instead simply refer readers to other references on the subject and proceed to the essence of the book without the burden of all those origins, insertions, courses, and functions? After all, how much can the body change from year to year to justify such duplication? Although I contemplated referring readers to other sources, I quickly rejected the idea. Why? Even though anatomy and physiology do not change significantly by evolutionary processes from year to year or even from decade to decade, what does change from decade to decade, year to year, and even month to month is our understanding of the details involved.

Anatomy and physiology are not static sciences. This is evidenced by the fact that the physiology books used as the primary references in the earlier editions of this text are not referenced in this fourth edition. The understanding of vocal fold physiology has significantly changed, and I have cited more recent sources, often written by the same authors I referenced in earlier editions. As this chapter was being written, libraries were undoubtedly receiving new reference materials that contain significant new information about the anatomy and physiology of voice. When does one stop reading and referencing and begin writing? Science moves forward, but the presses must roll. Such a dilemma is faced by every author of a reference book.

Because many readers probably are familiar with the information in this chapter from their basic anatomy and physiology courses, this chapter is intended merely as a review of the highlights.

ANATOMY AND PHYSIOLOGY OF THE VOCAL TRACT

The birth of a human infant usually is signaled by a loud cry. That cry constitutes the infant's first attempt to signal its presence in the world and in a basic sense to establish communication, as if to say, "I am here. Please take note of my existence." Although the birth cry is reflexive and unlearned, the anatomical and physiological functions of the structures involved are extremely complex. The birth cry could be considered the initial stage of speech and language development because it is the first time the infant uses biological structures in the nonbiological function of voice in communication.

The technical term for voice production is *phonation*. It is a process of sound generation that occurs when air exhaled from the lungs is interrupted by the closed vocal folds. As exhaled air is forced through the trachea, pressure is increased below the closed vocal folds, setting them into vibration and producing a sound wave. The sound produced by the vibrating vocal folds is resonated in the chambers above and shaped into the sounds of the particular language being spoken.

The vocal folds are housed in a complex valving structure called the larynx, which is situated immediately above the trachea. The larynx as a sound generator of voice constitutes the inferior or lowest structure in the human vocal tract. Figure 1.1 shows a sagittal section through the human head and neck regions demonstrating the structures that comprise the vocal tract. In a biological sense the vocal tract also could be considered the upper respiratory tract or part of the upper digestive tract, depending on which function is being studied: respiration (breathing) or deglutition (mastication and swallowing). The vocal tract is composed of regions called the nasal cavity, oral cavity, and the pharyngeal cavities (nasopharynx, oropharynx, and laryngopharynx).

The Nasal Cavity

The most superior aspect of the vocal tract is the nasal cavity. Its superior borders are composed of the bones that form the cranial floor, the lateral margins by the nasal turbinates (conchae), the anterior aspect by nasal bones and alar cartilage of the external nose, the floor by the bony hard and muscular soft palates, and the posterior border by the pharyngeal wall.

The pharyngeal orifice for each auditory (eustachian) tube is located on each lateral and somewhat posterior wall of the nasal cavity. This auditory tube connects

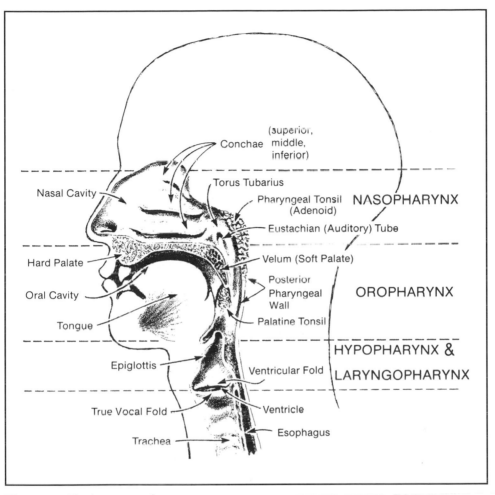

Figure 1.1. The human vocal tract.

the nasopharynx with the middle ear to maintain pressure equilibrium between the middle ear space and the external atmosphere. Also in the posterior nasopharynx is the mass of lymphoid tissue called the pharyngeal tonsils or adenoids. This tissue is often involved in velopharyngeal closure. The management of tonsil and adenoid tissue as it relates to voice and velopharyngeal closure is addressed in Chapter 8.

Biologically, the nasal cavity contains the sensory end organs from the bulbs of the olfactory nerve (cranial nerve I) for the sense of smell. During inhalation, the surface area of the nasal cavity regulates the temperature of the air and moistens and filters it. The nasal turbinates (conchae) provide an extensive surface in the nasal cavity for the accomplishment of these biological tasks.

In speech, the nasal cavity functions as a resonator when coupled to the oral and pharyngeal cavities. This coupling process occurs at the velopharyngeal port, which is located at the posterior entrance to the nasal cavity. (This process is discussed in detail later in this chapter.) Figure 1.1 shows the velopharyngeal port in an open position, as it would be during breathing and the speech production of the nasal consonants /m/, /n/, and /ŋ/. Essentially, the nasal cavity is completely separated from other cavities during the production of all speech sounds except these nasal consonants.

The Oral Cavity

The oral cavity is bounded anteriorly by the lips, anteriorly and laterally by the maxillary and mandibular dental arches, superiorly by the hard and soft palates, posteriorly by the faucial pillars and the posterior pharyngeal wall, and inferiorly by the muscular structures of the mandibular cavity and the tongue. The oral cavity is variable in its dimensions because of the movement potential of the tongue, lips, and oropharyngeal structures. In speech, the oral cavity functions as a resonator of sound produced by the larynx, and the structures contained in it serve as articulators to shape sounds into specific vowels and consonants. Biologically, the oral cavity functions in the mastication and swallowing of food and liquid.

The Pharyngeal Cavity

The pharyngeal cavity extends from the base of the skull to the lower aspect of the larynx at approximately the level of cervical vertebra number six (C-6). It is formed in a major sense by the three constrictor muscles (superior, middle, and inferior) that constitute a muscular tube or passageway from the nasal and oral cavities down to the opening to the larynx and esophagus. This passageway connects the oral and nasal cavities with the larynx, trachea, and lungs during respiration as well as with the esophagus during deglutition. In speech the pharyngeal cavity acts as a resonating cavity and forms the posterior and lateral borders of the vocal tract. The pharyngeal cavity is divided anatomically into the nasopharynx, oropharynx, and laryngopharynx (hypopharynx) as it connects these three cavities. The region above the soft palate described here as the nasopharynx has been called the posterior nasal cavity, and some authorities maintain that it should not be referred to as the nasopharynx (Cassell & Elkadi, 1995; Peterson-Falzone, Hardin-Jones, & Karnell, 2001).

Velopharyngeal Mechanisms

From a voice production standpoint, one of the most important mechanisms for resonance management in the vocal tract occurs at the velopharyngeal port. The soft palate or velum is a musculature extension from the bony hard palate that either separates or couples the oral and nasal cavities. During breathing the velopharyngeal port is open, allowing air to be drawn into and forced out through the nasal cavity. This port also is open during the articulation of the nasal consonants /m/, /n/, and /ŋ/. During deglutition and the production of all other English consonants, the velopharyngeal port essentially is closed.

The mechanisms involved in velopharyngeal closure are complex, involving different patterns and muscle groupings for deglutition and speech. The muscles include the superior constrictor, levator veli palatini, palatoglossus, palatopharyngeus (also called the palatothyroideus), and uvulas (musculi uvulae). Three additional muscles the tensor veli palatini, stylopharyngeus, and salpingopharyngeus—have origin and insertion in the area but are not directly involved in regulating the velopharynx. The tensor veli palatini primarily regulates the status of the middle ear cavity and is not considered a factor in velopharyngeal closure. Of the muscles, the levator veli palatini has received the most attention in the literature and is considered the primary muscle of velopharyngeal closure.

Superior Constrictor

The paired superior constrictor muscle (see Figure 1.2) originates from the general area of the pterygoid hamulus of the sphenoid bone and a raphe (tendon) that connects the pterygoid hamulus with the mandible (pterygomandibular raphe) continuous with the buccinator muscle anterior to the raphe. The course of the muscle is on a horizontal plane in a posterior and then medial direction to insert into the midline pharyngeal raphe. At this raphe, the fibers from the left constrictor connect to those from the right side. Upon contraction, the superior constrictor decreases the cross-sectional space of the upper pharynx. Below the superior constrictor are the middle and inferior constrictors, which complete the ring of muscles forming the bulk of the pharynx.

Levator Veli Palatini

The levator veli palatini is a paired muscle that forms the bulk of the musculature of the velum (see Figure 1.3). From a complex origin on the petrous portion of the temporal bone and lateral and posterior to the torus tubarius (the cartilage of the auditory tube), this muscle courses downward, medialward, and slightly anteriorly to enter the velum. As the muscle enters and forms the bulk of the velum, passing inferior to the uvulas muscles, a muscular sling is formed. Upon contraction of the levator muscles, the soft palate or velum is elevated and displaced posteriorly to achieve closure.

Palatoglossus

The palatoglossus is a paired muscle that influences the velum in an inferior direction. It also can be considered a muscle that lifts the posterior and lateral margins of the tongue.

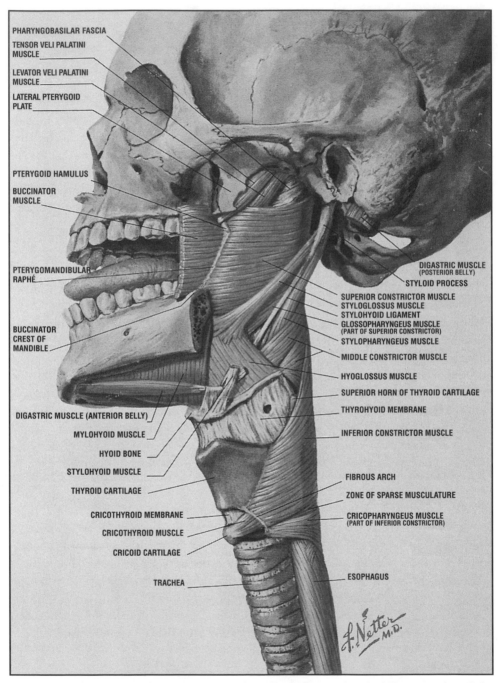

Figure 1.2. Pharynx musculature. *Note.* From *The CIBA Collection of Medical Illustrations* (p. 22), by Frank H. Netter, M.D. Copyright 1959 by CIBA-GEIGY Corporation. Reprinted with permission.

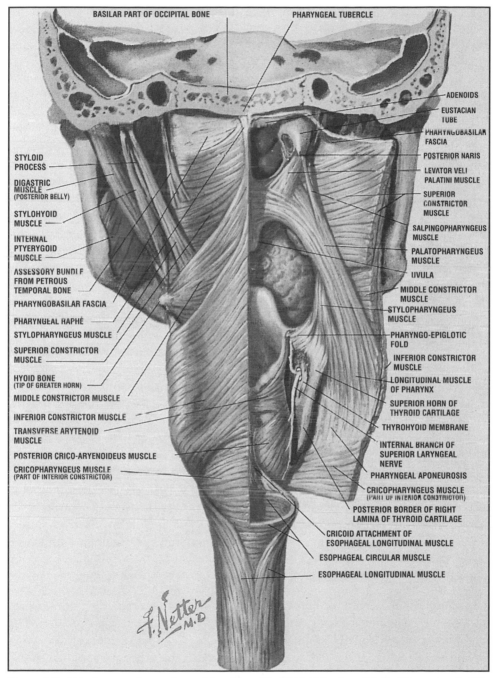

Figure 1.3. Velopharyngeal musculature. *Note.* From *The CIBA Collection of Medical Illustrations* (p. 23), by Frank H. Netter, M.D. Copyright 1959 by CIBA-GEIGY Corporation. Reprinted with permission.

It extends from the lateral margins of the velum in a downward and slightly anterior direction to insert into the tongue. The muscular basis of the anterior faucial pillar is formed by this muscle. During velopharyngeal closure, the palatoglossus is essentially passive because it works antagonistically to the levator veli palatini muscle group.

Palatopharyngeus

The palatopharyngeus is a paired muscle that can be considered a muscle of either the pharynx or the velum. It originates in the velum and courses in an inferior direction to form the muscular basis of the posterior faucial pillar. Some fibers of this muscle integrate with muscle fibers of the superior constrictor. Although not active in velopharyngeal closure in a major sense, the palatopharyngeus can function to regulate the degree of elevation of the velum in closure, acting antagonistically to the levator veli palatini. The primary functions of this muscle are to depress the velum, constrict the pharynx, or even elevate the pharynx and tonsils during swallowing. Some fibers of the palatopharyngeus course inferiorly to insert into the thyroid cartilage of the larynx, giving support for the additional name palatothyroideus (Cassell & Elkadi, 1995; Peterson-Falzone et al., 2001).

Uvulas

The uvulas muscle also is paired and forms the longitudinal midline of the velum. The origin of these paired muscles has been described as occurring on the posterior nasal spine and, generally, the posterior border of the hard palate. However, dissections have shown them to arise from the oral surface of the palatine aponeurosis, which is a band of connective tissue that binds and integrates the many muscles found in the velum. It is the palatine aponeurosis that is attached to the posterior nasal spine. The uvulas muscle courses posteriorly and then inferiorly along the superior aspect of the velum to terminate and form the bulk of the uvula. The uvulas muscle remains controversial in its contribution to velopharyngeal closure, although it most certainly contributes by adding bulk to the portion of the velum that is most directly involved in closure (Dickson & Dickson, 1982). The uvulas also can shorten the velum upon contraction.

Tensor Veli Palatini

The tensor veli palatini is a paired muscle of the velum that originates from the base of the skull, generally at the medial pterygoid plate and surrounding structures. The muscle courses vertically in an inferior direction, ending as a tendinous connection around the hamulus of the medial pterygoid plate of the sphenoid bone. From this hamulus the tensor becomes a fibrous sheet of connective tissue entering the velum. Some of the fibers attach to the posterior border of the bony palate, whereas others become continuous with fibers from the opposite side of the velum.

The tensor muscle functions more to open the normally collapsed auditory tube for middle ear ventilation than for any other activity during velopharyngeal closure.

Patterns of Velopharyngeal Closure

Examination of velopharyngeal closure processes from several angles (lateral, anterior, superior, and multiview projection), as well as by several different processes (lateral radiography, tomography, base view and Towne view projections, endoscopy, and ultrasound), shows clearly that velopharyngeal closure is accomplished by the synergistic involvement of several muscles when swallowing and speech are considered (Skolnick, 1996). The bulk of velar lifting is accomplished by the levator veli palatini. The mass of velar muscle is lifted upward and slightly posteriorly by action of this muscle.

According to most authorities, the superior constrictor muscle contributes to velopharyngeal closure. It contributes to the medial movement of the lateral walls of the pharynx and the anterior movement of the posterior pharyngeal wall. It is the muscle fibers of the superior constrictor that are involved in most instances of the Passavant's pad. Bulging of the muscle to facilitate velopharyngeal closure often seen dramatically in patients with velopharyngeal insufficiency from orofacial clefting and other etiologies (Peterson-Falzone et al., 2001).

There is little disagreement that lateral wall movement is an important part of most patterns of velopharyngeal closure. The patterns of closure were described originally by Skolnick, McCall, and Barnes (1973) and refined by Skolnick (1996). The most typical pattern appears as essentially sphincteric in nature (see Figure 1.4),

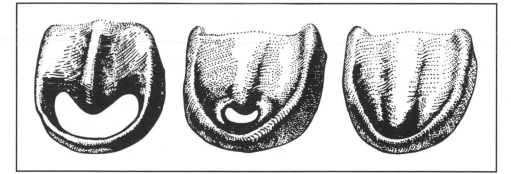

Figure 1.4. Velopharyngeal closure. Sphincteric closure of velopharyngeal portal in a normal subject seen from base view. Left: portal at rest. Middle: portal during partial closure (note that a coronal pattern is developing as velum moves posteriorly and pharyngeal walls contract centrally). Right: full closure has occurred, producing coronally oriented slit. *Note.* From "The Sphincteric Mechanisms of Velopharyngeal Closure," by M. L. Skolnick, G. N. McCall, and M. Barnes, 1973, *The Cleft Palate Journal, 10,* p. 288. Copyright 1973 by *The Cleft Palate Journal.* Reprinted with permission.

but sagittal and coronal patterns have been described and are commonly seen clinically (Peterson-Falzone et al., 2001). The pattern of closure is an important consideration for physicians who are involved in the physical management of velopharyngeal closure difficulties, because surgeries to correct abnormalities must accommodate the closure pattern present in a given individual.

Velopharyngeal closure has been studied using various technologies, including electromyographic (EMG) measurement of direct muscle activity, which provides important information regarding the muscular processes of velopharyngeal closure (Kuehn & Moon, 1998, 2000). It has also been studied using radiological examination techniques and endoscopic visualizations. Bell-Berti (1976) obtained EMG recordings from the levator veli palatini, superior constrictor, middle constrictor, palatoglossus, and palatopharyngeus muscles of three normal speakers of American English. The levator veli palatini was found to be the primary muscle of velopharyngeal closure for each of the subjects. This finding was corroborated by Moon, Smith, Folkins, Lemke, and Gartlan (1994), although they stated that an interaction exists between the levator veli palatini, the palatoglossus, and the palatopharyngeus muscles when all velar positions are considered.

Velopharyngeal closure is very complex in its normal function. For example, when a person with normal closure says, "I'll paint it," the soft palate or velum is closed for all sounds until the /n/ in "paint." The brain sends messages via the nerves innervating closure, directing the closure muscles to relax. This allows rapid opening of the velopharyngeal port and nasal resonation to occur on the /n/ sound. A reversal of this process is needed instantaneously, however, because the nasal sound /n/ is immediately followed by a nonnasal /t/. For the pressure for the /t/ sound to be released orally, complete velopharyngeal closure must occur. These rapid and precise movements are necessary to articulate accurately one word containing a nasal consonant (e.g., "paint"), and the complexity of the process is magnified in an ongoing stream of verbal behavior in which the nasal consonants /m/, /n/, and /ŋ/ are liberally disbursed. Dalston and Keefe (1988) described the reaction time of velopharyngeal closure using a photodetector system and determined an average reaction time of 206 msec among typical speakers. In participants ranging in age from the 20s to the 80s, Hoit, Watson, Hixon, McMahon, and Johnson (1994) found no age-related differences in nasal airflow.

An excellent overall description of the complex and interactive forces of all these muscles on velopharyngeal opening (for nasal respiration) and closing (for speech, voice, and swallowing functions) was provided by Berry, Moon, and Kuehn (1999). They projected a finite-element model of how the soft palate functions for a theoretical 10-year-old child based on previous histologic studies of muscles and tissues. Their model is complex, but the outgrowth description of how the soft palate functions during speech is very helpful. More information is provided on the complex process of velopharyngeal closure and concerns in clinical populations in Chapter 8.

ANATOMY AND PHYSIOLOGY OF THE LARYNX

The larynx is composed of one bone, five major cartilages, four minor cartilages, and several intrinsic and extrinsic muscles, all bound together by complex ligaments and membranes into a functional unit (see Table 1.1). The adult larynx is situated at the superior aspect of the trachea, just anterior to the third through sixth cervical vertebrae (see also Figure 1.1).

The Hyoid Bone

The single bone involved in the laryngeal region is the hyoid, which can be considered a bone of the tongue and pharynx because muscles of the tongue and pharynx attach to it from above, or of the larynx because structures of the larynx (muscles and cartilages) attach to it from below.

Figure 1.1 shows the relationship between the larynx (vocal folds) at the top of the respiratory tract and the esophagus leading to the stomach. During swallowing, the larynx is tilted and sphincterically closes so that food or liquid is channeled into the esophagus, avoiding the respiratory tract. This valving process during swallowing is controversial but likely occurs on three levels: inferior, the true vocal folds; middle, the ventricular folds; and superior, the epiglottis and aryepiglottic folds. This closure process most likely occurs from inferior to superior, and duration is increased

TABLE 1.1
Components of the Larynx

Major Cartilages	Minor Cartilages
Cricoid (unpaired)	Corniculate (paired)
Thyroid (unpaired)	Cuneiform (paired)
Arytenoids (paired)	
Epiglottis (unpaired)	**Bone**
	Hyoid
Intrinsics	
Posterior cricoarytenoids	**Extrinsics**
Lateral cricoarytenoids	Stylohyoids
Transverse arytenoids	Digastrics
Oblique arytenoids	Geniohyoids
Thyroarytenoids	Thyrohyoids
Cricothyroids	Sternohyoids
	Sternothyroids
	Omohyoids

as bolus size is increased. Swallowing is also accompanied by an elevation of the larynx and pharynx at the initiation of the swallow (Logemann, 1998a, 1998b).

The larynx can be seen and detected externally by palpating the laryngeal prominence in the middle of the neck. This prominence is more easily identified in adult males. During swallowing, the marked tilting of the larynx can be observed easily. The hyoid bone (body) can be palpated just superior to the laryngeal prominence; just inferior to the prominence, the anterior ring of the cricoid cartilage can be detected. Other than these significant landmarks, the intricate structures that compose the larynx are hidden from external view except through peroral inspection with a mirror, laryngoscope, or endoscope.

The Five Major Cartilages

The five major cartilages that comprise the larynx are the unpaired cricoid, the unpaired thyroid, the two paired arytenoid cartilages, and the unpaired epiglottis. Figures 1.5 and 1.6 show the functional relationships of these five cartilages.

The Cricoid Cartilage

The cricoid cartilage constitutes a superior extension of the top tracheal cartilage with an approximate diameter of the trachea. It is shaped similarly to a signet ring that would fit loosely on the typical little finger, giving perspective to its size dimensions. Its major landmarks include an anteriorly directed arch or ring and a large posterior quadrate (four-sided) lamina. Four articular facets (surfaces for articulation) are located on the cricoid: two on the lateral aspect of the quadrate lamina to which the thyroid cartilage attaches and two on the superior aspect of the lamina for arytenoid articulation. The cricoid cartilage attaches inferiorly to the superior ring of the trachea by means of the cricotracheal membrane or ligament (Zemlin, 1998).

The Unpaired Thyroid

The largest of the laryngeal cartilages is the unpaired thyroid, which consists of two rather large, flat plates called the thyroid lamina. These lamina are joined anteriorly to form the thyroid angle. Although Aronson (1990) and Citardi, Gracco, and Sasaki (1995) stated that the angle of the thyroid is significantly different between postpubescent males (90°) and females (120°) and that this angle difference is an important factor in pitch differences between the sexes, Kahane (1982) reported the angle difference to be much less (mean values of 84.2° for males and 92.5° for females). Kahane's findings are compatible with several studies of thyroid angles in males and females (Zemlin, 1998). Regardless of the angle, the superior aspect just below the thyroid notch forms the laryngeal prominence, or the Adam's apple, which

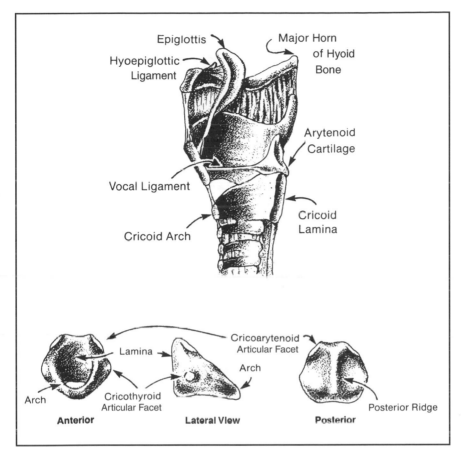

Figure 1.5. Laryngeal cartilages.

is easily identified in most males. This prominence is the most anterior aspect of the larynx.

Arising from the superior surface of each thyroid lamina is the superior horn, which indirectly attaches to the major horn of the hyoid bone. The remaining space between the superior aspect of the thyroid and the hyoid bone is filled with the thyrohyoid membrane. The superior aspect of each thyroid lamina depresses downward in front to form the thyroid notch just above the angle. This notch is easily palpated and helps in the identification of these laryngeal landmarks.

The essential landmarks of the thyroid cartilage are completed by the paired inferior horns that extend from the posterior and inferior aspects of each thyroid lamina to articulate on the lateral aspects of the posterior quadrate lamina of the cricoid.

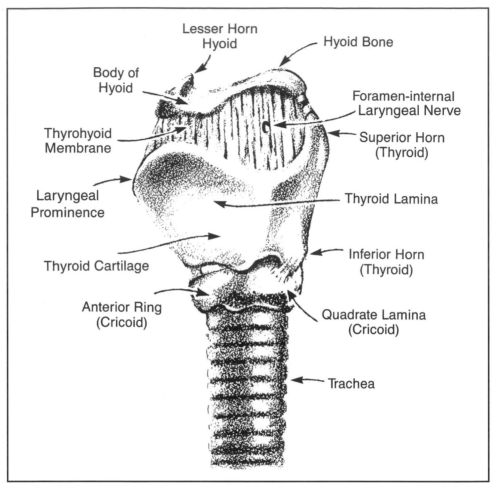

Figure 1.6. Laryngeal cartilages: lateral view.

This joint between the thyroid and the cricoid is the most significant factor in voice pitch adjustments. (The functional aspects of this joint relationship are discussed in detail later in this chapter.)

The Paired Arytenoid Cartilages

The tiny and complex paired arytenoid cartilages are responsible for most of the laryngeal valving processes involved in biological and phonation functions of the larynx. Each arytenoid is composed of three significant processes. From a posterior view, the apex and muscular processes are well defined. A lateral view of a sagittal section through an arytenoid cartilage reveals the vocal process directed anteriorly

thyroarytenoid when stained to distinguish fast twitch from slow twitch fibers. In humans, the vocalis region of the thyroarytenoid is composed of many slow twitch fibers, whereas the muscularis region is composed of high concentrations of fast twitch fibers (Sanders, 1995).

Posterior Cricoarytenoid

The posterior cricoarytenoid is a fan shaped paired muscle that originates on the posterior surface of the quadrate lamina of the cricoid. It courses and converges in a lateral direction to insert on the posterior surface of the muscular process of the arytenoid by means of extensive ligaments. Contraction of the posterior cricoarytenoid functions to rock and slide each arytenoid along a longitudinal axis on the cricoid. The effect of such contraction is to part the arytenoid cartilages and open, or abduct, the glottis. Upon contraction, the posterior cricoarytenoid functions to also slightly elevate, elongate, and thin the vocal fold by rocking the arytenoid cartilage in a posterolateral direction (Sataloff, 1998c). The converging nature of this muscle generates force at excellent mechanical advantage in abduction of the vocal folds. Laryngeal dilation or abduction occurs entirely by the function of the posterior cricoarytenoid (Figure 1.7).

The role of the posterior cricoarytenoid during speech is somewhat controversial, because its primary function is to abduct the vocal folds for respiration purposes. However, it is clear that during speech there are voiced and unvoiced segments, and the posterior cricoarytenoid is considered an important articulator in facilitating quick voiceless functions during speech. It is also likely that the posterior cricoarytenoid functions to counterbalance the tension of the vocal folds during high intensities of human voice, contributing to the fine-tuned mechanisms of phonation (Sanders, 1995).

Lateral Cricoarytenoid

The lateral cricoarytenoid muscle is paired and originates on the superior and lateral surface of the cricoid arch. It courses posteriorly and slightly superiorly to inset on the lateral aspect of the muscular process of the arytenoid in a plane almost directly antagonistic to the posterior cricoarytenoid. It functions to facilitate glottal closure by adducting, slightly lowering, and thinning the vocal fold. The primary function of this muscle is to help facilitate closure of the vocal fold tissue (Sataloff, 1998c; see Figure 1.7).

Transverse Arytenoid

The unpaired transverse arytenoid (also called the interarytenoid) muscle extends across the posterior surface of each arytenoid cartilage, entirely covering the surface. Upon contraction the transverse arytenoid functions to slide the arytenoid cartilages medially to adduct the glottis (see Figure 1.7).

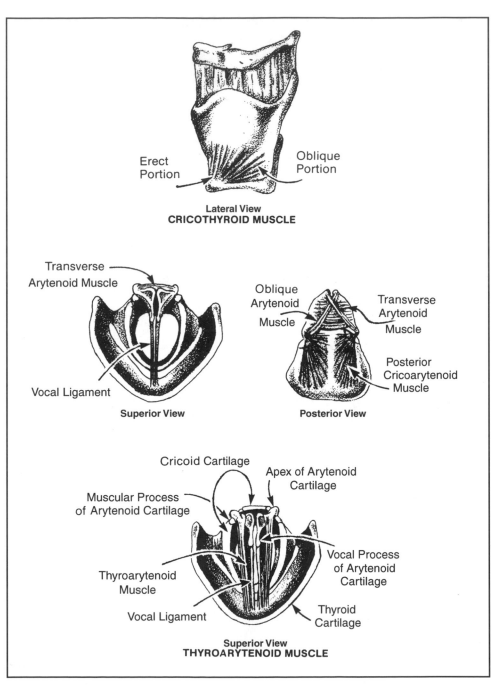

Figure 1.7. Intrinsic laryngeal muscles.

Oblique Arytenoid

The oblique arytenoid is a paired muscle that crosses superficially to the transverse arytenoid from the base of one transverse arytenoid cartilage to the apex of the other (see Figure 1.7.) In harmony with the transverse arytenoid, the oblique arytenoid functions to adduct the arytenoid and the glottis. Some of the fibers of this muscle extend beyond each apex and become the aryepiglottic muscle forming the aryepiglottic fold.

Cricothyroid

The cricothyroid is a paired muscle that is divided into erect and oblique portions (pars recta and pars oblique). The cricothyroid muscle directly influences the cricothyroid joint in such a manner that the cricoid arch is adducted in relation to the thyroid cartilage. The limit of this joint movement is determined by the restricting influence of the ligaments that connect the inferior horn of the thyroid to the cricoid on each side. Upon contraction of the cricothyroid muscle, either the cricoid is moved relative to the thyroid (A. E. Aronson, 1990) or vice versa (Dickson & Dickson, 1982; Seikel et al., 1997). In either case, the relative distance between the arytenoid cartilages positioned on the cricoid and the thyroid cartilage is increased when this muscle contracts. Thus the paired cricothyroid muscle is responsible for increasing the length of the vocal folds. This increase produces stretching of the vocal folds, which in turn causes an increase in longitudinal tension and a decrease in cross-sectional mass. Under these conditions the fundamental frequency of vocal fold vibration rises, which is heard as increased pitch. The cricothyroid muscle also adducts the vocal folds by generating longitudinal tension (see Figure 1.7). In addtion, the cricothyroid muscle is likely a significant factor in producing the changes in the vocal fold tension that result in normal jitter (cycle-to-cycle variation in frequency) measurements (Larson et al., 1987).

Membranes of the Larnyx

Several connective tissue membranes bind and integrate the cartilages and muscles of the larynx into a functional valving mechanism. The thyrohyoid membrane fills the space from the superior margin of the thyroid cartilage to the hyoid bone (see Figure 1.6). Another mass of connective tissue is the quadrangular membrane that binds the aryepiglottic folds superiorly and the ventricular folds inferiorly.

The conus elasticus is composed mainly of yellow elastic tissue and is divided into an anterior and two lateral portions. The anterior portion fills the space between the inferior thyroid margin and the anterior arch of the cricoid. The lateral portions are thinner and fill the lateral portions of the larynx close to the mucous membrane that lines the larynx. The superior border of the conus elasticus becomes the fibrous tissue that covers the vocalis muscle and acts as a cushion to protect the folds from mechanical damage that may be caused by the constant vibration of the vocal folds. This fibrous cushion is called the lamina propria (vocal ligament) and is divided into superficial, intermediate, and deep layers (Hirano, Kurita, & Nakashima, 1981; Sataloff, 1998c; Figure 1.8).

The Vocal Folds

The vocal folds constitute one of the valving mechanisms in the larynx that protect the respiratory tract. They also are the source of air impedance in phonation. They are composed of muscle, connective tissue, and epithelium. A coronal section through the larynx reveals these combination layers of tissue (see Figure 1.8).

The bulk of the vocal fold is composed of the vocalis muscle, which, as discussed previously, constitutes the medial portion of the thyroarytenoid. Surrounding the muscular portion of the vocal fold are the tissues of the lamina propria (superficial, intermediate, and deep layers). A basement membrane provides a transition from the epidermal cell layers and the superficial layer of the lamina propria and is a site for phonotrauma. This region and the superficial layer of the lamina propria are vulnerable to vocal abuse or misuse and resultant Reinke's edema. The layered structure of the lamina propria, which varies along the length of the vocal fold, is thickest at the midportion of the vocal fold and becomes thinner toward the anterior and posterior aspects. Variance in the relative contribution of the superficial, intermediate, and deep layers also occurs along the anterior and posterior dimensions of the vocal fold (Sataloff, 1998c).

The vocalis muscle and lamina propria are covered by stratified squamous epithelium, which also varies in thickness along the length of the vocal fold, with the greatest thickness in the middle region. The squamous epithelial layer differs from the mucosa of most surrounding tissues in the larynx that are involved in biological valving (e.g., the ventricular folds). These tissues are lined with columnar epithelium.

Although the structural layers of the vocal folds seem to vary between children and adults, little variance is seen between adult sexes. Titze (1994) stated that the vibrating tissue that constitutes the vocal folds is composed of the cover (epithelium and superficial layer of the lamina propria), the transitional tissue (intermediate and deep layers of the lamina propria), and the body (vocalis muscle).

The blood supply to the vocal fold is an important consideration for understanding normal and pathological larynges. The larynx is supplied by (a) the superior laryngeal artery, (b) the cricothyroid branch of the superior thyroid artery, and (c) the inferior laryngeal artery. These arteries are branches of the thyroid artery from the

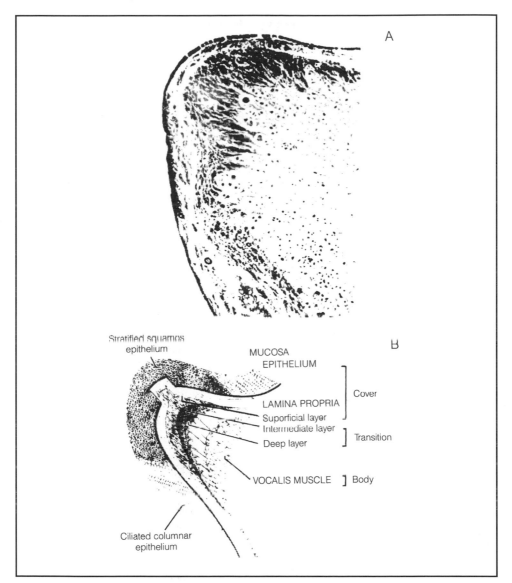

Figure 1.8. Larynx: coronal view through vocal folds. *Note.* From "The Structure of the Vocal Cords," by M. Hirano, S. Kurita, and T. Nakashima, in *Vocal Fold Physiology* (p. 34), by K. N. Stevens and M. Hirano (Eds.), 1981, Tokyo: Tokyo University Press. Copyright 1981 by Tokyo University Press. Reprinted with permission.

external carotid artery. Angiography of the vocal folds in fresh cadavers has revealed the following:

- Vessels of the free edge run parallel to the longitudinal axis of the vocal fold.

- The bloodstream on the free edge flows posteriorly from the anterior end and anteriorly from the posterior end of the fold.

- The blood vessels in the mucosal free edge are clearly differentiated from upper and lower mucosal surfaces of the vocal fold as well as from the vocalis muscle portion.

- A reticulated vascular network in the midportion of the vocal fold provides for blood distribution.

- The distribution and direction of blood flow are highly suitable for a structure undergoing constant mechanical vibration.

- The blood volume of the vocal fold decreases markedly during vibration. If this did not occur, the distribution and circulation of blood would be markedly disturbed during vibration. This blood reduction constitutes a fail-safe system to prevent abnormal hemorrhaging as a result of normal vibration (Titze, 1994).

- A slight rise in temperature of the vibrating vocal folds occurs during phonation as a result of viscous friction, which complements what would ordinarily be a drop in temperature with reduced blood flow during phonation (Cooper & Titze, 1985).

From a superior view (see Figure 1.9), the vocal folds appear as the most medial projection from the lateral walls of the larynx. Between the vocal folds is the variable fissure or chink called the glottis. The glottis is the space between the vocal folds formed by the rima glottis, which is the margin of the vocal folds medially. The anterior-to-posterior dimensions of the glottis are divided into the intermembranous and intercartilaginous portions. The intermembranous portion includes the glottal length from the most anterior point to the junction of the vocal processes and the muscular folds. The point where the vocal folds converge anteriorly is called the anterior commissure. The intercartilaginous portion is the remaining area formed by the vocal processes of the arytenoid. The posterior border of the glottis is often called the posterior commissure, but this is incorrect because it is merely the posterior aspect of the glottis.

Figures 1.10 and 1.11 show the vocal folds of a 25-year-old nondysphonic woman in two stages of vibration. Figure 1.10 shows the arytenoid cartilages in an adducted state bringing the vocal folds together at the closed phase of a vibratory cycle. There is a slight opening in the posterior aspect of the glottis, which is normal in females. Figure 1.11 shows the vocal folds as they are being opened by air pressure during phonation. The photo has captured an opening phase of the vibratory cycle; the arytenoid cartilages remain in an adducted or closed phase during phonation.

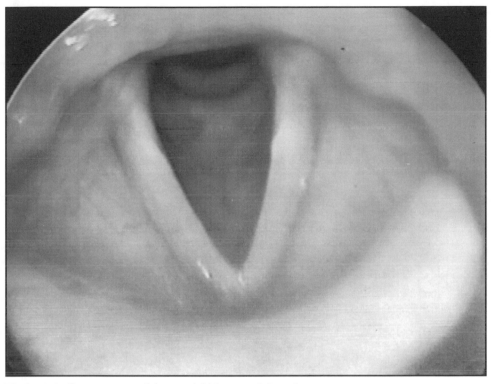

Figure 1.9. Superior view of the vocal folds in an abducted state.

Under light inspection the color of the vocal folds appears whitish compared with the pinkish tone of the surrounding tissues. This whitish appearance is caused by a reduced blood supply to the vocal folds and also by the tightly bound squamous epithelial covering of the vocal folds, which provides a highly reflective surface to the light. The white color is one indicator of healthy vocal folds.

PHONATION THEORY

Two theories of phonation have prevailed in the voice science literature: neurochronaxic and myoelastic–aerodynamic. The neurochronaxic theory holds that the vibration process of the vocal folds in phonation occurs in response to individual neural impulses, causing the abduction–adduction necessary to produce glottal pulsing. In direct conflict is the myoelastic–aerodynamic theory, which explains phonation as a phenomenon of passive vibration of the vocal folds in response to subglottal airflow and pressure.

Phonation is undoubtedly a myoelastic–aerodynamic phenomenon (Titze, 1994). The process of using airflow and pressure through a constriction to produce vibration

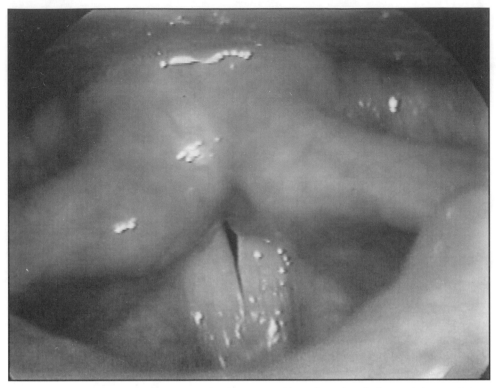

Figure 1.10. Superior view of the vocal folds in an adducted or closed phase of glottic closure. Arytenoid cartilages are adducted, bringing the vocal folds into this position. Slight opening in the posterior aspect is normal in this 25-year-old woman.

of tissue can be demonstrated through an analogy. Lips vibrate if they are relaxed in light approximation and air is forcibly blown from the lungs through the mouth. Horses do it all the time to generate the sound that can almost always be identified as coming from a horse. The lips vibrate in rhythmic response to airflow and oral pressure. In phonation, this same process occurs as the adducted vocal folds are blown apart in rhythmic sequence in response to airflow from the lungs and subglottal pressure.

It is important to understand the concept of normal variability in the anatomy and physiology of the normal larynx. We all notice variation in human faces, each composed of one nose, two eyes, and one mouth with lips, and each combination forms a unique but normal and recognizably unique pattern. Similar normal variation occurs in the form and function of the human larynx. Casper, Brewer, and Colton (1987) documented variations in configuration and movement patterns in selected laryngeal structures during a phonation protocol among men and women. They observed these variations using fiber optics. The authors concluded that, when no

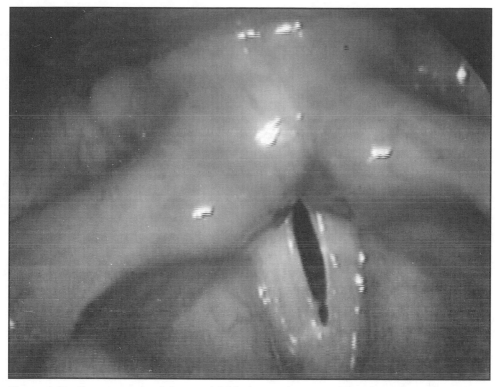

Figure 1.11. Superior view of the vocal folds during phonation. The photo shows the opening phase of the vibratory cycle.

clear tissue changes or lesions are observed, distinction between normal and abnormal variation is indeed difficult and at times impossible.

Although the process of phonation, as described, seems simple, it is actually very complex when studied in detail. Information on vibration patterns has been obtained by such research methods as fiber-optic endoscopy and stroboscopy (Cranen & de Jong, 2000), high-speed digital image recording (Kiritani, 2000), aerodynamic methodology (Hillman & Kobler, 2000), electroglottography (Fourcin, 2000; Scherer, 1995), and other methodologies that are less common (Kent & Ball, 2000).

PHASES OF PHONATION

Phonation has been considered on a continuum of difficulty, ranging from a simplistic view of an encyclopedic description to one of the most complex phenomena of human physiology. Titze (1994) described phonation as a process of vocal fold oscillation, which includes several mechanisms for self-sustained oscillation. The energy source for phonation is the exhaled respiratory airstream. The vocal folds function in simple harmonic oscillation because of the mass, stiffness, and internal interactive forces present when the aeromechanical forces stimulate vibration. Titze explained these factors from a descriptive and mathematical point of view. The following is a more general description of the various stages of a typical cycle of phonation. Although it is not very detailed, perhaps it is practical for the speech–language pathologist to use when describing phonation to a client.

Phonation can be described by detailing three phases of vibration: opening, closing, and closed. When a person initiates phonation by exhaling air, the vocal folds are set near the paramedian position. In this position, the mucous membrane of the vocal folds begins to move as a rippling wave. Several vibrations of this ripple effect occur before the glottis completely closes.

Complete closure of the glottis is effected by the adductive musculature moving the arytenoid cartilages into medial compression. As this is happening, air from the lungs through the trachea is forced through an increasingly narrowed glottis. According to Bernoulli's principle, as the glottis narrows, air is forced through the constriction with increased velocity, increasing the intermolecular space of the air molecules and causing a drop in pressure at the point of constriction. The final effect of these pressure-flow dynamics involved in Bernoulli's principle is complete medial compression of the vocal folds along their entire medial surfaces as a result of the suction created by the negative or dropped pressure.

It is difficult to imagine how airflow can generate such negative pressure. This can be demonstrated, however, by holding two pieces of typing paper close together and blowing air between them. The papers will vibrate and will be sucked together during portions of the vibration cycle. This same effect occurs in the larynx between the vocal folds. The main difference is that vocal folds are designed to respond to these forces and typing paper is not.

With the vocal folds in a closed state, one cycle can be analyzed further. The glottal closure causes an increase in subglottal pressure until it is sufficient to overcome glottal resistance. When this happens, the opening phase of vibration begins. In this phase, the vocal folds are blown upward in a traveling wave that undulates from the lower lip of each vocal fold to the upper lip.

After the pressure has forced the vocal folds apart completely, the closing phase begins. This closure process also undulates upward from this lower lip contact until the entire medial surface of the vocal fold is closed once again. This closed phase remains complete for a time that depends on the intensity of the sound being produced. After the duration of the closed phase, the cycle repeats itself in the same fashion. Each cycle involves this undulating traveling wave from the lower lip to the upper in both the opening and closing phases.

These rhythmic pulses produced by the vibrating vocal folds constitute the glottal tone. The frequency of the tone depends on the number of cycles occurring each second. The glottal tone or waveform represents a sound wave of compressed and rarefied air molecules. These sound wave vibrations then are resonated by the chambers of the vocal tract.

The sound that is present in the vocal tract under conditions of phonation is composed of the fundamental frequency of vibration and harmonics of the fundamental. The harmonics are multiples of the fundamental, so if the fundamental were a 100-hertz (Hz) tone, the multiples would be 200, 300, 400, 500 Hz, and so on. Thus a complex tone is present in the vocal tract, where it is resonated and shaped into the vowels and consonants of the language being spoken. Underlying these sounds of the language is the voice of the speaker. For details of how vocal tract resonance shapes various vowels and how movement of the speech articulators modifies the airstream and waveform into the consonants of speech, see Baken and Daniloff (1991), Orlikoff and Baken (1993), Kent (1997), and Kent and Ball (2000).

SPECIFIC CHARACTERISTICS OF VOICE

The basic sound produced by the vibrating vocal folds is characterized by parameters of frequency, intensity, and quality. Frequency and intensity are dependent on factors at the level of the vocal folds or below in the respiratory system. Vocal quality is a function of characteristics in the vibrating vocal folds coupled with factors of resonance.

Frequency

Voice frequency is determined by the rate of vibration, or cycles that occur each second. This value is expressed in hertz (Hz). If a person's vocal folds were vibrating 100 times each second, that individual's fundamental frequency (F_0) would equal 100 Hz. Frequency is a physical measurement expressed in hertz; its psychophysical or perceptual correlate is pitch. Frequency and pitch are roughly equivalent; the frequency is the specific hertz of the tone, and the pitch is what the listener hears or perceives. Frequency also can be expressed as a musical scale value. For example, the 100-Hz tone essentially corresponds to the note G_2, meaning two Gs below middle C on the musical scale.

Several factors determine the specific F_0 of vibration: (a) the length of the vocal folds, (b) the cross-sectional mass of the vocal folds, and (c) the longitudinal tension of the vocal folds. Subglottal pressure also influences frequency but in a less significant manner. Length, cross-sectional mass, and tension interact to account for intersubject and intrasubject differences in frequency or pitch. Longer and thicker vocal folds vibrate slower, producing a lower frequency. Adult males typically have longer and thicker vocal folds than females and thus have lower pitches. These sex differences in pitch do not occur until puberty.

In a study on voice frequency, Kempster, Larson, and Kistler (1988) found that stimulation of both the cricothyroid and the thyroarytenoid muscles produces elevation of vocal pitch. They reported that the thyroarytenoid muscle has a faster contraction speed than the cricothyroid, but both synergistically function to raise the pitch.

Factors in Frequency Fundamental Change

Changes in longitudinal tension of the vocal folds account for intrasubject increases or decreases in pitch. The anatomical and physiological mechanisms involved in altering longitudinal tension are found in the cricothyroid and thyroarytenoid musculature. Contraction of the cricothyroid muscle modifies the relationship of the cricoid relative to the thyroid cartilages, increasing the thyroarytenoid distance. Because posteriorly the vocal folds are attached to the arytenoid cartilages riding the cricoid, and anteriorly the vocal folds are attached to the thyroid, this increased distancing has the effect of stretching the vocal folds and increasing their longitudinal tension. Under this stretching condition the vocal fold frequency of vibration increases and the pitch rises. A similar phenomenon occurs when the tension is increased on a guitar or piano string: The frequency or pitch rises as tension is increased.

The increased longitudinal tension produced by cricothyroid contraction can be complemented by simultaneous contraction of the vocalis muscle. Vocalis contraction generates an isometric tension in the vocal fold when it occurs with cricothyroid contraction. Increased vocal fold tension results from this synergistic effect.

It can be confusing when trying to understand the relationship between greater *length* as being associated with lower frequency vibration in intersubject comparisons and greater *lengthening* as producing higher frequency vibrations in intrasubject changes. It is helpful to remember that greater lengthening within a subject is associated with a corresponding reduction of cross-sectional mass of the vocal fold and an increase in longitudinal tension, which accounts for the higher pitch.

As expected, vocal folds producing a low-frequency sound are thicker than vocal folds producing higher pitches. For example, in falsetto the vocal folds are sufficiently tense to decrease the vertical layer of the vibrating vocal fold, eradicating the influence of the upper and lower lips (Kent & Ball, 2000).

One significant factor involving frequency and pitch is pitch variability. Cycle-by-cycle frequency variation in a speech signal is called pitch perturbation or jitter (see Figure 1.12). Horii (1982a) defined *jitter* as the average period difference between consecutive cycles divided by the average period. The difference must be unintended, with the person under observation producing a tone that is as steady as possible. This

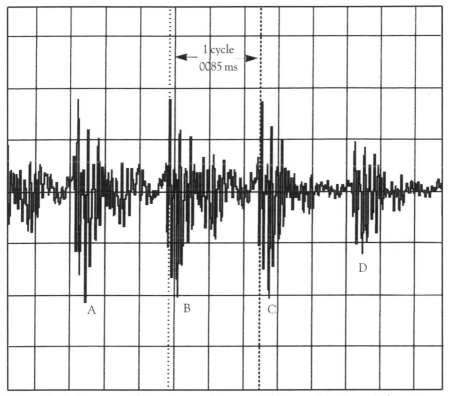

Figure 1.12. Spectrographic printout of jitter and shimmer. A to B to C shows jitter. C to D shows shimmer.

value can be expressed as a percentage by multiplying it by 100. Horii found an average jitter value of .75% among eight English vowels produced by 20 adult males with no laryngeal pathology.

Increased jitter is one vocal characteristic noted in the voice spectrum of persons with laryngeal pathology. Brown, Morris, and Michel (1989) reported data, summarized by Kent (1994b), that indicate that mean jitter ratio values (mean jitter in milliseconds divided by the period in milliseconds times 100) range between .50% and .90%. Perhaps the most significant finding of their study relates to the stability of jitter as a measure of normal phonation. Comparing jitter ratio (and other values not reported here) among healthy young and older female speakers, they found no significant change in jitter ratio as a function of aging. This conclusion was essentially restated by Kent and Ball (2000), with added insight into overall variability seen in the aging voice, which might be influenced by increased jitter, particularly when health and fitness issues are eliminated.

Another important concern in jitter analysis is the method of capturing the vocal signal for analysis. Doherty and Shipp (1988) found that jitter analysis is best obtained from live samples because recorded samples introduce abnormal jitter to the signal. The following indicates the descending order of adequacy for speech samples: direct sampling, digital audiotape (DAT) recordings, frequency modulation (FM) recordings, audio reel-to-reel recordings, and audiocassette recordings. The latter should be avoided.

Intensity

The intensity of a sound produced by the vocal mechanism is the physical measurement of sound pressure and is expressed in decibels (dB). The psychological correlate of intensity is loudness. Intensity and loudness are roughly equivalent: The intensity of a sound is a specific decibel level, and the loudness is the sound level perceived by the listener. Several factors are responsible for increases in the intensity or loudness of a vocal sound: (a) increased airflow from the lungs and (b) increased resistance to flow by the vocal folds, which together cause (c) increased subglottal pressure.

Increased resistance to flow is equivalent to greater medial compression by the vocal folds. If the vocal folds do not resist this increased airflow, the resulting sound merely sounds breathier. When resistance occurs, however, greater pressure builds below the closure for each vibration. The result is greater compression of air molecules in the trachea below the glottis. When this compressed air finally overcomes the laryngeal resistance and displaces the vocal folds, the compression wave released collides with the column of air in the vocal tract with greater energy, sending a more intense shock wave into the vocal tract. The result is a sound with greater intensity, which is perceived as louder. To sustain this intense sound, the greater airflow and glottal resistance must be maintained.

The intensity of the human voice must vary to sustain the prosodic factors of stress and intonation. A normal adult larynx is capable of generating a tone of 100 to 108 dB at a distance of about 1 meter from the mouth (Daniloff, Schuckers, & Feth, 1980; Kent, 1994b). This represents a remarkable amount of sound pressure. For very soft speech, as little as 2 to 3 cm H_2O pressure is sufficient to cause the vocal folds to vibrate and produce a soft tone. For loud speech, 15 to 20 cm H_2O pressure is needed, and 40 to 60 cm H_2O pressure is needed for a loud shout. The normal human respiratory system is capable of providing the needed laryngeal driving force to accommodate these extreme needs.

Increased subglottal pressure during louder phonation efforts must be met with increased laryngeal airway resistance. This resistance cannot be measured directly but can be calculated when pressure-drop factors from the trachea to the pharynx across the laryngeal valve are known and compared with translaryngeal airflow. Smitheran and Hixon (1981) demonstrated that laryngeal airway resistance can be calculated without physically invading the trachea to determine tracheal pressure. The peak oral pressure during the production of a voiceless stop-plosive can be taken as an estimate of the tracheal pressure existing at the corresponding moment. This value had been difficult to obtain in previous studies and required puncturing the trachea or having the client swallow a pressure transducer to locate it on a horizontal level to measure the tracheal pressure.

Testing 15 nondysphonic adult males, Smitheran and Hixon (1981) calculated mean laryngeal airway resistance values of 35.7 cm H_2O/LPS (liters per second). This method provides a reliable and valid method of analyzing laryngeal potential for airway resistance for producing voice in nondysphonic and dysphonic persons. The norms for laryngeal airway resistance provide speech–language pathologists and voice scientists opportunities for subject comparison. Intrasubject comparisons also can be made with this method to document improvement in laryngeal efficiency as a result of vocal management. Hoit and Hixon (1992) showed that laryngeal airway resistance does not differ significantly across the age span in women as it does in men (Melcon, Hoit, & Hixon, 1989). Additional data on aerodynamic factors in phonation, including a description of how such information can be helpful clinically, can be found in Hillman and Kobler (2000).

The three phases of vocal fold vibration (opening, closing, and closed) are modified in duration under conditions of increased intensity. The increased laryngeal airway resistance to increased flow and pressure is manifested by lengthened duration of the closed phase in a vibration cycle.

One significant factor related to intensity and loudness is variability. Cycle-by-cycle variation in intensity is called loudness perturbation or shimmer (see Figure 1.12), which Horii (1982a) defined as the average decibel difference between peak amplitudes of consecutive cycles. He reported a value of .17 dB shimmer across eight vowels produced by 20 adult males with no laryngeal pathology. Abnormal shimmer and jitter values often are present in dysphonic patients. The concerns expressed about jitter analysis reported previously also pertain to shimmer analysis (see Doherty & Shipp, 1988; Kent & Ball, 2000). It is also important to remember that these cycle-to-cycle differences must be unintended.

One should also keep in mind that vocal pitch (frequency) and loudness (intensity) are interactive, and it is difficult to modify one without an accompanying change in the other. This is fundamental to understanding good vocal hygiene. Gramming, Sundberg, Ternstrom, Leanderson, and Perkins (1988) reported that trained singers increase the frequency of their voices by about one-half semitone (half step) per decibel of increased intensity.

Vocal Quality

Vocal quality is much more difficult to describe than vocal frequency and intensity. Several terms are used in the literature to describe vocal quality. Most of the following terms have limited communicative potential: *mellow, rich, clear, bright, ringing, hollow, booty, smooth, harmonious, pleasing, velvety, sharp, heady, clangy, chesty, throaty, covered, open, breathy, balanced, coarse, crude, heavy, golden, warm, brilliant, cool, flat, round, dull, pointed, pingy, pectoral, shallow, deep, buzzy, reedy, whiney, orotund, light, toothy, white, dark, metallic, dead, cutting, constricted, strident, shrill, blatant, poor, faulty, whispery, thin, whining, piercing, raspy, guttural, pinched, tight, twangy, hard* (Boone, 1991).

Such terms, although not commonly used, would not contribute to understanding important parameters of voice quality. Even more-common terms, such as *harsh, hoarse, tense, spastic,* and *breathy,* have limited communicative potential. Most people can distinguish vocal quality in the extreme sense when it is either excellent or significantly defective but are less adept at analyzing the subtle voice quality factors heard in most persons. Speech–language pathologists must be competent in distinguishing vocal parameters of quality.

Several factors contribute to voice quality. Some occur at the level of the larynx and depend on the status of the vocal folds that generate the sound. Others are resonance phenomena that occur in the supralaryngeal structures of the vocal tract. Voice quality is a composite phenomenon of sound source and sound resonance and involves numerous physiologic and acoustic correlates (Kent & Ball, 2000).

The sound spectrum present in the vocal tract includes frequencies from the fundamental and its harmonics. A fundamental of 100 Hz could have multiple harmonics reaching as high as 3000 Hz in the typical male speaker (Lieberman, 1977). Although the intensity of each multiple harmonic decreases up the spectrum from the fundamental, the energy nevertheless is present in the vocal tract and available for resonance and articulation. For a higher fundamental, such as would be heard in a female or a singer, these values are increased proportionately.

The vocal tract functions as an acoustic filter that suppresses sound energy at certain frequencies, allows maximum sound energy to be maintained at other frequencies, and considerably amplifies the energy of other bands of frequency energy. The frequencies at which maximum sound energy is fostered and amplified are called *formant* frequencies. The terms *resonance* or *vocal tract resonance* apply to these regions of sound amplification. Acoustic filtering and resonance, as applied to the sounds of human speech, are described in detail by Lieberman (1977), Baken and Daniloff (1991), Titze (1994), and Kent and Ball (2000). However, the speech–language pathologist working with clients with voice disorders is not interested in the process of shaping the vocal tract to modify the acoustics of the glottal tone into a speech signal of the various vowels but rather in the process of shaping the sound produced by the vocal folds into a quality voice.

Because voice quality is a composite of sound source and sound resonance, several characteristics must be present in the spectrum to ensure good quality. The sound source factors include vocal folds capable of vibrating in phase with each other (i.e., the left and right vocal folds are vibrating at all times at essentially the same point in the vibratory cycle). When this occurs the vocal folds are vibrating periodically. For this to happen, the mass, length, tension, and approximation characteristics of each vocal fold must be equal. Under such conditions the waveform generated is periodic.

When pathology is present in the larynx, a high probability exists that one vocal fold will have mass, shape, tension, and approximation characteristics that differ from the other fold. In such a case, the glottal waveform generated is aperiodic. When the glottal waveform is aperiodic and abnormal, it does not matter how well the tone is resonated—it always sounds abnormal. Likewise, if the waveform is periodic and normal but the resonance is abnormal in some sense, the vocal quality sounds abnormal. (Several later chapters discuss voice qualities resulting from abnormal glottal wave generation, poor resonance factors, or combinations.)

Periodic glottal waves and certain aspects of normal resonance can be demonstrated objectively by means of spectrographic analysis. Figure 1.13 shows a narrowband spectrographic analysis of (a) a normal voice and (b) a dysphonic voice. The figure shows the clear harmonics of the normal voice and the obliteration of the harmonics, particularly the higher harmonics, which become nothing more than spectral noise in the dysphonic sample.

An additional factor related to vocal quality involves the supraglottal structures of the vocal tract, structures above the vocal folds that provide vocal resonance. Trained singers appear to be able to produce voice with a vocal tract setting that includes a low laryngeal height as well as moderately dilated, rounded, yet tense pharyngeal walls about the glottis. This supraglottal configuration appears to be related to the improved vocal quality heard in the trained singer. Pershall and Boone (1987) confirmed this vocal tract configuration by direct observation of supraglottal structures of the vocal tract by means of videoendoscopy.

In an attempt to somewhat quantify the notion of vocal quality, researchers have proposed use of the phonetogram. Phonetography, also called the Voice Range Profile (see Chapter 3), is the registration of the dynamic range of a voice as a function of fundamental frequency. For example, fundamental frequency (F_0) and sound pressure level (SPL) are measured simultaneously and plotted on an x–y diagram. From these measurements three additional acoustic voice quality parameters can be measured with the F_0 and SPL. The jitter value in the F_0 can be used as a measure of vocal roughness; the SPL difference among frequency bands (0–1.5 kHz vs. 1.5–5 kHz) can be used as a measure of vocal sharpness; and the vocal noise level above 5 kHz can be used as an index of breathiness (Pabon & Plomp, 1988; Titze, 1994).

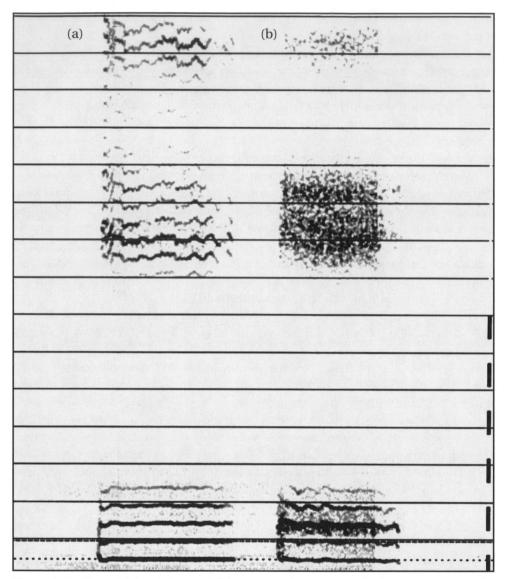

Figure 1.13. Normal (a) and abnormal (b) spectrographic patterns. The bottom cursor is at the fundamental frequency level (120 Hz), and the second cursor is at the second harmonic (240 Hz). Note the obliteration of the upper harmonics in the dysphonic voice, in which there are no harmonics, merely spectral noise.

Another acoustic index of vocal quality is the harmonic-to-noise ratio. Acoustic analysis provides a ratio of sound pressure of the vocal fundamental and its harmonics relative to any spectral noise between the harmonics. As shown in Figure 1.13, little spectral energy is seen between the harmonics in the normal voice portion, but considerable spectral noise is manifest in the dysphonic voice portion. The harmonic-to-noise ratio shown for the normal voice is 22.55 dB, indicating that the harmonics are, on average, more than 22 dB more intense than the spectral noise. In the dysphonic portion, the ratio is only 2.56 dB, indicating that the spectrograph is able to detect little intensity difference between the harmonics of the sound, which give the voice a clear pattern, and the surrounding noise, which gives the voice its hoarse or dysphonic quality.

Vocal Registers

One of the most confusing aspects of vocal quality from a resonance perspective is that of vocal registers. The terms *head voice, chest voice, midvoice,* and *falsetto* are only a few of the terms used by voice (musical performance) teachers, voice scientists, and speech–language pathologists to describe the laryngeal and resonance factors in voice production. As a person sings a tone from the lowest to the highest of his or her range, several shifts of laryngeal and resonance focus can be heard independent of pitch or loudness. These changes are labeled *vocal register shifts* and occur in speaking as well as singing. Although several registers are described in the literature of musical pedagogy and voice science, Titze (1994) maintained that three definite vocal registers exist for speaking: pulse, modal, and falsetto (or loft). The terms *chest voice, head voice,* and *falsetto voice* apply more to singing registers.

Pulse Register. The pulse register, also called the low-frequency register, corresponds to the vocal quality described as "vocal fry." It represents a pattern of vibration so slow that individual vibrations can be heard, from a low of 3-Hz to 50-Hz tone, but more typically from about 25 Hz to 80 Hz in men and 20 Hz to 45 Hz in women (Sataloff, 1998c). Pulse register tone can be produced under conditions of extreme glottal resistance (tension) or when the vocal folds are relaxed and floppy. There also is an increase in the closed phase of a vibrating cycle in pulse register.

Modal Register. In modal register, the entire vocal fold is involved in the vibration, and the thickness of the folds produces an upper and lower lip to the vibrating margins. This layered nature of the vocal folds is evident in vibration until the upper ends of the modal register are reached. Typical speaking and trained singing, and most of the tones in the vocal pitch range, are in the modal register. Within this register the larynx functions most efficiently, so tremendous potential for loudness increases (up to 110 dB) exists. The modal register refers to the most common frequencies used by typical speakers, from about 75 to 450 Hz in men to 130 to 520 Hz in women (Sataloff, 1999).

Loft Register. The highest register is the loft or falsetto. It is the opposite of the pulse register. As the upper end of the pitch range is reached, the shift into the loft register involves a laryngeal adjustment in which only the margins of the vocal folds are involved in vibration. The upper and lower lips of the vocal folds are essentially obliterated by the tension, and only tight phonating edges remain. The tension involved in this loft register also tends to stabilize the anterior and posterior aspects of the intermembranous glottis so that only the midregion of the folds vibrates. This reduced length factor also increases the frequency of vibration.

Many popular singers have learned to produce voice almost entirely in the loft register, and others can shift from modal to loft with little obvious transition. One goal of vocal performance training is to teach students to make smooth transitions from low to high tones without obvious breaks so as to use the voice's entire frequency range; however, significant intensity increase is possible mainly in the modal register. For more information on the basic acoustic and physiological bases for registers and shifts of register, see Titze (1994) and Sataloff (1998c).

Vibrato

One interesting and rather complex aspect of voice, particularly of the singing voice, is vocal vibrato. The perception of vibrato is that of periodic or regular modulations in pitch or frequency and loudness or intensity above and below modal levels. The frequency modulations are typically less than one-half semitone. When they become excessive, a "wobble" in the voice is perceived, and this condition is generally referred to as tremolo voice (Sataloff, 1998c). The repetitive nature of these modulations is between 5 and 7 Hz, but the range may be from 3 to 10 Hz. The loudness or intensity variations may range from a nearly nonmeasurable increase to several decibels. When intensity or amplitude modulations are identifiable, they are usually synchronous with the frequency modulations (Horii, 1989). Most singers consider vibrato to be a desirable aspect of the singing voice. If a vibrato-type sound is heard in the speaking voice, particularly on vowel prolongation, it is called vocal tremor and usually reflects an undesirable aspect, often neurological disorder. Ramig and Shipp (1987) compared vocal vibrato in opera singers and vocal tremor in individuals with neurological impairments (Parkinson's disease, amyotrophic lateral sclerosis, essential tremor, etc.) and reported that these vocal phenomena may be part of the same acoustic and physiological continuum. Vibrato has been studied electroglottographically (Hicks & Teas, 1987), acoustically and perceptually (Rothman & Arroyo, 1987), and in terms of vocal transition (Myers & Michel, 1987). These studies are described in an issue of the Journal of Voice that was devoted entirely to the study of vibrato in singing and speaking (Sataloff, 1987). A summary of factors related to vibrato can be found in Kent (1994a) and Kent and Ball (2000).

DIFFERENCES IN PITCH
RELATED TO AGE AND SEX

A person's first use of the larynx as a sound generator usually is the first cry after birth. Regardless of the person's sex, the frequency of the cry ranges between 400 Hz and 800

Hz, with the median frequency closer to the 400-Hz level (Kent, 1994b; Lieberman, Harris, Wooler, & Russell, 1971). Some researchers have claimed that different physical and psychological states can be discriminated in infant cries (Wasz-Hockert, Lind, Vuorenkoski, Partenen, & Valanne, 1968). Kent (1994b) provided excellent information about the vocal characteristics of infant cries far beyond the fundamental frequency of the cry, including data on minimal and maximal frequencies, durations, intensities, shifting patterns, and harmonic factors.

At birth the intermembranous length of a person's vocal folds is approximately 3 mm. The vocal folds of both sexes increase steadily and equally until around puberty, when the male larynx undergoes more dramatic enlargement than the female. These growth changes parallel modifications of the human voice across the age span, as reviewed by Case (1993). The distinguishing growth changes after puberty are well documented by Kahane (1982):

A high level of morphologic congruence appears in the male and female prepubertal larynx:

- Clear sexual dimorphism is manifested in laryngeal structures at puberty.

- Prepubertal female laryngeal dimensions are closer to adult size and weight than male counterparts, suggesting that the female larynx requires less growth per time unit to reach maturity.

- Laryngeal cartilage growth occurs through oppositional (external expansion) and interstitial (internal expansion) processes, so the basic shape is not changed in cartilage growth.

- Extensive regional growth characterizes the enhancement of the anterior aspect of the male thyroid cartilage. This growth, rather than the thyroid angles, produces the typical male Adam's apple. This growth produces a thicker thyroid lamina at the angle, and the prominence cannot be interpreted as indicating greater length of the male vocal folds.

- Male growth changes are two to three times those of females in almost every aspect, particularly in the thyroid cartilage, in which the mean increase from anterior to posterior is 15.04 mm for males and 4.47 mm for females.

- Growth of the vocal folds likewise is greater in males than females (mean = 11.57 mm [63%] in males and 4.16 mm [34%] in females).

- Vocal fold length and thickness grow independently, with data supporting the possibility that thickness continues to increase after length has reached adult dimensions.

The information available from the literature is often not very helpful with regard to pitch because of great variability from person to person and because of considerable variability in methodology used in obtaining the data. Therefore, I devised Table 1.2,

TABLE 1.2
General Data on Fundamental Frequency of Voice

Age	Gender	Expected Average Speaking Frequency
Infants	Both	413 Hz (average crying frequency)
7 Years	Both	Around 275 Hz
10 Years	Both	Around 250 Hz
11 Years	Female	Around 225 Hz (prepuberty)
11 Years	Male	Around 225 Hz (prepuberty)
14 Years	Male	Around 185 Hz (puberty proceeding)
15 Years	Female	Around 215 Hz (puberty proceeding)
18 Years	Male	Around 115 Hz (mature male)
18 Years	Female	Around 200 Hz (mature female)
30s	Male	Around 112 Hz
30s	Female	Around 196 Hz
60s	Male	Around 112 Hz
60s	Female	Around 189 Hz
80s	Male	Around 146 Hz
80s	Female	Around 200 Hz

from various sources, including my own experiences. It can be used in a general sense for clinical comparison in evaluating the pitch usage of a particular client.

THE AGING VOICE

Much information is now available regarding the changes that occur in voice during the aging process. Because aging often is accompanied by disease processes, the effect on voice must be analyzed. What is known about healthy male and female voices during the golden years?

Anatomical changes in the larynx include ossification and calcification of the laryngeal cartilages, making them more brittle and rigid. This is accompanied by slight erosion of the joint surfaces where cartilage articulates with cartilage. These changes affect the overall movement potential of the larynx for voice. There is also atrophy of the muscle tissues that comprise the vocal folds. Additionally, there is a thinning of the lamina propria and the subepithelial connective tissues. Most of these changes occur more dramatically in men than women (Hirano, Kurita, & Sakaguchi, 1989).

These anatomical and physiological changes in the tissues of the aging larynx are reflected in voice parameters, including speaking fundamental frequency (pitch), vocal intensity (loudness), stability of pitch and loudness as reflected in jitter and shimmer measurement, and respiratory support for voice and speech. Most listeners can judge the extremes of aging in voice parameters and accurately discriminate the characteristics that reflect aging. Linville (2000) provided an excellent chapter documenting aging factors in voice. Following is a summary of some of the voice changes that occur with age.

- *Fundamental frequency.* Whereas a clear divergence of vocal fundamental frequency between males and females occurs at puberty, it appears that a slight vocal convergence occurs in the menopause stage, with men's and women's voices becoming closer in pitch. This convergence occurs as the older male voice rises in pitch and the older female voice remains more stable until extreme old age (Hollien, 1987; Linville, 2000; see Table 1.2).

- *Vocal intensity.* The effect of aging on vocal intensity is not clearly understood. The stereotype of the older voice is that intensity is increased, perhaps due to hearing loss in older persons. However, the compensation for hearing loss must be understood in the context of reduced respiratory support and vital capacity for speaking. It is likely that older speakers have at least reduced capacity to significantly increase the intensity of their voices (Hollien, 1987; Linville, 2000).

- *Vocal tremor.* One commonly perceived aspect of the older voice is vocal tremor, a rather rhythmic fluctuation of pitch and intensity much like the quality of vocal vibrato in singing. Tremor is a rhythmical, involuntary oscillation of the vocal folds likely reflecting changes in the neurological status of the larynx more than reflecting normal aging. Barkmeier and Case (2000) reviewed the literature comparing adductor-type spasmodic dysphonia, vocal tremor, and muscle tension dysphonia and commented on the difficulty of distinguishing vocal tremor from other laryngeal pathologies. Hollien (1987) stated that, although vocal tremor accompanies the aging process, it can signal the neurological changes of clinical dysarthria.

- *Voice quality.* Voice quality abnormalities such as vocal roughness, aperiodicity, and breathiness are more prevalent in older people. For example, Linville, Skarin, and Fornatto (1989) studied 20 women ranging from 67 to 89 years of age. One significant finding they reported is frequently inadequate glottal closure during voice production. This would be correlated with increased breathiness in the voice as well as reduced loudness potential. Many of the acoustic changes associated with aging are reflected in changes in the tissues of the larynx. Kahane (1987) reported on the connective tissue changes that occur in the larynx as a result of aging and related those changes primarily to changes in vocal pitch.

One of the most complete studies of phonational frequency range for adult males and females was reported by Ramig and Ringel (1983). They studied 48 males in three age categories (25 to 35, 45 to 55, and 65 to 75) and compared vocal characteristics of those in good health and those in poor health. Their data indicate that the laryngeal mechanism reflects the aging process, but the changes are more significant when health is considered. Chapter 3 includes data on the changes of laryngeal function across the age span; these data should prove helpful in evaluating patients with voice disorders.

EMG DATA ON VOICE PHYSIOLOGY

Several electromyographic analysis studies of intrinsic laryngeal muscle activity have been completed. Every such muscle has been studied by use of hooked-wire electrodes placed in the muscle either percutaneously or perorally. The percutaneous approach generally is selected to reach the thyroarytenoid (TA; vocalis), lateral cricoarytelloid (LCA), and cricothyroid (CT). The peroral approach is used to reach the posterior cricoarytenoid (PCA) and interarytenoid (IA). Although the number of subjects generally is small in these studies, several consistent patterns of electromyographic activity seem apparent:

- Increases in pitch are accompanied by progressive increases in the activity of the CT and TA muscles (Gay & Hirose, 1972).

- Glottal abduction during inhalation is generated by sustained activity of the PCA with an accompanied reduction of activity of the IA, LCA, CT, and TA.

- Increased activity occurs in the CT, TA, LCA, and IA during adduction for phonation.

- Voiceless consonants are produced during running speech by quick bursts of PCA activity, which produces milliseconds of nonphonation. This is complemented by simultaneous suppression of the adductor muscles.

Zemlin (1998) emphasized that EMG tracings do not reveal the degree to which a measured muscle contributes to overall movement, but merely that a particular muscle or muscle group is active during a particular motor task.

An additional factor of laryngeal adjustment is necessary for proper control of human speech and singing. All verbal languages contain phonemes that are either voiced or voiceless. All vowels are voiced, as are many consonant sounds, such as /v/, /z/, /g/, and /d/. When a person is speaking or singing voiced phonemes, the brain controls the larynx and generates adduction of the vocal folds so that phonation or voicing can occur. However, when a voiceless consonant occurs, quick reciprocity and abduction must occur through the duration of the voiceless segment. This is occasioned by a quick posterior cricoarytenoid burst and a cessation of adduction activity, which opens the glottis and allows a voiceless sound to be produced. This reciprocity is illustrated in Figure 1.14.

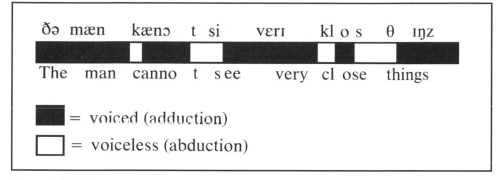

Figure 1.14. Phonation reciprocity.

Laryngeal control in singing is very delicate in vocal fold adduction, abduction, and quality control. It is marvelous how well these adjustments are controlled to produce, for example, the voice of a great singer or actor. Even nonprofessionals can communicate rather well with subtle nuances of pitch, intensity, and quality control that enhance and add meaning to the messages being communicated.

It is intriguing to contemplate the sensitivity of instant adjustment a singer must be capable of accomplishing in the larynx to match a note perfectly without trial-and-error feedback. These adjustments are produced as the singer is hearing the note to be sung while establishing in the larynx the longitudinal tension and medial compression adjustments necessary to match the pitch of the note to be sung. This must happen instantaneously as exhaled air hits the adducting vocal folds, causing them to vibrate in a specific frequency. If the adjustments are not right, the singer is out of the show.

Even in speech these same adjustments are made but with less serious consequences when errors occur. Fortunately, the adjustments are highly programmed in people's brains, and for the most part they require little conscious control. Otherwise, people would find themselves as confused as the proverbial centipede trying to control the action of leg number 39.

These fine-tuning mechanisms within the structure of the vocal folds are clearly understood. Wyke (1983) described this neuromuscular control of voice production as a system of intralaryngeal mechanoreceptors acting reflexively in response to aerodynamic forces from the lungs. Wyke described three types of mechanoreceptors: subglottal mucosal, laryngeal myotatic, and laryngeal articular. These mechanoreceptors, found in the mucosa, muscle spindles, and connective tissue joints of the larynx, provide sensory feedback to the brain regarding aerodynamic forces acting on the larynx. As a function of this feedback and the motor adjustments to it, vocal fold stability is maintained in a constantly changing aerodynamic system. This feedback also allows the speaker or singer to preset the vocal folds in a specific state of tension to allow a specific pitch to be produced. This occurs almost instantaneously in the case of great singing, and the perfect note is sung with little adjustment.

SUMMARY

This chapter has introduced many of the basic principles of voice science. Recent evidence on the anatomy and physiology of voice science has been presented to provide a basis for understanding principles of normal phonation. Details of intrinsic laryngeal structures, basic phonation theory, aspects of frequency (pitch), intensity (loudness), and quality control have been emphasized. These normal aspects provide a basis for understanding the deviations found in the various dysphonias presented in the remaining chapters.

Medical Aspects of Voice Disorders

The speech–language pathologist working with clients with voice disorders must be comfortable with medical relationships, terms, and procedures. The following sample of a physician's report on a patient referred for voice management is typical of the language used in such communications:

> I am referring the following patient for voice evaluation and possible therapy. He was biopsied with the following results:
>
> The specimen is stated to be the right and left vocal cord tissues from biopsy. The right part consists of an approximately 2 × 1 mm portion of somewhat translucent epithelially surfaced soft tissue. The left portion consists of a 5 mm aggregate of tissue similar to the right portion. Under microscopic analysis, multiple sections reveal a fragment of tissue surfaced by benign squamous epithelium that focally contains mucus-producing cells. No hyperkeratosis or dyskeratosis is noted. The underlying stroma contains a few scattered collections of mononuclear cells. Sections also reveal the presence of focal hyalinization with congested vascular structures present in the underlying stroma as well as a few small focal strands of skeletal muscle fibers.
>
> This patient also has probable neuromuscular deformity. There is no evidence of upper motor neuron signs.
>
> Please evaluate and advise on speech–language pathology finding. Thank you for seeing this patient.

No matter how well the speech–language pathologist is trained, physicians typically use language that may be unfamiliar to the speech–language pathologist, who then must search through a medical dictionary for definitions and clarification. The speech–language pathologist cannot hope to acquire, in the course of training in communication disorders, the necessary background in medical management to communicate equally with the physician and should not be expected to do so. Likewise, the typical physician is somewhat unfamiliar and perhaps uncomfortable with the language used by speech–language pathologists in describing communication disorders.

However, for competent management of patients with voice disorders, an understanding of terms and procedures involved in medical management can be helpful to the clinician providing behavior modification of abnormal voice habits.

This chapter introduces basic information regarding medical procedures in the treatment of voice disorder, including the background, training, and certification procedures for medical specialties commonly involved. General procedures of medical evaluation, drug therapy, and surgery for patients with voice disorders also are explained.

MEDICAL SPECIALTIES IN VOICE DISORDER

Although many medical specialties can be involved in the treatment of patients with voice disorders, the bulk of evaluation and treatment is done by specialists in otolaryngology, neurology, psychiatry, psychology, radiology, plastic surgery, and pathology. Speech–language pathologists working in medical settings may be overwhelmed by the jargon of the physician, medical procedures and processes, and the lexicon of health care. On-the-job training provides perhaps the only appropriate means to learn quickly what is needed for competency in medical settings, to become comfortable in interprofessional relationships with physicians, and to communicate easily with physicians. Johnson and Jacobson (1998) have edited an excellent book titled *Medical Speech–Language Pathology: A Practitioner's Guide*. The scope of medical speech–language pathology practice is clearly described for all topics, including those related to disorders of voice. Golper's (1998) *Sourcebook for Medical Speech Pathology* also includes information regarding health care professionals, specific settings where health care is provided, communication and record-keeping procedures, numerous terms used by health care providers, and the symbols of communication that are unique to the medical world. The speech–language pathologist working in medical settings is encouraged to consult these references. It would also be well for a speech–language pathologist working in a medical setting to have available a current medical dictionary. Also, Singh and Kent (2000) have generated a dictionary of speech–language pathology that includes most significant medical terms used by speech–language pathologists.

• *Otolaryngology: Head and Neck Surgery.* Otolaryngology is the medical specialty for ear, nose, throat, and head and neck surgery. Physicians in this field are trained in general medicine and have fulfilled a specialization residency of 5 years, the 1st year in general surgery and the remaining 4 years in surgical and medical treatment of diseases of the ears, nose, and throat. This is the discipline that works most closely with speech–language pathologists in the treatment of most voice disorders. Otolaryngologists manage most disorders involving the larynx and many involving the general vocal tract. Their certification of specialization is by the American Board of

Otolaryngology: Head and Neck Surgery, of the American Medical Association (AMA), under the accreditation auspices of the Accreditation Council for Graduate Medical Education. An advanced program beyond otolaryngology specialization is the Residency Education in Otology–Neurology (Otolaryngology), which provides advanced education in the diagnosis and management of disorders of the temporal bone, lateral skull base, and related structures. This is a 24-month program beyond residency in otolaryngology (*Graduate Medical Education Directory*; AMA, 2000). (The *Graduate Medical Education Directory* was referenced for all of the specialties that follow.)

• *Neurology.* A neurologist is a physician who specializes in the clinical evaluation and treatment of diseases and disorders of the nervous system. The clinical neurologist is certified by the American Board of Psychiatry and Neurology (AMA) and therefore has considerable background in the psychiatric condition of patients. The methodology used by the clinical neurologist includes general reflex assessment as well as administration and interpretation of diagnostic procedures, including roentgenologic studies, electroencephalography, electromyography, psychological testing, biochemical testing, and ophthalmological and otological procedures pertaining to the nervous system. In evaluating and treating patients with voice disorders, the neurologist is most helpful in assessing the integrity of the innervation of the larynx, pharynx, and general vocal tract anatomy and physiology. Several central nervous system disorders also can affect the voice and speech functions, making the clinical neurologist a valuable member of the treatment team.

• *Psychiatry.* The specialty of psychiatry includes training in a 3-year residency preparing the physicians for competence in the diagnosis, treatment, and prevention of all psychiatric disorders. Certification of training is from the American Board of Psychiatry and Neurology (AMA), so, in addition to the training in psychiatry, physicians obtain some experience in general neurology. Most medical procedures in psychiatry involve individual psychotherapy, family and individual counseling, crisis and stress management, pharmacological assessment and treatment as it pertains to mental illness, hypnosis, biofeedback of biological processes as they relate to mental states, and general behavioral management training. Psychiatrists are particularly helpful in managing patients with psychogenic (nonorganic) voice disorder.

• *Psychology.* The nonmedical discipline of psychology is highly correlated with psychiatry. The differences are centered on the fact that the psychiatrist is a physician and can treat patients with prescribed medicines, whereas the psychologist usually has a doctoral degree in clinical psychology and cannot directly prescribe medicines. Rather, psychologists treat mental illness and general psychological disturbance or maladjustment through counseling, group or individual psychotherapy, hypnosis, biofeedback, and so forth, without pharmacological support other than that prescribed by a physician.

• *Radiology.* The specialty of radiology requires 4 years of residency in diagnostic oncology and 3 years in radiation oncology. Certification is through the American Board of Radiology (AMA). Radiologists also receive some training in nuclear medicine. They use various methods to examine the human body to diagnose and sometimes treat disease. The therapeutic portion of training includes extensive experience in the treatment of malignant tumor disease by means of radiotherapy. Several of the specific radiological techniques used in the evaluation and treatment of patients with voice disorders are covered later in this chapter.

• *Plastic Surgery.* The plastic surgeon is certified by the American Board of Plastic Surgery (AMA) as having completed a minimum of 3 years of general surgery followed by at least 2 years of plastic surgery. Specific training supports medical competency in the treatment of traumatic defects requiring reconstructive surgery of the maxillofacial region and the general body and extremities, burns, aesthetic operations, plastic surgery of the hands, and treatment of congenital anomalies such as absence of external ear structures, cleft lip and palate, and other orofacial defects. The plastic surgeon works most closely with the speech–language pathologist in the management of cleft lip and palate patients who have velopharyngeal insufficiency. Some plastic surgeons have specialized fellowship training for surgical management of the cranium and have the additional title of craniofacial surgeon.

• *Medical Pathology.* The medical pathologist is a physician who is certified by the American Board of Pathology (AMA) as having completed a residency in microscopic analysis of normal and clinical tissues of the body. Several certification procedures can be followed to become board certified, including an emphasis on normal or clinical tissues. Each takes a minimum of 2 years of residency training. Medical pathologists analyze tissue removed in biopsies and in tonsillectomy, adenoidectomy, and tumor surgery. This pathological diagnosis confirms whether a tissue removed is benign or malignant and identifies the nature of the tissue. Although pathologists generally work directly with other physicians rather than with speech–language pathologists, the latter often receive medical reports containing pathology reports and therefore must have some familiarity with this specialty.

MEDICAL PROCEDURES IN VOICE DISORDER

The thorough examination and treatment of a person with voice disorder may involve several medical disciplines to clarify the etiological and treatment procedures necessary for competent management. The specific procedures covered here are those directly involved in the examination and treatment of laryngeal pathology, including the vocal tract.

Indirect (Mirror) Laryngoscopy

Perhaps the most common evaluation procedure in examining the status of the laryngeal structures is indirect mirror laryngoscopy. The procedure usually is done by the laryngologist and involves directing a light into the oral cavity to reflect off a laryngeal mirror to inspect the larynx and hypopharynx. Benninger and Gardner (1998) described the details involved in general head and neck examinations, including the specifics on mirror laryngology. Lucente and Joseph (1999b) also demonstrated with photos the proper technique for indirect laryngoscopy and the procedures for general oral cavity examination.

The patient's position is of great importance in maximizing the probability of success. The client should be seated in an erect manner with the jaw protruded a little. As the patient protrudes the tongue, it is wrapped with gauze and held firmly by the examiner. The patient then is asked to breathe gently through the mouth or pant like a dog. After warming the surface of a laryngeal mirror, the examiner inserts it into the oropharynx region over the tongue. Often the back of the mirror touches and elevates the velum. Light is directed against the mirror by a headlight system. When the mirror is positioned properly, the light is reflected off the mirror into the regions of the larynx for examination. Once the examiner can see the structures of the larynx, including the vocal folds, the patient is asked to phonate and say an "ee" sound to help elevate the epiglottis so that the even anterior commissure can be observed more readily.

This indirect inspection method permits general examination of the larynx. Tissue mass changes, movement disorders, growths, infections, and phonation abnormalities generally can be discerned by indirect laryngoscopy. Some patients are difficult to examine by this means. Anatomical variations or a strong gag reflex can make the procedure ineffective. Even when a topical anesthetic is used to lessen the gag, some patients, particularly children, are difficult to examine. Patience and an explanation that no pain is involved may be helpful. Figure 2.1 demonstrates indirect laryngoscopy.

Endoscopy

The prefix *endo-* refers to "within," so laryngeal endoscopy refers to any procedure that allows inspection within the confines of the larynx. Several variations of laryngeal endoscopy have been used in the history of laryngology.

Laryngoscopy

A number of instruments allow direct inspection within the larynx. With the patient asleep under general anesthesia, a laryngoscope can be placed into the throat to allow

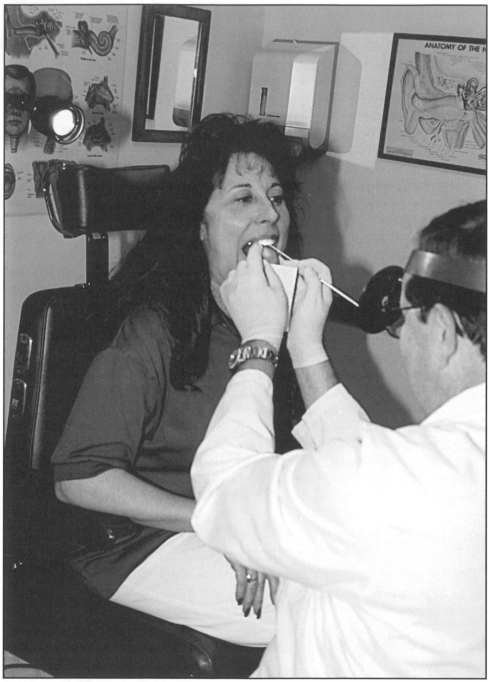

Figure 2.1. Indirect laryngoscopy.

direct inspection of the larynx. Lighting is provided and the view is direct rather than from mirror reflection. This technique allows direct inspection and surgical access to the tissues of the larynx. Microlaryngoscopic microscopes with binocular magnification now enable the surgeon to see fine changes in the status of laryngeal tissue. These changes and general details revealed can be documented by video or still photography (Yanagisawa & Driscoll, 1995).

Many laryngoscopic procedures can be accomplished at the physician's office, obviating hospitalization. Patients must be carefully selected for office medical procedures, and there should be detailed control of medications typically taken. Blitzer, Pillsbury, Jahn, and Binder (1998) provided excellent details of procedures involved in office-based surgery and laryngeal treatments, including vocal fold augmentation and biopsy.

Fiber-Optic Endoscopy

The development of fiber optics ushered in endoscopic examination through flexible tubing. Light travels along hair-thin fiber-optic bundles from a cold light source, providing illumination at the end of the bundle. Another bundle of fibers carries the image being investigated back into a magnifying scope. Machida America, Pentax, Flexview, and Olympus are companies that have developed flexible nasopharyngolaryngoscopes that allow direct inspection in close proximity of the nasal cavity, pharynx, or larynx, depending on how deeply into the body cavities the scope is inserted. Each manufacturer's product varies in cross-section width (3.3 mm to 4.0 mm; newer models are even smaller) at the distal end of the scope. The light and image potential of each model also vary. However, each provides excellent views of the structures involved. Comparisons of images from various models have been reviewed by Shprintzen (1989), and Karnell (1994) has provided photographs showing how various placements of the flexible scope reveal different areas of the nasopharynx and larynx as the scope is inserted. A patient being examined with the flexible fiber-optic endoscopy and an internal view of structures are shown in Figures 2.2(a) and 2.2(b), respectively.

Once the nasopharyngolaryngoscope is in place at the point of desired investigation, the examiner can manipulate the tip several degrees in an upward or downward direction. This flexibility permits careful inspection of tissue at close proximity. The device is designed to be inserted into the nasal cavity, through the velopharyngeal port, into the pharynx, and finally into the laryngeal cavity. During the insertion process, inspection can take place along the entire route. Attachments are available for 35-mm single-lens reflex photography as well as video cameras.

Yanagisawa, Isaacson, Kmucha, and Hirokawa (1989) reported on the merits of various endoscopic techniques, including rigid and fiber-optic methods. They strongly recommended video recording of the examination process, whichever method is used: "The addition of the video camera in nasopharyngeal observation greatly enhances

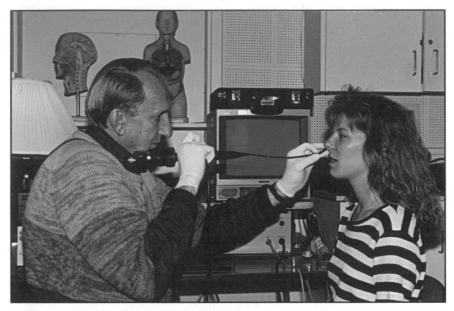

Figure 2.2(a). Flexible fiber-optic endoscopy.

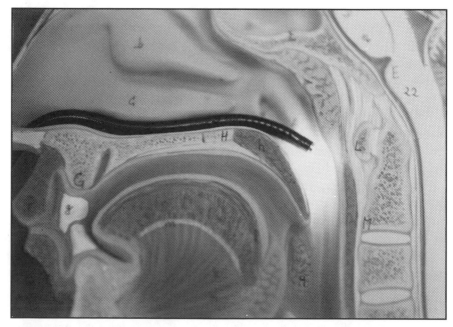

Figure 2.2(b). Model showing one placement of nasopharyngolaryngoscope.

the examiner's ability to assess structure, function, and disease by permitting review and comparison of images that once were preserved only in the examiner's memory" (pp. 17–18). These thoughts were confirmed by Koufman (1995), Karnell and Langmore (1998), and Woodson (1998).

Fiber-optic videolaryngoscopy is not without its pitfalls and limitations. Casper, Brewer, and Colton (1988) presented evidence of distortions in the video image and cautioned against making judgments of anatomical or physiological integrity on the basis of fiber-optic examination data alone. Shaw and Lancer (1987), Gulya and Wilson (1999), Handler and Myer (1998), and Sataloff, Hawkshaw, and Spiegel (1999) all provided marvelous color atlases of upper respiratory tract structures in normal and pathological states, and the reader is encouraged to use these excellent references to become familiar with the look of various pathologies that might affect voice.

Stroboscopy

The stroboscope permits an observer to view moving objects as though they are stationary or in slow motion. When a beam of light is focused on a moving object and interrupted in regular pulses, the observer views only the phase of movement exposed by the light. Movement patterns occurring between light pulses are not seen. The effect of stroboscopic light can be seen in nightclubs where the beats of light illuminate the dancers' movements.

The vibrating vocal folds can be viewed in the same manner as each light pulse illuminates a point in the vibratory cycle. A microphone is placed on the client's neck to conduct laryngeal sound to a stroboscopic generator that filters and amplifies the sound and then determines its fundamental frequency (F_0). The fundamental frequency is transmitted from the generator via electronic pulses to a lamp that emits an intermittent beam of light at the identical frequency. This light beam is introduced into the larynx via an endoscope or laryngeal mirror (indirect laryngoscopy) for examination. The endoscope can be attached to a video camera for videotape storage (videostroboscopy). If the light beam frequency is exactly the frequency of vocal fold vibration, the vocal folds will be seen at the same phase of vibration and will appear stationary. If the light beam is altered slightly out of frequency phase, then the vocal folds will appear to move in slow motion. If the phase frequency is kept equal to zero, the same point in the vibratory cycle can be visualized because the vocal folds appear stationary. When the phase angle at which the flash is generated is adjusted slightly, a specific portion of the vibratory cycle can be examined.

Stroboscopy (strobovideolaryngoscopy, laryngostroboscopy, laryngovideostroboscopy) facilitates examination of the details of vocal fold movement that are not apparent under traditional indirect or direct laryngoscopy. It documents patterns of abnormal vibration and the sites of lesions. The assessment of the following vocal fold parameters has been discussed by Hirano (1996), Hirano and Bless (1993), Karnell (1994), and Cranen and de Jong (2000):

- The nature of vocal fold edges during phonation
- Width of the open glottis and amplitude of vibration
- Fundamental frequency (F_0)
- Phases of vibration (opening, opened, closing, closed)
- Open quotient, speed quotient, speed index
- Regularity or periodicity of successive vibrations
- Symmetry of movement between the vocal folds
- Vibration of the mucosal tissue covering the vocal fold muscles
- Vibration patterns of the lower and upper lips of the vocal folds
- Extent of contact area between the vocal folds during closed phase

Use of the stroboscope and videostroboscopy of laryngeal structures is becoming a standard in otolaryngology. Its value as a diagnostic tool is well documented in the literature. Sataloff et al. (1987) reported that in 161 of 515 cases examined by videostroboscopy, its use established or altered the diagnosis or management of the patients involved. Among the disorders diagnosed or altered were arytenoid dislocation (7 patients), hemorrhage (22), nerve paralysis (25), nodule (10), scar (33), and web (3). Numerous additional categories of diagnosis were presented. The videostroboscope was also used by Izdebski, Ross, and Klein (1990), McFarlane and Watterson (1990), and Woodson (1998) to document laryngeal function in various forms of voice disorder.

As with any instrumental approach to evaluation, training and experience are key elements in accuracy. It is within the scope of practice of speech–language pathologists to use stroboscopy, but training at the typical master's degree in communication disorders will seldom provide it. Case (1998) discussed the use and misuse of videostroboscopy in a national telerounds sponsored by the National Center for Neurogenic Communication Disorders at the University of Arizona. (A video of this presentation is available by contacting the University of Arizona.)

In 1998, the American Academy of Otolaryngology Voice and Swallow Committee and the Special Interest Division on Voice and Voice Disorders of the American Speech-Language-Hearing Association issued a joint statement regarding the use of strobovideolaryngoscopy. This joint statement approved use of strobovideolaryngoscopy, including both rigid and flexible endoscopy, by speech–language pathologists with expertise in voice disorders and with specialized training in its technology and usage. The statement included the caveat, however, that physicians are the only professionals qualified and licensed to render medical diagnoses related to the identification of laryngeal pathology as it affects voice. Speech–language pathologists are to use this procedure only to assess voice production and vocal function or as a therapeutic aid and biofeedback tool. Nonmedical professionals who use strobovideolaryngoscopy should follow these well-defined guidelines (American Speech-Language-Hearing Association, 1998).

Stroboscope documentation of visual aspects of voice disorder coupled with acoustic information is used throughout this book in the case studies presented. State-of-the-art clinical management of voice requires this visual and acoustic documentation. (Figures 2.3 and 2.4, show, respectively, the equipment for stroboscopy and an actual examination.) Chapter 3 details evaluation procedures in videostroboscopy.

Radiologic Examination

Several radiologic techniques, traditional as well as advanced, are available for investigating the status of the vocal tract for voice production. These techniques range from standard lateral radiograms to advanced scanning forms. Silva, Muntz, and Clary (1998) reported on the importance of conventional radiography in the diagnosis and management of pediatric patients presenting with possible airway obstructions. They recommended use of radiographic imaging only as a supplement to surgical intervention to investigate the obstruction.

Roentgenography

A standard means of photography of the body is by roentgen rays, more commonly called radiography or X ray. Still or in-motion pictures can be taken. Motion picture radiography is called cineradiography when standard motion picture film is used and videoradiography when the image is stored on videotape, the common procedure today. Fluoroscopy is a radiologic technique that uses a fluoroscope, which shows the image on a fluorescent screen covered with crystals of calcium tungstate. Videofluoroscopy is a common technique in radiologic motion study stored on videotape.

Ultrasonography

Diagnostic ultrasonography has been used widely in the clinical medical fields of vascular surgery, cardiology, neonatology, ophthamology, gynecology, urology, and obstetrics but is seldom used in the treatment of head and neck lesions. Gluckman (1998), however, recommended its use by physicians who treat many patients with head and neck lesions. It is a procedure based on the pulse–echo principle, in which an ultrasound beam is generated by a transducer that also serves to detect the returning echo from tissues. Tissues of different densities provide varied degrees of impedance to these transmissions and alter the returning echo. The echoes are transduced into electrical signals for amplification and image processing. Ultrasonography provides dynamic 2-D images on the monitor screen, permitting an accurate evaluation of the tissues being inspected.

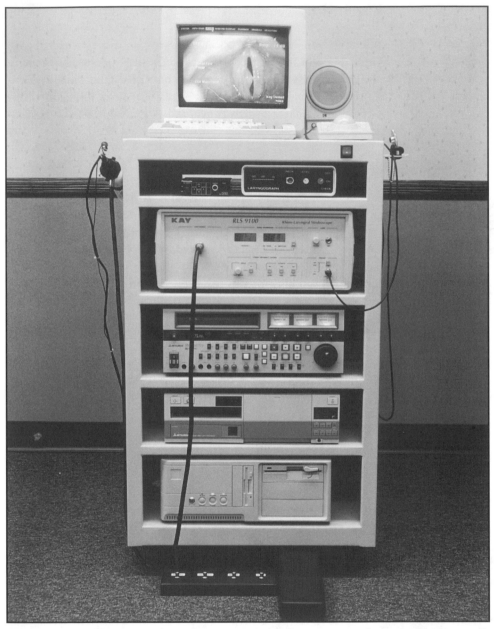

Figure 2.3. Kay Elemetrics videostroboscopic system with computer analysis setup. Laryngograph is also shown. (Photo courtesy of Kay Elemetrics.)

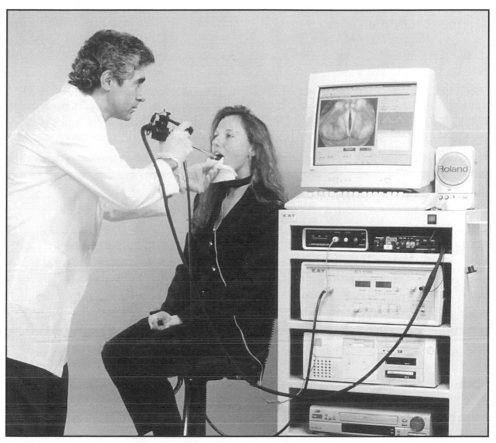

Figure 2.4. Videolaryngoscopic examination with stroboscope. (Photo courtesy of Kay Elemetric.)

Computed Tomography

Computed tomography (CT) is a scanning technique based on the physical principle that various normal and pathological soft tissues have slightly different radiation absorption coefficients. These differences do not show up in standard radiography, in which all of the tissue appears as only one shade of gray.

In CT scanning, the X-ray photons entering and exiting the patient are measured by crystal or gas detectors, and multiple density readings are taken as the X-ray source shifts and rotates around an axis. The computer then solves the equations of relative density detected as a result of the relative absorption factors of the various tissues. The results are displayed in two dimensions on a cathode ray tube for direct interpre‐ tation or photographic recording.

Magnetic Resonance Imaging

The application of nuclear magnetic resonance physics to anatomical imaging has had a significant effect on medical practice. The designation *nuclear magnetic resonance* has been replaced by the less threatening designation *magnetic resonance imaging (MRI)*. Underlying this technology is the notion that various elements (including human tissues) contain randomly spinning protons that tend to align within a superimposed magnetic field. The process of magnetization enables tissue differences to be detected and used to generate maps (images) of those difference values in gray-scale–coded images. The images provide clear distinctions of various tissues along a gray-scale continuum.

MRI, which has been used to image laryngeal and surrounding structures, provides definite advantages over CT scanning techniques for diagnostic purposes. According to Hoover, Wortham, Lufkin, and Hanafee (1987), "MR surpasses CT, especially in ability to differentiate subtle differences in soft tissue boundaries and tumor extension in the head and neck" (pp. 245–246). Moore (1992) used MRI to study vocal tract resonance volumes and found these volumes to predict well the acoustic resonance frequencies of the voice. MRI techniques have also been used extensively in craniofacial management of patients who have, among other anomalies, orofacial clefting that affects the velopharyngeal and other speech-related structures.

Over the past few decades, CT and MRI scanning have enabled professionals to study *in vivo*, which means it can be done in the living person (as compared to *in vitro*, which describes a biological event that occurs in a laboratory or artificial environment). More recently, further advances in imaging have allowed the study of movement in physiologic processes, as opposed to static images. Such processes as single-photon emission tomography, positron emission tomography, functional magnetic resonance imaging, and "three-dimensional" imaging of the larynx and other body structures provide unique visualization of the structures of voice (Yumoto, Sanuki, & Hyodo, 1999).

These imaging technologies are not used by the speech–language pathologist but often are presented in team meetings for professional discussion. The experienced medical speech–language pathologist often becomes competent in reading with the physician the implications of certain images for patient management. Most of the imaging technologies are used by radiologists and otolaryngologists to identify laryngoceles and carcinomas, including evidence of metastasis from the laryngeal area. An excellent reference for the medical speech–language pathologist on the general use of radiological imaging, particularly in the brain, has been provided by George, Vikingstad, and Cao (1999) and, pertaining to the laryngeal area, by Weismann and Curtin (1995). Ong and Stone (1998) used MRI, ultrasound, and electropalatography to measure vocal tract shapes in subjects producing various speech sounds and confirmed information regarding how the vocal tract is modified to perform speech functions. Additionally, Fisher, Xu, and Parish (1999) reported on the usage of MRI to assess hydration levels in the vocal folds and recommended this technique to monitor large water changes in these delicate tissues.

DRUG TREATMENT IN VOICE DISORDER

Several pharmacotherapeutic treatments are used in the medical management of patients with voice disorders. These include antibiotic treatment of infections, symptomatic treatment of upper respiratory conditions in the form of antihistamines, anti-inflammatory and antidematous treatment in the form of adrenocorticosteroids for tissue swelling, psychological or mood-modifying drugs, moisteners for dry mouth and throat and nasal crusting, and local anesthetics to eliminate gagging or nerve transmission.

It is beyond the scope of this book to cover the many drugs that are used by physicians in treating voice disorder. The speech–language pathologist will find that nearly every client is treated with pharmaceutical medications under the direction of the referring physician. I have consulted the *Physician's Desk Reference* (PDR; Walsh, 2000; also www.pdr.net) for most evaluations. The typical speech–language pathologist has insufficient background in biochemistry to understand the pharmacologic effects of various medications and can get into trouble when attempting to explain such effects to a client. Although it is tempting to comment on the medications' effects on voice, I believe that such comments should be left to the physician.

It is appropriate to ask about the medications being taken when taking a case history. Most clients can provide a list, often with correct spellings. The speech–language pathologist should write down each medication in generic or trade form and consult the PDR for further information about the drug. The PDR often mentions possible effects of a specific medication on the voice. In such instances the referring physician should be asked to clarify the effect the medication might have on the voice.

Often a speech–language pathologist working in a medical setting or directly with a physician becomes, through experience, familiar with the usage, dosage, and voice sequelae of various medications. Until such experience is gained, it is best to recognize that some medications can affect the voice and to the use the PDR to investigate each reported medication. Vogel, Carter, and Carter (2000) investigated how various drugs affect patients with communication disorders. Their book covers such topics as neuroscience and drugs and how drugs affect specific disorders such as Parkinson's disease, myasthenia gravis, amyotrophic lateral sclerosis, multiple sclerosis, dementia, and spasmodic dysphonia. It also addresses the issue of aging as it is affected by medication. Additional references covering drugs and vocal function include books by Martin (1988) and Sataloff (1998b).

Sataloff (1991, 1998b) has also written fine tutorials on drugs and vocal function, covering such topics as basic principles of drug action, biological variation, dose-response relationships, multiplicity of actions, placebo effects, and specific pharmaco-logic medications as they relate to the voice. The tutorials also discuss drugs for vocal dysfunction and include chapters on medications for voice professionals and traveling performers. This information was reinforced by Sataloff, Hawkshaw, and Rosen (1998) in a chapter titled "Medications: Effects and Side-Effects in Professional Voice Users."

SURGERY AND THE VOICE PATIENT

Speech–language pathologists who treat patients with voice disorders must be cog-nizant of surgical considerations, including principles of anesthesia, laryngoscopic examination, biopsy, intubation and extubation, microsurgery, traditional "knife" surgery, and laser surgery. Specific forms of surgery involved include thyroplasties, tumor or benign growth removal, and various techniques in cancer management. Only general surgical considerations are discussed here.

Phonosurgery

A growing and positive change in the attitude of many physicians who treat patients with voice disorder is that they should treat the voice as well as the larynx. When a physician examines a patient and discovers an abnormal change in the tissues of the larynx, particularly on the vocal folds, several treatment choices are available. One is to investigate surgically the nature of the tissue change in the form of biopsy. In some cases this is an important course to take. From a voice disorder perspective, it is help-ful when the physician realizes that surgery on the larynx is also surgery on the voice. Care must therefore be taken to determine whether the surgery needs to be done or whether a more conservative approach might be in order. Should surgery be neces-sary, it is helpful when the surgeon approaches the larynx from a concept of phono-surgery (voice surgery) rather than laryngeal (structure) surgery.

Phonosurgery has been defined by von Leden, Abitbol, Bouchayer, Hir-ano, and Tucker (1989) as "surgery designed primarily for the improvement of the voice. . . aesthetic surgery for the vocal system" (p. 175). If this definition of surgery is accepted, such procedures as the surgical removal of vocal nodules, polyps and other tumors, and Reinke's edema, whether done by knife or laser, would not be con-sidered phonosurgery unless the surgeon realizes that altering the vocal fold has the potential of altering the voice, a concern that should be primary in the mind of the surgeon. Procedures that fit directly into the concept of phonosurgery are those designed to shift the vocal folds into a better position for phonation; those used to alter the position or tension of the arytenoid cartilages and thus the vocal folds; various forms of cancer surgery, including tracheoesophageal puncture (see Chapter 7); the diverse forms of thyroplasty (Blaugrund, 1995; Gross, 1999; Tucker, 1999); and injection techniques such as BOTOX for treatment of spasmodic dysphonia (Blitzer & Brin, 1992b; Ludlow, 1995). Much of the surgery on the larynx is done with lasers (see Abitbol, 1995, for more information on laser voice surgery).

Concomitant with the increased acceptance of the concept of phonosurgery, there is a trend in laryngology to document the patient's voice prior to any surgery that has the potential to alter the voice. This documentation can be done by a laryngologist or by a speech–language pathologist or voice scientist who has the necessary equipment. This documentation should include at least a high-quality audio recording of the voice and preferably an additional video recording of phonation. Additional documentation is available using the equipment described in Chapter 3 and in Debruyne, Ostyn, Delaere, and Wellens (1997) and Murry, Abitbol, and Hersan (1999).

When a physician determines that laryngoscopic inspection with possible biopsy is necessary, in most cases a general anesthetic is necessary. The physician in charge of this process is the anesthesiologist, who produces the general anesthetic effect by introducing into the patient one of several possible pharmacologic agents. Respiratory control is necessary and is accomplished by oral or nasal intubation involving a plastic tube that is inserted through the larynx into the trachea. A ballooning device on the tube allows the anesthesiologist to inflate it to protect against aspiration during the surgery, because the normal reflexive potential of the larynx is lost under anesthesia. A respirator is attached to the intubation device, and respiration is thus controlled.

Visualization of the status of the larynx through the laryngoscope is aided by the attachment of a binocular microscope. The surgeon can inspect the tissue of the larynx and insert instruments through the laryngoscopic tube for tissue manipulation and possible removal. Instruments that may be used, depending on the purpose of the surgery, include forceps, scalpels, probes, scissors, suction tip instruments, fiber-optic probes for transillumination, needle holders for suturing, and special staining instruments. Each of these instruments is attached to a long handle so that it can be introduced through the laryngoscope to reach the larynx. With these instruments the surgeon can remove the tissue that will be sent for biopsy to the pathologist, who will determine its nature under microscopic analysis. If the purpose of the surgery is endolaryngeal removal of pathological tissue, rather than biopsy, this can be accomplished by using the same general surgical procedures.

Laser Microsurgery

Laser microsurgery is a technique involving use of the CO_2 laser and is employed in the treatment of many laryngeal diseases. The CO_2 laser beam has a thermal effect that evaporates the water content and rapidly destroys soft tissue. The amount of destruction depends on the power setting of the beam and the duration of application.

The CO_2 laser has advantages over traditional surgical techniques involving scissors and scalpels in that it produces minimal bleeding and no visible postoperative edema or scarring. The CO_2 laser allows more critical demarcation of tissue because it is coupled to a surgical operating microscope. A leading reference on laser surgery is Abitbol's (1995) *Atlas of Laser Voice Surgery*, which provides information on microlaryngoscopy, anesthetic techniques, and laryngeal pathology management, as well as 475 color photographs of pathologies and surgical management.

SUMMARY

This chapter has presented general descriptions of medical treatment for patients with voice disorders. Most such patients are involved in significant medical treatment. The chapter has covered the nature of medical specialties pertinent to voice as well as general examination procedures available, including techniques of laryngoscopy, endoscopy, and various forms of radiologic and ultrasound examination. General information regarding the importance of pharmacotherapeutic treatment and material on surgical techniques were also discussed.

Evaluation Procedures in Voice Management

Technology enables visualization of aspects of the world that we were unaware of not long ago. On television screens we see electron microscopic images, for example, that show how filthy and contaminated carpets and bed sheets are even after they have just been washed. Under the electron microscope, we see microorganisms that appear to be escapees from Jurassic Park, looming large and angry enough to actually eat us. In fact, they are so tiny that we never see these creatures, and we likely eat *them*.

Luckily, human characteristics such as voice are not submitted to the scrutiny of the electron microscope or everyone would be found "filthy and contaminated," ready for the "voice junkyard." When one does scrutinize vocal habits, one finds that many individuals have such pleasing voice characteristics that they attract attention and enhance a communication message. Others have such abnormal voices that listeners' attention is focused on the differences and abnormalities at the expense of communication. Between these extremes lie the majority of persons. The professional responsibility of physicians and speech–language pathologists who work with patients with voice disorders is to identify and discriminate the voice characteristics that are sufficiently abnormal to require some form of treatment. This chapter is designed to help speech–language pathologists in this evaluation.

The voice evaluation process is made more difficult because some normal parameters cannot be measured easily or objectively, as mentioned in Chapter 1. Pitch, loudness, suprasegmentals such as inflection and stress, oral–nasal resonance balance, laryngeal valving functions of the glottal waveform, and general vocal tract resonance functions are some of the many parameters that the speech–language pathologist can measure precisely. Other aspects, such as vocal quality, are more elusive to objective measurement and are subjected to perceptual judgments. The voice-oriented speech–language pathologist must be concerned with both measurement and perceptual evaluation. Therefore, the state of the art in voice evaluation and therapy remains a combination of science and perceptual judgment.

The speech–language pathologist often becomes involved in the management of a patient with voice disorder by referral from a physician who has diagnosed the problem, done whatever was medically possible to alleviate abnormal symptoms or characteristics, and finally passed the client on for speech–language pathology services. In some cases, a physician refers a client for special testing, such as stroboscopy or aeromechanical analysis, to assist in the diagnostic process. In other cases, for example, in schools, a child is screened out as having voice characteristics that appear abnormal, and a chain of events is begun to determine whether the disorder is significant enough to warrant management. In all types of cases, the speech–language pathologist must conduct a proper and thorough diagnosis or evaluation.

MEDICAL REFERRAL

One of the most troublesome concerns for speech–language pathologists is knowing whether or when to refer for medical consultation when the client has not been evaluated and referred by a physician. This problem occurs often in schools. Many speech–language pathologists have been trained never to work with a voice case until there has been a medical examination of the larynx and the physician has referred the patient for voice therapy. In schools, this can become frustrating to the speech–language professional because medical referral requires parental support and usually a significant amount of money. A student may be identified as having a voice disorder and the referral process begun, only to be stopped by a parent who is not willing to take the child to a physician, or the child may be referred to a physician who reports "nothing wrong." Parents then ask, "Why the referral? Why the expense?" There is also the difficulty of passing through the medical gatekeeper known as the "primary care physician." This physician holds the key to obtaining, in most instances of medical insurance and health maintenance organization (HMO) politics, the likelihood of having a potential client seen by a specialist who can examine the larynx and report on its status. This gauntlet of referral processes often discourages the school speech–language pathologist, thwarting treatment processes for a child who may need them.

Although there is no easy solution to this problem, some recommendations are possible. Medical referral is an important part of voice management, and when deliberate and carefully thought-out processes are followed, significantly more referrals will be handled properly. However, this management of referrals requires hard work in developing professional relations with referral physicians.

Although some physicians are happy to work closely with speech–language pathologists, others may not be as cooperative. Thus, it is wise to seek doctors with a cooperative attitude or attempt to change the opinion of those with less cooperative attitudes. Moran and Pentz (1987) surveyed otolaryngologists in five geographic regions of the United States and found that most have a positive attitude about the role of voice therapy for their patients. Most are happy to work with a competent speech–language pathologist and will provide medical support for the voice therapy process. Cordero (1999) discussed the importance of good medical referrals in the management of voice-disordered patients and stressed that the physician should be aware of the communication and voice needs for each age group.

A speech–language pathologist seeking a good relationship with a physician should obtain an appointment with one (typically an otolaryngologist) to whom referrals are likely. The speech–language pathologist should explain that, because referral is important in the management of voice clients, the purpose of the meeting is to discuss how this can best occur. Explain to the physician the difficulties of screening schoolchildren who seem to have dysphonia. The following are typical questions that could be asked of the physician:

- How do you feel about referring all persistently hoarse children for laryngoscopic examination?

- Who should not be referred?

- What happens when you examine a student who is persistently hoarse and your examination does not identify any vocal fold pathology?

- What do you say to the parents and child about the hoarseness? Does this disturb you?

- How do you feel that children with vocal nodules should be handled? With surgery? Vocal therapy? Both? In what order? How could I as a speech–language pathologist help?

- What should I do with a child who has been screened as having a hoarse voice but whorse parents will not take him or her to a physician for examination because of expense? Are there clinics where these services can be obtained? Do you ever see patients pro bono or at reduced fees?

The issues raised by these questions are controversial, and both professions are somewhat divided over the answers. Focused position statements on the issue of voice therapy in the public schools were presented in *Language Speech & Hearing Services in Schools* (Kahane & Mayo, 1989; Sander, 1989). The speech–language pathologist should understand the polemics involved by reading these articles and forming an opinion prior to meeting with the physician but should be open to the physician's opinions. In any regard, this communication process between the two professionals should form the foundation for a good relationship and can help the speech–language pathologist decide which physicians are receptive to voice referrals. Open communication is essential for developing rapport but is difficult over the phone; most physicians would be happy to meet for lunch or dinner to discuss professional matters.

Parental support of the medical referral process is most important. Many problems must be overcome to gain support, and, again, communication is essential. A note sent home usually produces success in only a few cases. A telephone call is much better. A personal appointment is best and is critical for referral follow-up. The speech–language pathologist should call the parents, set an appointment, and be prepared to convince them that their child has a voice disorder and that medical referral to establish etiology is necessary. It is hard to do this with words alone, and it is recommended that the speech–language pathologist use pictures, models, and tape recordings when possible. Using good audiovisuals, the speech–language pathologist should explain to parents and significant others, including the child involved, the nature of the voice disorder. At the end of the presentation, those involved should understand what constitutes a voice disorder, what its long-term and short-term consequences are, what the causes may be, why the medical referral is necessary to determine the specific reason, and whether medical treatment might be necessary before or during therapy. This communication process greatly increases the probability of a successful referral, particularly when good rapport has been established with the physician.

School or clinic policy often forbids referral to a specific physician. Instead, a list of all available doctors in the area who can provide the service is given to the parents or client, who then must decide whom to call. This makes little sense and can only lead to disappointing results. It would be preferable to provide the names of several physicians who are likely to respond well and then let the parents or client decide. In such cases, there is no bad choice. It is also necessary in most instances of medical insurance to obtain the support of the primary physician in a managed care organization or HMO before a referral can be obtained for laryngeal examination. This can also complicate the referral process.

SCREENING AND IDENTIFICATION IN SCHOOLS

Students with voice disorders usually are identified in screening by a speech–language pathologist early in the school year or by teacher referral. To identify these students accurately, the teacher must have a general working knowledge of what normal voice is and is not. It is appropriate for the speech–language pathologist to hold a short workshop early in the school year to teach the faculty basic listening skills to help in the identification process. Many teachers have little understanding of the voice and the bases of its disorders. A voice disorder workshop should be directed at developing the general listening skills necessary to help identify the two most common areas of voice disorder found in schools: hoarseness and excessive nasality.

Many other voice concerns could be taught, but it is wise to keep the instruction process simple and manageable. The lecture should cover one disorder that causes hoarseness (e.g., vocal nodules) and one that produces excessive nasality (e.g., cleft palate). It is a good idea to show slides to illustrate the laryngeal and pharyngeal bases of these disorders, play taped samples of voice and speech characteristics, and provide practice in listening and judging recorded samples. The presentation should encourage considerable dialogue between the teaching staff and the speech–language pathologist and improve the process of teacher identification of students with voice disorders.

Problems in Voice Screening

When screening children in school, the speech–language pathologist should keep in mind that voice patterns and larynx conditions are highly changeable and capricious. Many severe voice disorders are a result of temporary conditions. A child may have a severe cold or allergic reaction that causes changes in the laryngeal structures and produces hoarseness. It is inappropriate to enroll such a child in voice therapy until more is known about the persistence and etiology of the vocal pattern. Because the same voice characteristics can be caused by temporary as well as by more persistent conditions, it is necessary to follow up on screening to ensure that the child has a condition that requires remediation.

Questions that should be asked of the child at the screening include, "Does your voice always sound as it does today?" "Do you have a cold?" and "How long has your voice sounded like this?" The reliability of the answers may be questionable, but they can provide some insight into whether the voice disorder is temporary or persistent. These same questions should be asked of the child's classroom teacher.

Regardless of the information thus gained, the speech–language pathologist should screen the child again 2 weeks later. Comparison of vocal patterns 2 weeks apart requires that at the initial screening a sample be taped. The student should state name, date, school, and count from 1 to 20. This is the only sample needed.

When to Refer to a Physician

When the persistence of voice disorder has been determined and the vocal pattern judged abnormal, the next question is whether medical referral is necessary. To be on the safe side, the speech–language pathologist could refer every child with any kind of persistent voice disorder for medical clearance before initiating therapy; however, such a blanket approach is unnecessary. The primary concern is that a child might have a serious medical condition in the laryngeal structures requiring surgery or medicine rather than therapy. Such conditions do exist commonly and the concern is legitimate.

A question often asked is whether speech–language pathologists should be concerned about laryngeal cancer in children. The answer is simple: This condition is so rare in children that one need not refer voice cases simply to be sure that the youngsters do not have cancer. However, other medical conditions that are not rare can be progressive and interfere with breathing, and the speech–language pathologist should be aware of these possibilities.

Juvenile papillomas (see Chapter 8), for example, are wartlike growths in the larynx that can obstruct the airway. The vocal symptoms are not easily distinguished from those produced by a less threatening condition, such as vocal nodules, but the treatment is radically different and entirely medical. Other conditions, such as laryngeal web, polyps, laryngeal paralysis, and trauma, can produce similar voice symptoms. Medical examination of the larynx thus is necessary to determine the exact cause of the vocal symptoms.

Therefore, a safe and reasonable position on referral is that any child with a voice disorder stemming from abnormal functioning of the vocal folds that produces a difference in voice quality, or in any way makes breathing difficult, should be evaluated medically before management by a speech–language pathologist. Laryngeal symptoms of persistent breathiness, tension, hoarseness, diplophonia, strain, aphonia, stoppage of phonation in the middle of a word or phrase, or any combination of these factors require medical attention before voice management when not associated with a cold or upper respiratory infection (discussed in detail in other sections).

Other characteristics, such as high-pitched voice, slight nasality that probably is not associated with velopharyngeal insufficiency, a soft (insufficiently loud) voice, or an excessively loud voice not associated with other laryngeal symptomatology usually can be managed without medical referral as long as improvement occurs rather quickly. When progress is not rapid, the speech–language pathologist should refer the client to a physician to rule out organicity. Experience with persons having voice disorder can help one determine when medical referrals should be made. Until obtaining sufficient experience, a speech–language pathologist should perhaps be more inclined to initiate medical referrals. It is better to err on the side of overreferral.

THE CASE HISTORY

The process of taking a case history in evaluating persons having voice disorders is very important. Information can be obtained that can help the speech–language pathologist determine factors related to organicity that require medical attention or to stress or emotional maladjustment requiring psychological or psychiatric referral, as well as factors that provide prognostic value and insight about which therapeutic approach might be most successful. Taking case histories requires excellence in interviewing so that the client is made to feel comfortable in sharing information that might be considered private. Several excellent case history forms have been published (Andrews, 1999; Boone & McFarlane, 2000; Colton & Casper, 1996). However, merely having the proper form to guide the questioning is not sufficient for obtaining an excellent case history; much more is necessary.

Emerick and Hatten (1974) pointed out that the speech–language pathologist who has been trained to think objectively and scientifically often may find talking with a client or the parents of a child so difficult that case history forms replace personal interaction. They described a case history interview as "essentially a process, not an entity—a process of verbal and nonverbal intercourse between a trained professional worker and a client seeking . . . services" (p. 25). They discussed many of the mistakes commonly made by clinicians and offered constructive suggestions. Hutchinson, Hanson, and Mecham (1979) suggested that a good interview should begin with open-ended, unambiguous, but not too specific questions. In a voice case history, such questions might include, "What is the problem you are having with your voice? Tell me how it developed." Excellent guides to general case history procedures are provided in Tomblin, Morris, and Spriestersbach (1994) and Deem and Miller (2000).

The next important task for the speech–language pathologist is to listen to the information provided so that pertinent follow-up questions can be asked. One of the most common mistakes beginning clinicians make in the case history process is to ask a general question listed on some form but not respond to the information provided; rather, they merely proceed to the next listed question. Listening and responding by comment or further questioning to tease out all concerns demonstrates mature and well-developed skills in interviewing.

If the speech–language pathologist follows a form in taking a case history, it should be used toward the end of the interview to ensure that all specific questions have been asked. The speech–language pathologist should begin the interview with general questions such as those suggested earlier. Next should come specific follow-up questions regarding the background of the disorder; onset and treatment history; related illnesses and medical aspects; day-to-day variability; social, vocational, and educational considerations; and finally the effect it has on the client. The speech–language pathologist then can go back over the case history form to ask specific questions that might have been overlooked. The form can be introduced thus: "Let me go over this form to see if we have missed anything of importance. Let me see. . . . Oh yes, what medications are you taking?"

The following specific areas should be investigated in any voice disorder case history:

- Nature of the disorder

- Date of onset

- Etiology

- Progression since onset

- Treatment sought

- Success of any previous treatments

- Client's general health and history of previous illnesses

- Association of onset with any physical ailments, emotional stress, or psychological disturbance

- Variation of vocal parameters throughout the day

- Voice fatigue factors

- Vocal habits during a typical day

- Leisure-time vocal habits

- Stability in vocational, social, and familial life

- Significant aspects of stress in vocational, social, familial, and marital life

- History of significant medicine usage, including current usage

- History of tobacco and alcohol consumption

- Litigation matters arising from treatment of the disorder

- Pain associated with the disorder

- Disorder's effect on vocational, social, familial, and marital life

- Aspects of voice most distressing: pitch, loudness, quality, durability, stability

- Fluid intake each day, particularly water

- Other considerations not specifically covered that the client feels might be important

These questions and areas of concern pertain to a general voice disorder case history. Obviously, many clients are referred for an evaluation because of a specific disorder, and much of this information would not be relevant. Examples include a person who is seen shortly after a laryngectomy, or one referred because of vocal nodules, contact ulcers, or some other specific disorder. In such cases only questions pertaining to that problem would be appropriate, and additional questions are provided in chapters pertaining to those disorders.

The relevance of some of the listed topics of investigation in the case history is self-evident; others may need clarification. One such area is the client's history of tobacco and alcohol consumption. If the client is merely a social drinker, there is little concern. Excessive alcohol consumption, however, should raise concerns about control of behaviors that might be considered vocally abusive. The relationship between smoking and laryngeal pathology is so clearly delineated that to ignore the evidence is foolish. I am so convinced of smoking's deleterious effect on voice that I would likely not enroll a client in voice therapy if he or she continued to smoke. The specific evidence for such a position is provided in Chapter 4.

Another area of concern is litigation. Laryngologists are facing an increase in medicolegal cases involving the voice. von Leden (1988) reported that the most common areas of litigation involve aggressive surgery for vocal nodules, failure to diagnose a malignant tumor, injudicious injections of Teflon and other prosthetics, and iatrogenic injuries of the laryngeal nerves. He cautioned his otolaryngology colleagues to take elementary precautions, keep good records, obtain informed consent, be precise in surgery for benign lesions of the vocal cords, and make pre- and post-surgery audio recordings of patient voices. It is important that any speech–language pathologist working with patients involved in litigation recognize the importance of good record-keeping practices and voice recording documentation.

EVALUATION OF SPECIFIC VOICE PARAMETERS

Following the case history interview, the speech–language pathologist must evaluate specific parameters of phonation to determine which, if any, are abnormal and contribute to the voice disorder. The evaluation process includes a description of the instrumentation involved.

Hearing Status

In voice evaluation it is important to determine the status of a client's hearing. Although hearing screening should be part of every voice evaluation, regardless of age, it is critical for older clients. Hearing loss has been shown to have an impact on several aspects of voice, including resonance, nasal characteristics, increased laryngeal or phonatory flow, increased subglottal pressure, and increased glottal resistance to flow (Higgins, Carney, & Schulte, 1994). The importance of documenting hearing status in vocal performance clients was stressed by Sataloff and Sataloff (1998), who stated, "Singers depend on their hearing almost as much as they do on their voices" (p. 145).

Pitch (Frequency)

The pitch of a human voice is a psychological or perceptual correlate of the physical dimension of the frequency of vocal fold vibration. When exhaled air from the lungs reaches the closed vocal folds, pressure builds until it is sufficient to blow the vocal folds apart, causing them to vibrate. The frequency of vibration establishes the perceived pitch. Stated more simply, a person's voice is high, low, average, appropriate, or inappropriate for a given age and sex depending on how many times per second the vocal folds vibrate when activated by exhaled air. There are complex anatomical, physiological, and acoustical bases for this process, as explained in Chapter 1 (see also Andrews, 1999; Colton & Casper, 1996; Orlikoff & Baken, 1993; Titze, 1994).

Frequency of vocal fold vibration is determined by the critical variables of (a) vocal fold length, (b) vocal fold mass, (c) vocal fold tension, (d) shape of the resonance system, and (e) airflow and subglottal air pressure factors. These variables interact in complex fashion to determine voice pitch. Age and sex differences are apparent and are reflected in pitch. The speech–language pathologist is not capable of determining the status of the vocal folds with regard to length, mass, and tension except by analyzing the pitch of the voice; only subjective judgments about the actual size characteristics of the vocal folds can be made. Therefore, the client's pitch is critical to evaluate. Key questions to ask include the following: Is the pitch appropriate for the person's age and sex? Is it too low? Too high? Monopitched? Is there sex confusion when others hear the voice without seeing the speaker? Is the pitch a factor of vocal abuse or misuse?

Essentials of Pitch Evaluation

To be comfortable with pitch evaluation, the speech–language pathologist should be generally knowledgeable about the pitch spectrum of the human voice and how it relates to the musical scale. The following are some basic concepts relating to these two areas:

- The range of tones produced by the human voice can be compared to the musical tones (notes) on a piano, pitch pipe, or any musical instrument.

- Piano notes, for example, range from 27 Hz (lowest note) to 4186 Hz (highest note).

- All of the notes (tones) between these frequency values on the piano can be divided into octaves.

- An octave represents a doubling of the frequency of vibration, so a tone of 100 Hz doubled to 200 Hz constitutes an increase of one octave.

- Each octave is divided into eight whole tones, with each tone represented by a letter of the alphabet: CDEFGABC. Each C begins a new octave.

- From C to D is one whole tone step. C-sharp (C#) represents a half step (semitone) up. That same tone can be represented as a half step down from D, in which case it would be designated as D-flat (D♭).

- The octave in the middle of the piano scale contains the commonly known note of middle C, which corresponds to a frequency of 262 Hz. (It is called middle C because it is the note that divides the treble and bass clefs and is common to both clefs.)

- The C in the octaves below middle C is designated as C_1, C_2, or C_3, depending on the octave in which it is found. C_1 is the note one octave below middle C, D_2 is two Ds below middle C, and so on.

- A note above the octave in which middle C is found carries the designator above the letter, for example, C^2, F^3, or A^1. These examples are, respectively, C two octaves above middle C, F three octaves above the F in the middle C octave, and A one octave above the A in the middle C octave.

- Each note or tone in the musical scale can be indicated by its alphabetical note (CDEFGABC) in the octave it represents, such as A_2 or B^2, or by its actual numerical frequency, such as 110 Hz or 1975 Hz, respectively.

Table 3.1 compares tones with the frequency and musical scale values in the human voice range.

In pitch evaluation, the speech–language pathologist's task is to determine the client's habitual pitch level, or speaking fundamental frequency, and how it relates to the person's overall pitch characteristics. The habitual pitch is the modal or average level heard in a continuing sample of speech, the level around which normal pitch

TABLE 3.1
Frequency (Hertz) and Musical Scale Values

Note	Frequency[a]	Note	Frequency	Note	Frequency
A_3	55	A_1	220	A^1	880
B_3	62	B_1	245	B^1	988
C_2	65	C	262	C^2	1046
D_2	73	D	294	D^2	1175
E_2	82	E	330	E^2	1318
F_2	87	F	349	F^2	1397
G_2	98	G	392	G^2	1568
A_2	110	A	440	A^2	1760
B_2	123	B	494	B^2	1975
C_1	131	C^1	523	C^3	2093
D_1	147	D^1	587	D^3	2349
E_1	164	E^1	659	E^3	2637
F_1	175	F^1	698	F^3	2794
G_1	196	G^1	784	G^3	3136

[a]All decimal points are rounded.

inflections occur. This frequency could also be considered the one heard most commonly as a person talks, essentially the central tendency of pitch. Under normal circumstances, the habitual pitch is the pitch best suited for the length, mass, and tension factors in the client's larynx and is the level at which the larynx functions most efficiently. Under the best of conditions, the habitual pitch level should be around a frequency that is comfortable and physiologically appropriate for the client. Sometimes it is not, and the person's pitch is inappropriately high or low, causing a physiological mismatch. The speech–language pathologist must evaluate the habitual speaking level to determine whether pitch change would be clinically relevant.

Pitch can be evaluated with complex and elaborate equipment or with a simple pitch pipe, which can be purchased for a few dollars at any music store. One commonly used instrument is Kay Elemetrics Corporation's Visi-Pitch II for personal computer interface (see Figure 3.1). The instrument provides a digital readout of the fundamental frequency (F_0) of vocal fold vibration and an oscilloscopic rendering of phonation. When the client speaks into a microphone attached to the Visi-Pitch, the F_0 of the voice is extracted; up to 15 seconds of voice can be stored on the oscilloscope, and more can be stored in extended memory. Cursors can then identify the specific voice sample to be evaluated for any point along the sample. These measurements also

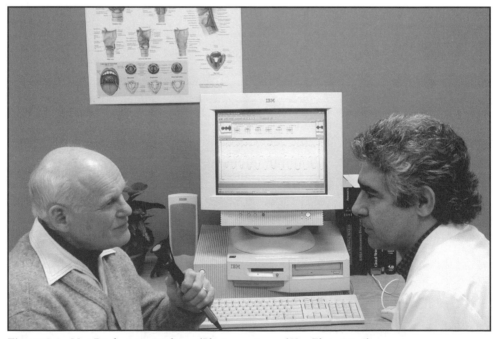

Figure 3.1. Visi-Pitch voice analyzer. (Photo courtesy of Kay Elemetrics.)

can be obtained from a quality tape recording. The Visi-Pitch instrument provides analyses of habitual pitch, basal (lowest possible) frequency, ceiling (highest possible) frequency, relative intensity (average loudness of the sample), maximum and minimum loudness or intensity levels, voice onset time, quality variations, glottal attack patterns, intonation patterns, timing and stress functions, and vibrato. (Many of these functions are described later.) Additional pitch measurement instruments include the Kay Elemetrics CSL and Multi-Speech 3700 system, discussed later in this chapter.

Measuring Pitch

The accuracy (validity) of measurement of voice tones using the Visi-Pitch or similar instrument depends on the instructions given to the client for obtaining the voice sample. Kent (1994a) discussed the importance of verbal instructions to clients in obtaining motor–speech samples, including voice. Many of the clinical processes presented in this section generally reflect Kent's recommendations.

When one is measuring extreme vocal usage, as in basal and ceiling frequencies, it is helpful to use the concept of "vocal idle" as a guide to the voice sampled and measured. Vocal idle is the least-effort usage of the voice. A good metaphor for vocal idle is the mechanical tuning of an automobile engine. To determine how well a car's engine is tuned, one does not drive it down the freeway at full speed. Even a poorly tuned engine can run fairly well at full acceleration. A better measurement would be obtained by evaluating performance when the engine is idling. Voice is similar. Even an inefficient larynx can produce voice when enough effort is applied; a better measure of vocal efficiency is to evaluate performance on vocal idle. This is an important concept for the speech–language pathologist to remember when evaluating various aspects of voice performance.

Habitual Pitch

After the speech–language pathologist has listened long enough in conversation to recognize the client's habitual pitch level, the next task is to isolate the habitual (modal) pitch so that it can be measured. An instrument such as the Visi-Pitch is used to isolate the pitch of the voice. The clinician usually begins by asking the client to count quickly from 1 to 10 and models the behavior. The modeling must be natural, not too fast and especially not too slow, because counting in individual numbers would provide an artificial sample. After one or two repetitions of this task, the instrument can be used to isolate the sample to be measured. After the speech–language pathologist determines that the isolated sample is representative of the client's typical speaking voice, the digital readout or the average on the computer readout is the habitual pitch.

Basal Pitch

To determine the basal (lowest possible) pitch, the speech–language pathologist can ask the client to produce a vowel (such as /á/) around the determined habitual pitch and hum down the musical scale until a tone is produced that is low, steady, and devoid of extreme tension or vocal breakage. This low pitch also should not involve glottal fry. One method to elicit the basal sound is to watch the Visi-Pitch screen and ask the client to do a glissando (rapid slide) down two or three times starting near the bottom of his or her range; the voice will be clear and steady until the basal is approached and then will break up and become fragmented on the screen. The horizontal cursor on the Visi-Pitch can then be placed at the point where breakage begins. If the client can sustain voice alone at that point, the basal has been obtained. The value of the basal frequency can be read off the screen where the horizontal cursor is placed. Voice in the glissando should not be averaged using vertical cursors, because they represent changing frequency.

Ceiling Pitch

To determine the ceiling (highest possible) pitch, the speech–language pathologist can ask the client to hum up the musical scale until the highest note emerges that does not sound strained. Most clients have varying ceiling frequencies depending on vocal effort. The client can be asked to produce a glissando or sliding pitch as high as possible, as modeled by the speech–language pathologist, who follows the procedures described for obtaining the basal frequency to determine the ceiling. At the point at which the voice stops on repeated glissando measurements upward, the client should be asked to sustain voice. If the client finds the pitch easy, the speech–language pathologist moves the cursor on the Visi-Pitch until a ceiling is reached. The frequency value on the cursor is used as the ceiling frequency.

Range

The speech–language pathologist can subtract the ceiling frequency from the basal frequency to determine the vocal range in frequency. The best way to present range data is in octaves or semitones (STs). There are 12 STs in each octave. Also, remember that each doubling of the frequency of vibration is one octave. A normal range for a healthy larynx is in the order of two to three octaves, or between 24 and 36 semitones.

STs constitute the most common basis of comparison and can be figured with the following formula:

$$ST = 39.86 \times \log (f_2/f_1),$$

where f_2 is ceiling frequency and f_1 is basal frequency. For example, if a 36-year-old woman can sustain tones as low as 147 Hz (f_1) and as high as 752 Hz (f_2), what is her range in STs? Simple subtraction indicates that she has a range of 605 Hz. That datum is not meaningful, however, because it does not allow comparison. To figure the STs, use a calculator with exponent and logarithm functions to do the following calculation:

$$ST = 39.86 \times \log{(752/147)}$$
$$= 28.2$$

Once the range in STs has been obtained, the woman's range can be compared with that of other women in her age category. The speech–language pathologist can provide positive feedback on the status of the larynx when the range is between 24 and 36 STs, which is compatible with the norms provided by Kent (1994b). When the range is between 36 and 48 STs, the potential for pitch usage is exceptional. It has been my clinical experience, however, that few persons other than trained singers have a pitch range more than 24 semitones, and such a range would not be considered unusual or inadequate.

Range measurement provides an index of laryngeal health for voice, because rarely does a nonprofessional voice user need much of the range potential for normal speaking. The professional voice user (e.g., the professional singer) is very concerned about range, however, because he or she must often sing notes that approach the upper and lower extremes of vocal range.

Optimal Pitch

The concept of an optimal (best) speaking pitch is found in the literature on voice beginning in 1940 when Grant Fairbanks introduced the concept (Fairbanks, 1960). The concept, which is not discussed as much today as when it was first introduced, is controversial, particularly the notion of measuring the entire vocal range and finding the pitch that represents one fourth or in some instances one third of the way up from the bottom of the range. Optimal pitch is based on the notion that the larynx performs best at a certain pitch (or near a certain pitch) and that speech–language pathologists would do well to train clients with voice disorders to speak at that pitch. Colton and Casper (1996) discussed the research attempts to validate the concept of optimal pitch, and they rejected the notion as it is defined by most authors who describe and use it.

Is optimal pitch a dead concept, however? If a speech–language pathologist interprets optimal pitch as a challenge to find a habitual pitch level that is less abusive, less effortful, and more efficient, then the concept is not dead as long as that pitch change is viewed in an overall evaluation of vocal fold physiology and vocal acoustics. The goal is to find pitch a that is *closer to* the pitch that might be considered optimal. Voice evaluations *often reveal* pitch patterns that require some attention. Some clients have habitual pitches that are too high, and some, too low. These pitch factors are often independent of overall physiological functioning of the larynx and stand out as independent parameters of voice. If, however, the interpretation of optimal pitch is that most clients with dysphonia have vocal pitches that are too high or too low and these factors are causal to the voice pathology, I would discourage this view. In my experience, however, there are some patients in whom changing the pitch of the voice helps trigger improved general physiological functioning, so it is appropriate to do so.

When pitch is identified as a factor that requires change, whether for improved physiology, efficiency, gender-related self-image, or improved vocal hygiene and physiology, specific steps can be taken to facilitate that change, as discussed in Chapter 4. As part of the evaluation process, however, it is important to attempt modification of pitch when one is concerned about pitch as a component of dysphonia. A trial period of pitch modification is appropriate as part of the evaluation proceedings, and it is usually easy to do.

In attempting pitch modification with the Visi-Pitch, the speech–language pathologist places the horizontal cursor slightly above the level of the client's habitual pitch (or slightly below if the pitch should be lowered). Then the clinician asks the client to count using a pitch that matches the cursor level. This visual feedback usually makes change easier than matching a tone or the clinician's voice. The clinician then evaluates whether the client's quality and ease of voice production are improved by the change in pitch. Also, the speech–language pathologist should ask the client how he or she feels about the difference. Different levels can be explored by moving the cursor and allowing the client to attempt normal pitch inflection around the cursor. This short trial period of change can add significant information about recommendations to make at the end of the evaluation.

In pitch evaluation it is important to remember that normal pitch usage involves voice that is close to the bottom of a person's pitch range. A typical adult has around two octaves (24 STs) of voice range and usually speaks a few whole tones above the bottom of the range. When a person speaks too near the bottom of the range, whether the pitch is (a) one component of an overall tense and hyperfunctional physiological pattern of voice production or (b) an isolated variable, the voice is generally less efficient in production. Often, if the client is encouraged to produce voice with less tension and appropriate tone placement (see Chapter 4), the pitch of the voice will emerge appropriately and naturally and specific attention to pitch will not be necessary. At other times, however, pitch is a variable that is independent of other physiological variables and must be evaluated and managed independently.

One of the most significant aspects of vocal pitch to be evaluated when investigating most dysphonias is vocal range or fundamental frequency range (FFR). FFR has been used extensively as an index of vocal health. The fundamental frequency (F_0) difference between the lowest and the highest tones produced constitutes the range, which can be expressed in absolute frequencies, tones or semitones, or octaves. Several authors (Kent, 1994b; Reich, Mason, Frederickson, & Schlauch, 1989; Stemple,

Glaze, & Klaben, 2000) have reported clinical evaluation processes that determine the pitch range of a patient. I have found that the typical range of adults is between 24 and 36 STs. Variables that affect range data include number of trials, time of day, general health of the subjects, presence of allergies, and numerous additional factors. Zraick, Nelson, Montague, and Monoson (2000) compared two methods of obtaining phonational frequency range—the glissando, or pitch sliding, method and a technique that uses discrete steps to obtain the range—and found both to elicit similar results.

VOCAL QUALITY

Chapter 1 describes the parameters of normal voice quality, including characteristics of the glottal waveform and resonance contributions. This section deals with voice quality in the clinical sense. It demonstrates how the speech–language pathologist can evaluate a person's voice quality with instruments, as well as through listening skill and perceptual judgment. Vocal quality is an inclusive concept that must be viewed as a combination of auditory–perceptual judgments and objective measurements of acoustic aspects of voice. It is not an easy task to delinieate or integrate these factions of voice quality, as indicated by an entire book's being devoted to the topic (Kent & Ball, 2000).

Voice quality is a confusing dimension for many clinicians. Certainly voice quality is influenced by numerous anatomical, physiological, psychological, sociological, cultural, multicultural, and pathological factors. Voice quality is also influenced by factors that can be isolated and measured separately, such as pitch, intensity, and resonance. In this chapter these measurements are considered as separate issues of voice evaluation.

Voice quality is determined either at the vibrating vocal fold level or by the shaping and resonating of sound produced by the vocal folds in the chambers of the pharyngeal, oral, and nasal cavities. When quality is affected negatively at the vocal fold level, it is because the folds are not vibrating properly as a result of some organic or functional condition in the larynx. Resonance processes cannot mask the negative effect produced by the vocal folds when they are vibrating abnormally. The voice quality will be perceived as abnormal regardless of resonance factors.

Hypofunctional and Hyperfunctional Voice

A common perception about the human voice is whether it has too much or too little tension. For normal voice quality to occur, the vocal folds must be able to meet at the laryngeal midline to approximate along their entire length, with just enough medial compression to impede the exhaled airstream, causing the folds to vibrate. There is a delicate balance between this approximation and resistance to airflow and the subglottal air pressure necessary to produce voice vibrations. Several conditions in the larynx might affect this balance negatively. The vocal folds might vibrate with too little approximation, allowing excessive air to escape through the glottis, in which case the voice sounds excessively breathy, meaning there is excessive airflow through the glottis during phonation. On the other hand, too much approximation can result in a voice marked by excessive tension. These conditions, respectively, cause voice qualities to be hypofunctional (too little approximation) or hyperfunctional (too much approximation).

Hypofunctional and hyperfunctional extremes occur often. An extreme of hypofunctional approximation is no voice at all, a condition called aphonia. An extreme of hyperfunctional approximation produces a voice quality so tense that airflow from the lungs cannot overcome the resistance of the taut vocal folds, producing a quality that sounds spastic. Between these extremes is a continuum of the gradients of laryngeal vibration. The voice qualities reflected in this continuum are described next in sufficient detail to allow the speech–language pathologist to be comfortable with each one. Figure 3.2 illustrates this continuum of vibration function at the vocal fold level.

Aphonia

The hypofunctional condition aphonia is heard in some forms of psychogenic (nonorganic) voice disorder in which nothing is structurally wrong with the vocal folds but the client produces no voice or sound. It also is found in recently laryngectomized persons. Other than laryngectomees, aphonic individuals are those who for psychological reasons make no attempt to produce voice or are so weak from illness or neurological disease that voice production is not possible.

Whisper

Whisper, which is on the hypofunctional end of the continuum, is easy to understand and identify because everyone has had an occasion to use it deliberately, for example, in the library, in church, or behind someone's back. However, the person who at all times can only whisper has a serious voice disorder. It could be caused by organic disease or psychological maladjustment.

HYPOFUNCTION	NORMAL FUNCTION	HYPERFUNCTION
Aphonia . . . Whisper . . . Breathiness . . . Normal Tension . . . Excessive Tension . . . Spasticity		

Figure 3.2. Continuum of vocal fold approximation. *Note.* From *Clinical Management of Speech Disorders* (p. 114), by D. E. Mowrer and J. L. Case, 1982, Austin, TX: PRO-ED. Copyright 1982 by PRO-ED, Inc. Reprinted with permission.

The quality described as whisper voice is produced by vocal folds that are so far apart during speaking attempts that only articulated airstream is heard. This can also occur when the vocal folds are fairly approximated but there is a significant posterior opening in the larynx. This articulation of sounds without voice support is the distinguishing characteristic between whisper voice and aphonia. In other words, the consonant sounds articulated by the tongue, teeth, or lips are heard in the whisper quality, but no voice supports them.

I believe that that whisper quality usually is a psychogenic voice disorder because an organic condition seldom produces true whisper other than in cases of severe and advanced neuromuscular disease. In most instances, whisper represents a functional turnoff of phonation when the client is otherwise healthy.

The glottal and supraglottal configurations supporting whispering have been generally described for clinical purposes (A. E. Aronson, 1990; Boone & McFarlane, 2000) but objectively delineated only by Solomon, McCall, Trosset, and Gray (1989), who used fiber-optic endoscopy on 10 nondysphonic persons under various conditions of whispered speech. They described vocal fold configuration, glottal size, and airway constriction of supraglottal structures and found significant differences between low-effort and high-effort whispering. Individual participant differences, however, tended to be considerably larger than any systematic patterns of whisper type. One significant finding pertains to the recommendation of whisper to accomplish vocal rest: The authors generally found vocal fold approximation during running speech whispering, which would be counterproductive to the recommendation of whispering as a form of vocal rest.

Colton and Casper (1996) reviewed much of the literature on glottal configurations during whispering and came to the conclusion that whispering is likely not harmful to laryngeal tissues and should not be avoided should clinical opinion indicate it might be helpful. They stressed that decreased laryngeal approximation might require increased effort in other areas of the vocal production system, which might be counterproductive. Care should also be taken to maximize hydration factors because whispering might have a drying effect on laryngeal tissues. Chapter 4 gives information about whispering as a recommendation for vocal rest.

Breathiness

Breathiness is a mixture of voice and excessive escape of air during speaking attempts. On the low end of the continuum, it is almost like a whisper except that slightly more voice is heard. Breathiness ranges from the near whisper to nearly normal voice. The significance of these subtle degrees of breathiness and an understanding of their causes are important factors in the clinical management of many voice disorders. Breathy voice quality correlates with other characteristics of voice quality, as indicated by Hillenbrand, Cleveland, and Erickson (1994), who determined that acoustic periodicity measures and relative amplitude of the first harmonic measures provide the most accurate predictions of perceived breathiness.

Excessive Tension

On the hyperfunctional side of the normal vibration pattern (described in Chapter 1) is phonation that includes excessive overadduction or medial compression of the vocal folds. This quality is heard perceptually as excessive tension. Like breathiness, tension exists on a continuum from slight (beyond normal approximation) to a degree that essentially stops the passive vibration of the vocal folds.

Tension is a common factor in many organic and nonorganic voice disorders, and the subtle variations often heard from client to client are important in distinguishing various voice disorders. Tension is a factor of excessive glottal resistance to airflow and subglottal pressure and often is described as a factor of overpressure. The greater the tension or overpressure, the greater the airflow and subglottal pressure needed to cause vibration.

Spasticity

When vocal tension from too much approximation of the vocal folds or overpressure is so great that even increased effort is not sufficient to overcome the resistance, voice is stopped and vocal spasticity occurs. In most cases, vocal spasticity is an intermittent phenomenon during voice production rather than a complete stoppage at all times. Typically, the person with a spastic voice quality manifests periods of excessive tension with periodic episodes of spasticity. Most patterns of spasticity indicate a neurologically based voice disorder known as adductor spasmodic dysphonia (see Chapter 5), which must be medically managed (Blitzer & Brin, 1992a, 1998).

The preceding categories of vocal fold approximation from hypofunctional to hyperfunctional aspects have been described perceptually. Hillman, Holmberg, Perkell, Walsh, and Vaughan (1989) are among many who have attempted to quantify vocal characteristics. Using noninvasive aerodynamic and acoustic recordings, they obtained measures of transglottal pressure, average glottal airflow, glottal resistance, vocal efficiency, vocal intensity, and fundamental frequency on 15 voice patients with nodules, polyps, contact ulcers, and nonorganic dysphonia. The results from these patients were compared with normative data on 45 participants from an earlier study by these same authors. They were able to objectively discriminate various conditions of hyperfunctional voice and correlate them to specific disorder conditions. Organic manifestations of vocal hyperfunction from nodules and other pathologies were accompanied by abnormally high values for the glottal waveform parameters of airflow, which reflected high vocal fold closure velocities and collision forces that produced vocal trauma. The opposite flow and acoustic parameters were found among the nonorganic voices, resulting in increased unmodulated airflow, a force less likely to cause vocal trauma. Other researchers have obtained surface EMG signals in an attempt to quantify the vocally hyperfunctional patient (Redenbaugh & Reich, 1989).

Hard Glottal Attacks

Hyperfunctional voice can involve excessive collision forces of the arytenoid cartilages. The perception is voice with abrupt onset called hard glottal attack. Hard glottal attack at the initiation of voice is generally considered a behavior that should be avoided. Andrade et al. (1999) studied the frequency of hard glottal attacks in patients with laryngeal masses and muscle tension dysphonia, comparing the findings with those for a control group of professional speakers and singers who did not demonstrate any laryngeal pathology or dysphonia. Those subjects with voice disorder demonstrated higher frequencies of hard glottal attack than the control group. Intuitively, one would assume a gender factor, suggesting that males are more likely to demonstrate increased instances of hard glottal attack. However, findings in this study indicated that females with dysphonia and laryngeal pathology were more likely to demonstrate instances of hard glottal attack.

COMBINATION OF FACTORS IN DYSPHONIA

In addition to the voice quality parameters representing variances along the phonation continuum from hypofunction to hyperfunction, several characteristics involve combinations of factors. These include hoarseness and diplophonia.

Hoarseness

Many different organic conditions affecting the vocal folds can produce the perceptual quality described as hoarseness. Hoarseness is a voice quality characterized by a rasping, grating, sometimes husky sound, frequently accompanied by voice breaks or diplophonia (double pitch). This description is typical of the perceptual usage of this term. Yanagihara (1967), who attempted to quantify acoustically the perceptual quality of hoarseness using a spectrograph, reported the following characteristics to be correlated with perceptions of hoarseness:

1. Noise components in the main formant of each vowel sampled
2. High-frequency noise components above 3000 Hz
3. Loss of high-frequency harmonic components

The greater the severity of hoarseness, the more prominent and exaggerated these factors become. From these findings Yanagihara advocated a classification of four types of hoarseness using sonogram tracings:

Type I. The regular harmonic components in the sonogram are mixed with the noise component, chiefly in the formant region of the vowels.

Type II. The noise components in the second formants of /ε/ and /i/ predominate over the harmonic components, and slight additional noise components appear in the high-frequency region above 3000 Hz in the vowels /ε/ and /i/.

Type III. The second formants of /ε/ and /i/ are totally replaced by noise components, and the additional noise components above 3000 Hz further intensify their energy and expand their range.

Type IV. The second formants of /α/, /ε/, and /i/ are replaced by noise components, and even the first formants of all vowels often lose their periodic components, which are supplemented by noise components. In addition, more intensified high-frequency noise components are seen.

Wolfe and Steinfatt (1987) used, among other measures, Yanagihara's sonogram tracing types to objectively discriminate normal from abnormal phonation among 51 patients with diverse laryngeal pathologies and found spectrographic noise to be the best single predictor of abnormality. Sasaki, Okamura, and Yumoto (1991) compared the total acoustic energy of the voice to the energy of the noise component present in the signal. Voice samples thus analyzed using a digital sonograph were correlated with perceptual judgments, producing high correlations (male sample, $r = 0.79$; female sample, $r = 0.81$).

An additional method of acoustically documenting the perceptual qualities of hoarseness is found in the harmonic-to-noise ratio, a measurement of the relative intensity of the vocal harmonics in a voice signal (acoustic multiples of the fundamental frequency) compared with the intensity of any surrounding spectral noise. Figure 1.13 shows a narrow-band spectrogram comparing a normal voice with a hoarse voice. Notice the obliteration of the harmonics in the upper frequencies of the spectrum as the magnitude of hoarseness is measured spectrographically.

It seems clear from the descriptions of hoarseness that many different characteristics are involved that have been described perceptually and acoustically. Many different organic conditions affecting the vocal folds can produce that quality. When a person has a cold and accompanying laryngitis, the voice becomes hoarse. Hoarseness also is caused by upper respiratory infections; allergies in the larynx; growths on the vocal folds, including cancer; vocal abuse and misuse; and numerous other conditions. Because the etiologies of hoarseness are so varied, the patterns of voice quality described as hoarseness similarly are varied. This is merely one reason why the terminology of voice disorder is controversial and researchers have recommended an international coordination of the terms used to describe various aspects of the voice (Sonninen & Hurme, 1992). By 2001 this recommendation had not been realized, and determination of vocal quality dimensions such as hoarseness remains a process of objective measurement of the bases of hoarseness transposed on that which can be perceived by a listener and evaluator (Kreiman & Gerratt, 2000).

Breathiness in Hoarseness

Most varieties of hoarseness result when some condition of the vocal folds prevents normal approximation and symmetrical vibration. For example, folds swollen from an infection usually are not affected uniformly. The mass characteristics of each fold therefore are different. In addition, the vibrating edge of each fold may be rough and uneven, resulting in incomplete approximation while speaking. This results in increased unobstructed airflow through the glottis during phonation, and breathiness is the primary perceptual characteristic heard. Some types of hoarseness involve a wet quality caused by excessive mucous secretions on the tissue of the folds. Other forms sound excessively dry because of insufficient lubrication of those tissues. Hoarseness can range from slight to severe. As recommended by Woo, Colton, Casper, and Brewer (1991) and Andrews (1999), the stroboscope works well to document these tissue differences in hoarse patients.

Perturbations

Cycle-to-cycle variations of voice production have been described as vocal perturbations. The speech or voice scientist can generate synthetic voice that does not vary and in which the cycles of frequency and intensity are exact and repetitive. Although computers can do that, the human larynx cannot. Even the greatest of singers cannot match the steadiness of bits and bytes. When vocal unsteadiness becomes apparent to human perception, dysphonia to some degree is the result. These variations of perturbation can be dichotomized into those that vary in (a) jitter (frequency) and (b) shimmer (intensity).

Jitter. Because the human voice is naturally unsteady when precisely measured, the degree of variation determines when the perception of abnormality has occurred. If a person is attempting to produce a tone such as a vowel prolongation as steadily as possible, the cycle-to-cycle variation of frequency can be measured and quantified. The value obtained is called jitter or jitter perturbation. A typical speaker without laryngeal disorder should be able to generate a vowel prolongation with very little jitter, usually less than 1%. As jitter values increase beyond this 1% level of normalcy, the voice appears increasingly dysphonic or rough. Therefore, jitter is a precise measurement of unintended frequency unsteadiness, which is one acoustic component of overall voice quality perception. Zraick, LaPointe, Case, and Duane (1993) presented data on jitter measurements of patients with the focal dystonia of torticollis and found that dystonic patients had, among other variables, significantly higher values of jitter than did typical controls. Jitter can be measured with a variety of instrumentation, including Visi-Pitch and laryngographic and spectrographic analysis. Figure 1.12 shows an acoustic waveform with time resolution demonstrating the cycle-to-cycle variation of jitter.

Shimmer. The perturbation information on jitter compares closely to the unsteadiness factor of vocal amplitude or intensity. Shimmer refers to the cycle-to-cycle variation of intensity. A typical speaker producing a prolonged vowel as steadily as possible should have little variation in intensity with each cycle of vibration. A larynx with functional or organic-based dysphonia will present significant unsteadiness of vocal parameters, including intensity. The value I use in determining whether a shimmer value is within normal limits is 1 dB. More than 1 dB of variation across the cycles would sound dysphonic, particularly when interacting with abnormal jitter values. Figure 1.12 shows a waveform display with indications of shimmer variation.

Many authorities appear to stress paying less attention to the precise perturbation measurements of jitter and shimmer and relying more on global and perceptual judgments of voice as an indication of dysphonia. This is apparent in the relative attention given to evaluation processes other than instrumental perturbation measurements (Andrews, 1999; Boone & McFarlane, 2000, Stemple et al., 2000). The science of voice measurement will continue to describe and use the acoustic algorithms of voice (Buder, 2000), but the voice clinician will more likely focus on perceptual characteristics, which are more clinically meaningful and potentially modifiable. In many years of evaluating and treating patients with dysphonia, I cannot remember a time when clinical decisions of management were based on a single measurement of jitter or shimmer. The measurements were obtained, that is certain, but only as a component for explaining overall judgments of vocal quality and stability. Such measurements have added greatly to our understanding of many aspects of normal and dysphonic voice, but it is unlikely that they will ever eliminate the need for more global and perceptual factors. The entire book *Voice Quality Measurement* (Kent & Ball, 2000) seems dedicated to integrating acoustic measurement with perceptual judgments, describing features that correlate for speech scientists and voice clinicians.

Tension (Strain)

Tension is often heard perceptually in hoarseness. Vocal tension is often described in the context of overall musculoskeletal tension and is one of the more difficult aspects of voice to evaluate and modify. It is often accompanied by pain when the larynx is manipulated or massaged, and that pain sometimes will refer to the ear. Musculoskeletal tension is often introduced into voice production when a person attempts to overcome the inefficiency of dysphonia and overdrives the system. However, it also can be etiologically related to various dysphonias as a form of vocal abuse (see Chapter 4). Roy and Leeper (1993) and Roy, Bless, Heisey, and Ford (1997) employed an extensive program of manual circumlaryngeal tension reduction and related voice change to perceptual and acoustic measures. Details of this process are reported in Chapter 4.

Diplophonia

Another characteristic heard in a few forms of dysphonia is double pitch, also called diplophonia. Authors of voice textbooks acknowledge the possibility of diplophonia but minimize its importance in the overall profile of voice seen in the dysphonias (Colton & Casper, 1996). Possible causes for diplophonia include the following:

- One vocal fold has different mass characteristics from the other fold and therefore vibrates at a fundamental frequency that is sufficiently different to produce the perception of two pitches.

- The action of the ventricular folds in vibrating simultaneously with the true vocal folds produces two pitches. (I believe this would be a rare finding.)

Diplophonia often is heard in cases of unilateral vocal fold paralysis in which the nerve supply to one vocal fold is disrupted for some reason. Without innervation, the approximation potential of the paralyzed fold is disrupted, which after a considerable period of time causes tissue atrophy. The lessened mass of the paralyzed vocal fold causes it to vibrate faster when it is in a position to be influenced by exhaled air. The faster rate of vibration is perceived as a higher pitch being produced by the paralyzed vocal fold than by the normal one. Diplophonia has not been well documented visually and acoustically in the literature.

INSTRUMENTATION IN VOICE QUALITY EVALUATION

Some instruments available for the speech–language pathologist in evaluating voice parameters that determine quality include the spectrograph, the electroglottograph, aeromechanical (flow and pressure) instrumentation, and a good audio recorder. The clinical voice laboratory is becoming an expected facility in training programs in speech–language pathology as well as in the clinical offices of otolaryngologists. Excellent general references for the basic instrumentation needed for such a laboratory are Gould (1987) and Sataloff (1991, 1998c). Kent (1997) and Baken and Orlikoff (2000) provide a complete description of how to interpret the information obtained from instrumental measurement. Kent (1994a) provided a scholarly discussion regarding the basic interpretation of vocal tract acoustics for the voice scientist, speech–language pathologist, or music teacher, information elaborated upon by Kent and

Ball (2000). All of these authors agree that in clinical relationships, effective management occurs when the scientific basis of vocal tract acoustics can be applied to the modification of dysphonic voices in practical and understandable terms. It becomes a challenge to maintain accuracy and objectivity in a forum of clinical communication to patients, a challenge faced by every clinician working with dysphonic individuals. Patients who receive a copy of their written clinical report after an evaluation do not understand much about jitter, shimmer, spectrographic details, and harmonic-to-noise ratios. Sometimes an attempt to impress with measurement merely causes confusion. Regardless, the speech–language pathologist must be comfortable with the instrumentation of measurement to competently treat patients with dysphonia.

Spectrograph

The sound or speech spectrograph has been described by Lieberman (1977) as probably the single most useful device for the quantitative analysis of speech. It was developed at Bell Telepone Laboratories in connection with work on analysis–synthesis speech transmission systems. Since those early days, extensive research and clinical applications have appeared in the literature and the laboratories. Baken and Daniloff (1991) and Baken and Orlikoff (2000) compiled much of that literature in these documents.

A powerful spectrographic instrument is Kay Elemetrics Corporation's Digital Sona-Graph 5500, a DC-16 kHz Spectrum Analyzer, which produces spectrograms, fast Fourier transforms, waveform displays of frequency and amplitude, and other analysis displays in real time (see Figure 3.3). The Sona-Graph's memory stores 2 megabytes of sampled data, which translates to about 50 seconds of speech sampled at 20 kHz. These same acoustic analyses are possible on the Computer Speech Laboratory (CSL), also manufactured by Kay Elemetrics Corporation, which has largely replaced the freestanding sonograph. The CSL turns a personal computer into a powerful speech acoustics laboratory.

Computer Speech Laboratory

The CSL is a comprehensive PC-based system for speech acquisition, analysis, editing, and playback. It has a large array of easy-to-use acoustic analysis routines that provide complete spectrographic detail, spectral information, pitch and intensity displays and analysis, long-term average spectrum, and numerous additional programs. The sampling rate potential of the CSL (50 kHz per channel with 16-bit resolution) provides excellent support for the most sophisticated acoustic analysis requirement. The CSL also provides extensive speech-editing capability, including mixing, subtracting, digital filtering, adding, and splicing of sound to be analyzed. The CSL is an ideal tool for professional use in the clinic or the speech science laboratory. Baseline measurements before therapy or surgery provide excellent

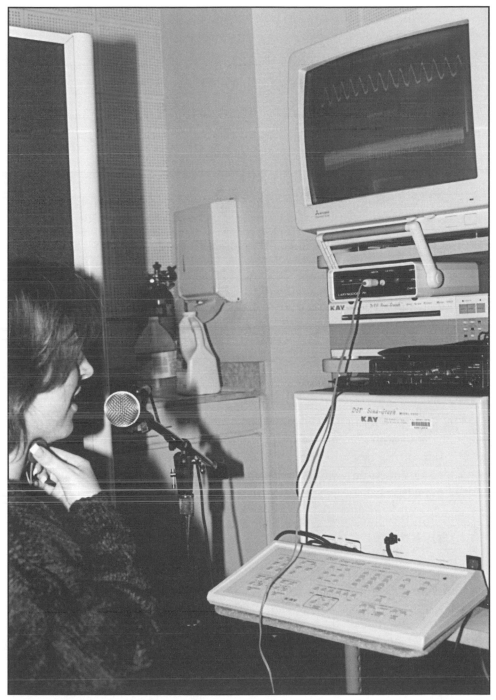

Figure 3.3. DSP 5500 Sona-Graph and Laryngograph.

documentation of a patient's voice, which can be compared to later measurements to chart decline or improvement. These objective measurements can be stored in patient files on the computer or printed out for medical documentation and record-keeping processes.

Some of the common uses of the CSL in clinical and voice science laboratories include the following:

- Immediate access to CD-quality playback of voice samples, which can be used to describe or monitor the voice quality for a patient or client.

- Spectrographic analysis of voice patterns to demonstrate to a patient clarity or abnormality of formant regions.

- Delayed auditory feedback can be used to provide feedback to a patient working on obtaining a certain voice quality.

- Real-time pitch and loudness contours can be used to help a client modify voice performance to match a targeted level established by the speech–language pathologist as more appropriate.

- The Multi-Dimensional Voice Program, with more than 22 parameters of voice that can be graphically and numerically represented and compared to a built-in database of voices.

- The Voice Range Profile, which portrays pitch and loudness contours of the human voice.

The CSL provides comprehensive support for the voice clinician to provide essentially any information needed in the clinical management of voice other than visualization of the larynx. Figure 3.4 shows a screen from the CSL demonstrating many acoustic data from a waveform. Figure 3.5 shows the screen from the CSL Voice Range Profile.

Electroglottograph

One of the most precise instruments available for glottal waveform analysis is the electroglottograph (EGG), also called the laryngograph. An example of such an instrument is the Kay Elemetrics Laryngograph (see Figure 3.3). The laryngograph transducers, positioned on the surface of each side of the user's neck at the level of the vocal folds, detect changes in voltage across the vocal folds during the vibratory cycle. The tiny current passes back and forth between the sensors.

In the larynx, vocal fold activity in vibration creates a variable resistance to the flow of electricity, which can be detected and quantified. Human tissue is a moderately effective conductor of electricity; air or space, by comparison, generates

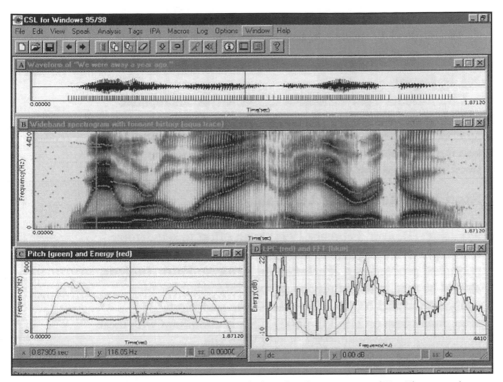

Figure 3.4. CSL (Computer Speech Laboratory). (Used with permission of Kay Elemetrics.)

increased impedance to the flow of electricity. Therefore, if a current of electricity were passed directly across laryngeal tissue, for example, to be detected by a special sensor, the relative conductance or resistance of that electrical flow would vary depending on whether the vocal folds were in a contact position, providing little resistance or impedance, or a noncontact position, providing increased impedance. These tiny variations can be quantified and represented graphically. From this, the opening, open, closing, and closed phases of vibration can be charted.

However, recent research indicates that the (laryngeal) Lx signal transduces only the vocal fold contact area and manifests little information about the open status of the glottis (Baken & Orlikoff, 2000). The duration, velocity, and degree of closure of the vocal folds are visually represented. Thus, the laryngograph provides accurate and objective representation of vocal fold movement and contact patterns. The results (Lx waveform or laryngograph waveform) are displayed on a monitor, oscilloscope, or graphic printout. The laryngograph system works with Visi-Pitch, IBM PC, CSL, or Kay 5500 Sona-Graph. It can also be used as part of videostroboscopy measurement, in which the Lx waveform can be superimposed on the monitor screen for analysis and printout capability. The waveform data can be compared

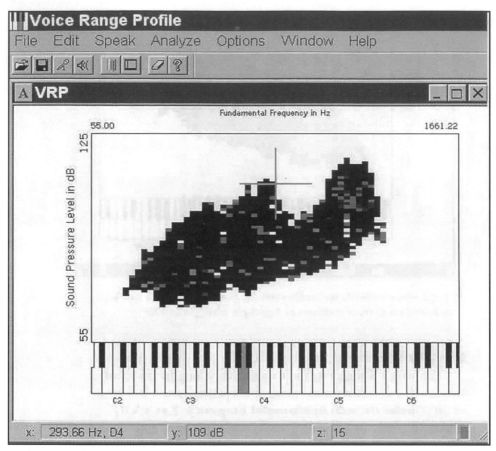

Figure 3.5. CSL—Voice Range Profile. (Used with permission of Kay Elemetrics.)

with acoustic, visualization-of-laryngeal-structure, and airflow data for further quantification of vocal parameters. An example of how the Lx waveform can be displayed with stroboscopic analysis is shown in Figure 3.6.

The EGG is commonly used in most clinical evaluations of voice when instrumentation is an important aspect of the process. Many clinics now have this technology and use it routinely. It is important that its use be moderated by many factors of concern, particularly in terms of interpretation of the EGG or Lx waveform. Colton and Conture (1990) and Titze (1990, 1994) provided significant guidelines for EGG usage, including cautions about interpretation. One concern is electrode placement, which Titze indicated should be as reduced as possible in interelectrode distance. Electrode size and angle can also affect the quality of the Lx obtained. Only a small portion (less than 1%) of the total current flows through the glottal area; therefore, much of the signal variability results from other tissues in the neck area. The total glottal signal, called the Gx, must be filtered to detect the Lx signal. This filtering process adds an additional independent variable to the accuracy of the dependent Lx signal. Colton and Conture warned that, although correctly placing the electrodes in the middle of each thyroid lamina is easy for large males, correct placement is difficult for children and smaller women. The tester should try variable positions until the best signal is obtained.

Additional concerns expressed by Colton and Conture include the following:

- It is usually more difficult to obtain good Lx signals in women than men because of women's smaller vocal folds, slightly larger angle (more obtuse) of lamina, and more-adipose tissue in the larynx area.

- The foregoing concern is somewhat countered by data on neck size circumference, which indicate that larger necks generate greater impedance. Therefore, caution is necessary when interpreting the Lx through the neck of, for instance, a tackle on a professional football team; a lot of impedance is likely.

- EGG is less reliable on patients with mass lesions on the vocal folds or with unilateral adductor paralysis.

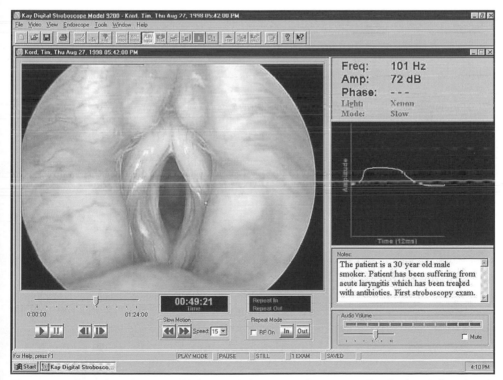

Figure 3.6. Digital strobe view of larynx with laryngographic tracing also displayed. (Used with permission of Kay Elemetrics.)

- Mucous strands can complicate the EGG picture by generating a current bridge across the glottis. Asking the subject to gently clear the throat and swallow prior to measurement might preclude this possibility.

- The Lx is somewhat imprecise in showing the cycle of vocal fold vibration, so caution is needed in interpretation.

- The EGG signal is a simple, noninvasive procedure for measuring some aspects of vocal fold vibration but, again, as long as caution is exercised in the interpretation process.

Some of the concerns listed are somewhat eliminated by the use of multichannel EGGs, as recommended by Rothenberg (1992). He wrote that multichannel EGG recordings can help eliminate the interpretation of Gx and Lx separation. Considerable additional discussion has occurred in the literature regarding how to interpret the Lx waveform signal (Baken & Orlikoff, 2000; Fourcin, 2000; Orlikoff, 1998), and the speech–language pathologist who uses this technology should consult these references. Notwithstanding, the clinical process of Lx usage remains essentially as it has for the past decade.

Aeromechanical Instrumentation

Basic to understanding phonation under normal and abnormal conditions is the concept of how airflow and air pressure relate to vocal fold vibration. Several attempts have been made to measure the efficiency of the vocal folds in opposing the flow of air through them to cause vibration, a process called laryngeal airway resistance.

Smitheran and Hixon (1981) described a method of calculating laryngeal airway resistance from the ratio of translaryngeal pressure to translaryngeal airflow. The aeromechanical instrumentation necessary to measure these factors includes an air pressure transducer coupled to an amplifier; a filter and storage oscilloscope system for pressure measurements; and a pneumotachometer coupled to a second but matched differential air pressure transducer, amplifier, and storage oscilloscope system for the measurement of airflow. From measurements obtained through these channels directed through a mask, the ratio representing laryngeal airflow resistance can be calculated. The authors reported data on 15 nondysphonic persons, with a mean laryngeal airflow resistance of 35.7 cm H_2O/LPS (liters per second).

Smitheran and Hixon's (1981) data compared favorably with earlier studies of laryngeal airway resistance that involved puncturing of the trachea with a hypodermic needle to measure tracheal pressure. Their method is noninvasive and therefore superior.

Airflow and air pressure during phonation can be measured with commercially available instruments, such as the Kay Elemetrics Aerophone II, Voice Function Analyzer (see Figure 3.7). The Aerophone II consists of hardware and software for computer-based phonation analysis. The hardware consists of a hand-held transducer

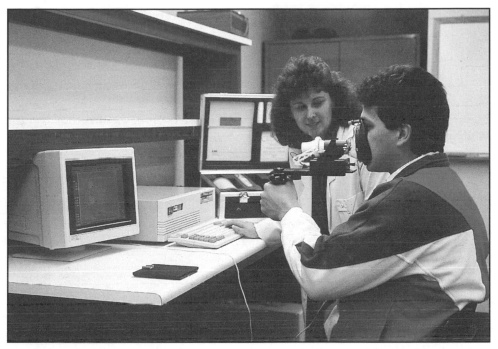

Figure 3.7. Kay Elemetrics Aerophone II Voice Function Analyzer, Model 6800. (Photo courtesy of Kay Elemetrics.)

module with different-size masks and disposable tubes for running speech and sustained vocalizations. The computer printout provides more than 22 voice and speech calculations, including airflow, air pressure, and sound pressure.

Woo, Colton, and Shangold (1987) used phonatory airflow with 150 patients having various laryngeal diseases and compared them with 60 persons with normal voices. They were able to discriminate categories of dysphonia etiology (paralysis, polyp, cancer, vocal nodules, etc.) on the basis of mean flow (unphonated) compared with alternating flow (modulated by vocal folds in phonation), as well as other frequency spectra data.

Normal values of laryngeal airflow are between 100 and 150 cc/sec (or ml/sec), typically toward the higher end of that range. The values for males are also typically a little higher than for females, but that is often determined by effort levels. Laryngeal pathology also significantly alters normal values. For example, a patient with laryngeal paralysis manifests poor laryngeal valving, and excessive air escapes during phonation, producing airflow values from 300 to 400 cc/sec. The perceptual correlate of excessive airflow is increased breathiness in the voice.

It is clear that phonatory airflow values are affected by several independent variables, such as age, gender, respiratory drive, degree of laryngeal valving at the vocal fold level, frequency and intensity of the sound being measured, and whether a vowel is used for sustained production as opposed to mean values obtained from continuous speech. When using these measurements, one should compare a patient's values to normative data, keeping in mind these variables.

Kent (1994b) summarized the flow data from several sources compiled by Kent, Kent, and Rosenbek (1987) and provided an excellent chart of data for adults and children. The data are reported in means and standard deviations by study and age group. Most adult flow rates are between 100 and 150 cc/sec, and values above 150 cc/sec should be considered at least borderline abnormal for excessive flow. Child flow rates appear only slightly lower. Kent's chart provided data on nondysphonic participants who were asked to whisper as flow measurements were taken. The mean flow rate of 413 cc/sec, with a standard deviation of 72 cc/sec, is only slightly higher than the value reported for a patient with vocal fold paralysis. Kent and Ball (2000) and Baken and Orlikoff (2000) provide a complete description of aeromechanical principles associated with voice production.

When a pneumotachometer or flowmeter is not available, an estimate of laryngeal airflow can be obtained using a measure called the phonation quotient, which correlates quite well with actual measurements of flow. The phonation quotient is calculated by dividing the vital capacity by the maximum phonation duration. Normative data from this procedure suggest a phonation quotient of around 145 ml/sec for males and 137 ml/sec for females (Prator & Swift, 1984).

INSTRUMENTATION FOR LOUDNESS MEASUREMENT

With many disorders of phonation, it is necessary to quantify the intensity or loudness potential of the voice. The Kay Visi-Pitch Voice Analyzer (see Figure 3.1) has a loudness (intensity) function as well as pitch analysis function and can measure the two simultaneously. In the intensity-only mode, the Visi-Pitch displays voice intensity variations on the screen. A horizontal cursor can be placed on the screen to match the intensity pattern, and a digital readout of the cursor level indicates the relative intensity. The clinician also can obtain a voice sample and use the vertical cursors to mark a section for computer analysis of relative intensity. This measurement is of relative intensity only. The distance between the microphone and the mouth must be kept stable for comparative measurements because the instrument provides no absolute value of sound pressure. Absolute intensity can be measured with a sound level meter (see Figure 3.8).

What is normal with regard to intensity of the voice? Certainly the speech–language pathologist must consider this issue during the evaluation process. The

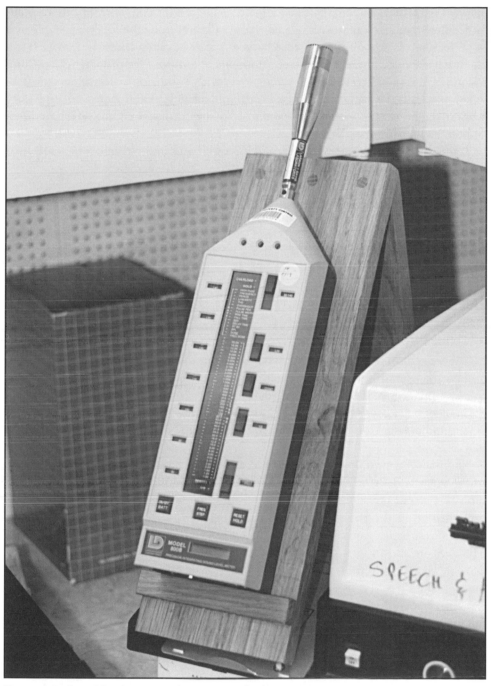

Figure 3.8. Sound level meter used to measure absolute intensity.

answer depends on the circumstances. Loudness levels for conversations in a restaurant differ from the loudness levels of pillow talk and from the loudness levels in a large lecture classroom. The normal larynx accommodates these extremes. For a client with a voice disorder, however, variations of loudness control might constitute a significant clinical concern. When a person with Parkinson's disease is evaluated, loudness control focusing on increased vocal fold adduction and increased respiratory support might be the most significant issue to be managed (Ramig, Countryman, Thompson, & Horii, 1995).

According to Colton and Casper (1996) and Kent (1994b), values typically used to determine whether a client has a vocal loudness concern are as follows:

- Conversation levels are typically around 60 dB (SPL around 1 meter).
- Maximum levels are around 100 to 110 dB (SPL around 1 meter).
- Minimum levels not involving whispering are around 40 dB.

INSTRUMENTATION FOR RESONANCE EVALUATION

Many voice disorders involve functional or organic dysfunction of the velopharyngeal mechanisms, resulting in abnormal vocal tract resonance. When velopharyngeal dysfunction occurs in speech, the vocal quality usually involves excessive nasal resonance, called hypernasality. Devices and instruments have been developed to detect and measure the airflow, air pressure, and sound pressure bases for this abnormal resonance.

Perhaps the most commonly used instrument for measuring the nasal component to the voice is the Kay Elemetrics Nasometer (see Figure 3.9). The Nasometer separates oral sound pressure from nasal sound pressure during running speech or vowel prolongation. It is computer interfaced, and large samples of speech or voice can be analyzed. Statistics can be calculated for voice samples and compared with norms. The data are shown by a score called *nasalance*, which is the ratio of nasal and oral acoustic SPL. This term is used to distinguish it from perceived nasality. The ratio is multiplied by 100 to convert it to a percentage.

Three sets of phonetically manipulated words and phrases have been used to obtain norms for nasalance. The Zoo Passage (Fletcher, 1978) is a short passage that excludes nasal consonants. The Rainbow Passage (Fairbanks, 1960) is a phonetically balanced passage that contains 11.5% nasal consonants. The Nasal Sentences (Fletcher) are five sentences in which 35% of the phonemes are nasal consonants. Using these readings, Fletcher, Adams, and McCutcheon (1989) derived normative data for the Nasometer:

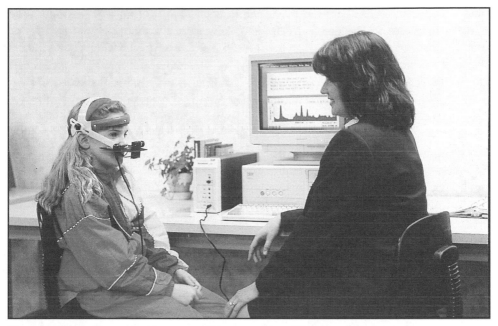

Figure 3.9. Kay Elemetrics Nasometer. (Photo courtesy of Kay Elemetrics.)

Reading	Mean Nasalance	Standard Deviation
Zoo Passage	15.53%	1.86
RainbowPassage	35.69%	5.20
Nasal Sentences	61.06%	6.95

These norms are for 117 children ages 5 through 12, but similar results should be expected with adults.

In the evaluation process, the speech–language pathologist would be interested in correlating the presence of high nasalance scores on the Nasometer with the condition of the velopharyngeal mechanism. Dalston, Warren, and Dalston (1991) compared nasalance scores from the Nasometer with aeromechanical estimates of velopharyngeal insufficiency and found nasalance scores to highly predict significant velopharyngeal openings. They concluded that the Nasometer is an appropriate instrument for assessing nasality and its physiological basis, the velopharyngeal mechanism. Similar results have been reported by Nellis, Neiman, and Lehman (1992) regarding velopharyngeal assessment after pharyngeal flap surgery and by Hardin, Van Demark, Morris, and Payne (1992) regarding comparison of listener judgments of hypernasality and hyponasality with nasalance scores. Dalston (1992) compared the Nasometer with an evolving method of assessment, the acoustic rhinometer, and found good correlations between the instruments. In terms of material used for sampling of the voice for nasalance, Watterson, Lewis, and Homan-Foley (1999) found that valid assessments of nasalance can be achieved with speech samples as short as six syllables, but Lewis, Watterson, and Quint (2000) cautioned that nasalance scores can be altered by the type of vowel context used, stressing that high vowels, for example, produce higher nasalance scores. Most clinical assessments, however, involve considerably more samples than a few syllables and a variety of vowel–consonant contexts. Watterson, Lewis, and Deutsch (1998) also provided information indicating that stimulus materials containing either low-pressure (vowels, glides, and liquids) or high-pressure speech items (stops, fricatives, and affricates) can be used in assessments without affecting measurement accuracy. Additionally, from a multicultural perspective, Nichols (1999) provided data on nasalance scores using the Nasometer for two populations of Mexican participants (two cities in central Mexico and three ages across childhood and into adulthood), and Doorn and Purcell (1998) provided data for nondysphonic Australian children. These studies all demonstrated the effectiveness of the Nasometer in measuring factors related to perceived hyper- and hyponasality under a variety of conditions.

Bressmann et al. (2000) described an additional system of obtaining measurements of nasalance using the NasalView, a PC-based system for computerized measurement of nasalance developed by Awan (1997) and manufactured by Tiger Electronics. They described how this system can be used in the clinical measurement of nasalance and also how it differs from the Nasometer.

INSTRUMENTATION FOR RESPIRATION MEASUREMENT

The speech–language pathologist must be prepared to evaluate the respiratory system as part of a voice evaluation. In most cases, the dysphonic client has more than sufficient respiratory support for phonation, and any abnormality in respiration involves coordination of breathing patterns for speech rather than sufficiency of air supply. The exception to this statement is when a patient with some form of dysarthria is being evaluated, in which case respiratory sufficiency becomes a primary issue. Disorders that cause dysarthria are discussed in Chapter 5. Respiration is considered so important to speech and singing that nearly an entire issue of the *Journal of Voice* (Sataloff, 1988) was devoted to this topic, and nearly every issue since that one has contained articles dealing with respiration and voice.

Kent (1994b) compiled norms for many aspects of respiration, including standards of measurement, appropriate instrumentation, capacities by age and gender, respiration rates by age and gender, physiological requirements for speech production, body size factors related to respiration, flow–volume relationships, and the effects of effects of smoking on the respiration tract. Many of these concerns relate to most voice evaluations, whereas others apply only to evaluations of special populations.

Determining which respiration tests to perform is a clinical decision that the speech–language pathologist must make in each instance of voice evaluation. The following are some of the pertinent questions: Is the vital capacity sufficient for this patient? Do the patterns of respiration show efficient use? Are speech and voice prolonged toward the end of respiratory cycles? Must attention be directed objectively toward respiration sufficiency and patterns in the clinical management process? Many evaluations of voice require little attention other than respiratory screening. As stated earlier, however, when evaluating patients with dysarthria, such as that found in Parkinson's disease and amyotropic lateral sclerosis, the clinicians must direct major attention to every aspect of respiration.

Sufficiency of Respiration

Under normal conditions, the human respiratory system provides more than sufficient air for normal phonation. The vital capacity (VC), often referred to as forced vital capacity (Kent, 1994b; Zemlin, 1998), of a person's lungs is measured by the amount of air that can be exhaled after as deep an inhalation as possible. To obtain this measurement, the client is placed before an instrument of respiratory measurement, such as a spirometer, and given the following instructions: "Take as deep a breath as possible. When you have achieved maximum inhalation, place your mouth onto this mouthpiece and blow all of your air into the tube [or mask]. Don't stop until all of your air is out. Let me demonstrate."

The normal VC value for individuals depends on body size, which correlates with age. For females, the displaced air in VC measurements ranges from 1,365 ml when height is 3 feet 8 inches and age is around 6 years, to about 4,447 ml when height is 5 feet 9 inches and age is around 18 years. For males, the VC ranges from 1,418 ml when height is 3 feet 8 inches and age is around 6 years to 4,927 ml when height is 5 feet 9 inches and age is around 18 years. These data indicate that there are gender differences beyond the size of the body. VC data for mature adults are similar to those given for 18-year-olds. A reasonable mean VC value for female adults (ages 18 to 30) would be around 3,500 to 4,000 ml, and for male adults (ages 18 to 30) around 4,500 to 5,000 ml. For research purposes, the exact range of data reported by Kent (1994b) for comparison purposes would be necessary; for most clinical evaluations, general comparisons should be fine. If proper support processes are engaged, a woman with a vital capacity of around 3,500 to 4,000 ml and a man with a VC of about 4,500 to 5,000 ml will have plenty of respiratory support for typical voice and speech purposes.

Although the vital capacity is used as an index of lung capacity for speech and voice functions, a person does not use the entire vital capacity in functional, quiet respiration or for speech. Other volumes are also useful in respiratory evaluation. Tidal volume is the amount of air inhaled and exhaled during any single respiration cycle during quiet, nonspeech breathing. Zemlin (1998) stated that 750 cc is a typical mean tidal volume value for young male adults, with a 95% range from 675 to 896 cc. For young female adults, the tidal volume range is from 285 to 393 cc, with a mean value of 339 cc. Thus, one can see that only a small percentage of total vital capacity is used in quiet breathing. The same is true for speech. Kent (1994b) reported that between 25% and 40% of vital capacity is used in speech by typical adults.

Two additional respiration values are important in the phonation evaluation process. Inspiratory reserve volume is the amount of air that can be inhaled after a tidal volume inhalation; expiratory reserve volume is how much can be exhaled after a tidal exhalation. These inspiratory and expiratory reserve volume values are large in healthy adults, ranging from 1,500 to 2,500 cc and from 1,500 to 2,000 cc, respectively. All of these respiration values exceed the minimal requirements for normal phonation.

In phonation, these volume respiration values must be translated into pressure and flow values to be meaningful. In other words, the respiration system must be able to generate sufficient pressure and flow to drive the vocal folds in vibration. During conversational speech the level of this pressure typically ranges between 5 and 10 cm H_2O.

Airflow through the glottis during phonation is around 100 cc/sec; the exact value depends on the magnitude of subglottic pressure and the opposition that the larynx provides to the flow (Netsell & Hixon, 1978). Netsell, Lotz, Peters, and Schulte (1994) compared developmental data for three groups of children (preschool, early school, and preadolescence) with adult norms on subglottal pressure, glottal resistance, and airflow. Their data indicated that pressure and resistance tend to decrease with increases in airflow as children mature. They accounted for these trends by noting the increased changes in laryngeal airway with aging. Younger children apparently have increased expiratory muscle forces behind their respiratory efforts for speech to compensate for smaller airway structures. Adult patterns involve improved coordination of inspiratory and expiratory muscle forces during speech breathing. Children move developmentally toward these adult patterns. No significant gender differences were noted in the child populations.

How can the speech–language pathologist measure these values in the voice evaluation? Hixon, Hawley, and Wilson (1982) have provided a simple method if only a simple screening procedure is needed to ensure that a client has minimal respiration support for phonation and elaborate instrumentation is not available. It requires a tall (12 cm or more), transparent drinking glass nearly filled with tap water, a regular drinking straw held to the inside of the glass by a large paper clip, and a strip of common surgical adhesive tape with centimeter markings on it and about as long as the glass is tall. The straw is submerged 10 cm into the glass. The subject blows into the straw. If bubbles are produced and can be sustained for 5 seconds, the minimum of 10 cm H_2O pressure over time has been obtained, and the client passes the screening test.

Chest and Diaphragm Movement

Several researchers have studied respiration volumes by measuring changes in chest wall, rib cage, abdomen, and lung dimensions during breathing. Hoit and Hixon with additional collaborators have written extensively about breathing patterns and volumes in speech and singing. They have investigated the speech breathing of children and adolescents (Hoit, Hixon, Watson, & Morgan, 1990), people of various ages (Hoit & Hixon, 1987), women (Hoit, Hixon, Altman, & Morgan, 1989), and actors (Hixon, Watson, & Maher, 1987). In most of these studies, electromagnetic transducers (magnetometers) were placed on the body so that one sensing coil could sense the strength of a magnetic field generated by a coil mate. Two generator-sensor pairs were used, one pair to sense rib cage diameter changes, the other abdominal diameter changes. These magnetometers provided the data that allowed analysis of respiratory patterns and volumes during various aspects of phonation and speech.

Hixon and Hoit (2000) provided an extensive worksheet to be used by speech–language pathologists in evaluating the rib cage during various activities of respiration, including many practical ones during speech. They used this article as a summary statement regarding their previous articles on specific attention to the diaphragm (Hixon & Hoit, 1999) and the abdominal wall (Hixon & Hoit, 1998). The worksheet provides guidelines of breathing evaluation that investigate, among other processes, resting tidal breathing; running speech production; maximum inspiration and rib cage expansion; maximum expiration and rib cage compression; various processes after total lung capacity inhalation, including voicing a soft vowel; and practical control processes such as panting, catching breath, gasping, and blowing out a candle. Observations are evaluated on an ordinal scale from 0 to −4 degree of abnormality (0 = *normal judgment*, −1 = *mild abnormality*, −2 = *moderate abnormality*, −3 = *severe abnormality*, −4 = *profound abnormality*). The worksheet also provides a space for additional comments.

It is difficult to summarize such extensive research efforts in a manner that is practical for the working speech–language pathologist who evaluates children and adults with dysphonia and who wishes to competently identify salient respiratory concerns. Here, however, are a few general conclusions:

- Expiratory effort in the upright body position during conversational speech involves both rib cage and abdominal regions, and in the supine position it involves only the diaphragm region.

- The abdomen occupies an especially important role during running conversation by supporting and increasing the diaphragm's inspiratory efficiency so that interruptions for inspiration during speech are minimal.

- Speech breathing patterns become adultlike quite early in life, around the end of the first decade, regardless of sex.

- Regardless of the attention the diaphragm has received in studies on breathing, it appears that younger subjects use rib cage changes to accomplish volumes necessary for speech.

- Attention must be directed toward the relationship between age and respiratory patterns of clients being studied for voice production. Younger people tend to use less capacity in speaking, take breaths more frequently, and terminate breath groups with remaining higher volumes of air in the lungs.

Another instrument that uses diameter changes in the rib cage and abdominal regions to quantify respiratory volumes is manufactured by Respitrace. This is a plethysmographic (size measurement) system consisting of two coils of wire (called respibands) that encircle the rib cage and abdominal compartments. The expansion and contraction of these coils during breathing causes changes in the oscillating frequency of the circuits within the electronic system. After the signals are calibrated for volume, recording values are equivalent to air volumes inhaled and exhaled.

More information regarding training of improved respiration for speech is provided in Chapter 4. Excellent general references for understanding respiration patterns in women and men, respectively, are by Hodge and Rochet (1989) and Hixon, Watson, Harris, and Pearl (1988).

MAXIMUM PHONATION DURATION

The ability to sustain phonation to a maximum duration is clinically relevant information as part of a voice disorder evaluation. Data on maximum phonation duration (MPD) across the age span from 3 years through geriatric years are provided by Kent (1994b) and shown in Figure 3.10. Kent's data indicate that a 3-year-old child can sustain a vowel just under 10 seconds, with a range from 2 or 3 seconds to just over 10 seconds. These data become clinically meaningful around school age, when children's mean duration is not much longer than that of 3-year-olds but the ranges increase. Adult norms indicate that men can sustain a vowel for more than 20 seconds and women for just under 20 seconds. These values go down for both male and female geriatric subjects.

MPD studies include an attempt to compare speech durations on voiced and voiceless phonemes to indicate phonatory efficiency. Boone and McFarlane (2000)

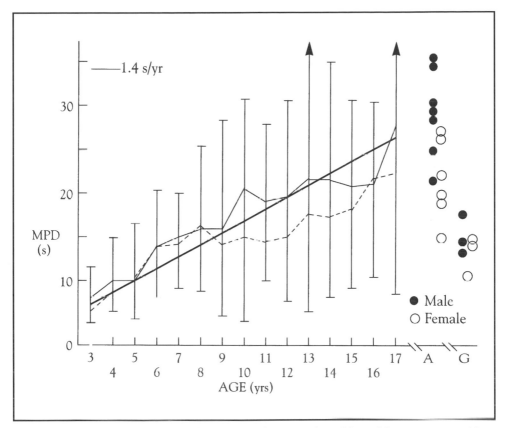

Figure 3.10. Maximum phonation duration as a function of age. Vertical lines are ranges. *Note.* From *Reference Manual for Communicative Sciences and Disorders*, by R. D. Kent, 1994, Austin, TX: PRO-ED. Copyright 1994 by PRO-ED, Inc. Reprinted with permission.

discussed the rationale for the *s/z* ratio procedure. They indicated that, regardless of age or gender, the durations of the voiceless /s/ should be similar in length to the durations of the voiced cognate /z/, providing a ratio of 1.0 (*z* duration divided into *s* duration). In actuality, these norms provide typical ratios less than 1.0 because an efficient and normal phonatory system provides voiced durations that are slightly longer than voiceless durations, so the ratios will likely be closer to 0.90 in typical speakers. When vocal pathology is present, the /z/ durations are negatively influenced by the pathology, shortening the durations. Boone and McFarlane reported ratios greater than 1.4 in patients with laryngeal pathology.

The strength of this procedure in evaluating phonatory efficiency depends on the validity and reliability of performance. Great variability is common in the duration performance of children and adults, and several efforts would be necessary to obtain an accurate measurement. The *s/z* ratio is relevant only when the data obtained reflect a client's maximum effort potential. This concern was expounded on by Stone (1983), who found that maximum phonation durations, which he called maximum phonation times, are highly variable under conditions of pitch level, presence of performance feedback, and number of trials. In fact, Stone's subjects continued to increase maximum phonation times up to 15 trials. Stone's data should at least caution the speech–language pathologist to limit the significance of MPDs and s/z ratios when viewed as isolated measures. The concern is also reflected in the high standard deviations of data reported by Kent et al. (1987). The reports that follow provide additional data on the s/z ratio and elaborate on this concern about test validity.

Tait, Michel, and Carpenter (1980) provided data on children 5, 7, and 9 years of age, using /s/ and /z/ prolongation as the database. They found no distinct pattern of MPD differences between boys and girls in 5- and 7-year-olds. However, boys consistently produced longer MPDs than girls in the 9-year-old group. Unlike sex, age appeared to have an influence on MPD values, which increased with years. In addition to MPD values, s/z ratios were figured and reported in mean and median form.

Eckel and Boone (1981) also provided data on s/z ratios of dysphonic patients with laryngeal pathology, dysphonic patients without laryngeal pathology, and nondysphonic persons covering a wide age range and including both sexes. Although they reported no statistical difference among the three groups in ability to sustain /s/, those with pathology had lower duration times for /z/ than persons in the other two groups. Also, the computed s/z ratios were significantly higher for the dysphonic subjects with laryngeal pathology (ratios of 1.40 were obtained 95% of the time, compared with approximate ratios of 1.0 for the nonpathology and nondysphonic groups). Eckel and Boone concluded that the s/z ratio has clinical relevance in determining laryngeal efficiency.

The reliability of the s/z ratio was tested by Fendler and Shearer (1988), who tested 78 nondysphonic children on occasions separated by 1 week. Two clinicians each tested half of the children and then the opposite half 1 week later. Test–retest statistics indicated no significant differences between the testers and subject performance. In other words, children who tended to have either longer or shorter s/z durations did not vary in the retest condition. Test–retest reliability of the s/z ratio was found to be consistent between tests and clinicians doing the testing.

An additional caution should be expressed about the use of the s/z ratio and MPDs. Hufnagle and Hufnagle (1988) reported data on 123 dysphonic children, 69 with vocal nodules and 54 with no obvious vocal fold pathology but with vocal dysphonia. No significant difference was found between the ratios of children with nodules and those with no obvious pathology, and the ratios tended to be similar to values expected in typical persons (range, 0.84 to 1.03). However, the durations of /s/ and /z/ were shorter than expected for nondysphonic children (range for /s/, 4.69 to 5.74 seconds; for /z/, 5.94 to 6.53 seconds). The authors cited respiratory support as a significant factor in their findings but concluded that the s/z ratio did not discriminate the presence of mass lesions in dysphonic children.

Schmidt, Klingholz, and Martin (1988) reported similar variability of MPDs among singers as a function of pitch, sound pressure, and vowels used. Therefore, even trained singers who knew how to control the voice well demonstrated variability in MPDs. Lee, Stemple, and Kizer (1999), as one aspect of a study investigating consistency of performance on several acoustic and aerodynamic measures, found that MPDs were variable when subjects were free to choose the intensity of the voice being tested.

Perhaps the most significant independent variable to consider in evaluating an MPD score clinically is whether the client expended near maximum VC (vital capacity) of the respiratory system. It is common for a clinician to ask a patient to take in a deep breath, as deep as possible, and hold a vowel sound as long as possible. These results are measured using a stopwatch to determine durations. If these instructions are given without determining whether maximum VC was used, the results are meaningless. It is clear that if only 65% of a client's VC has been used, essentially only 65% of MPD potential has likely been measured. Another important variable is the nature of vocal fold vibration during the task. Specifically, laryngeal airway resistance must be considered. Laryngeal airway resistance as a variable was evaluated by Solomon et al. (2000). They found no systematic relation between MPD and VC, because their subjects tended to use 90% of the VC for their best MPD trial. However, laryngeal airway resistance was strongly correlated with MPD values for men but not for women.

The MPD data and s/z ratios reported in these studies seem to support the notion that considerable information can be gained about a client's laryngeal efficiency from these simple tests. The conclusion one must reach when reviewing these many reports is that MPDs must be used only as one component of vocal efficiency measurement. When used, careful and specific instructions to the client to ensure maximum performance must be provided, and interpretation must occur with caution in the context of additional findings. Under these constraints, these simple measures can be most helpful in the evaluation process.

PERCEPTUAL RATING SCALES

No technology will ever make human perception obsolete. Many clinicians with years of experience in voice treatment remember clearly the time when the only voice measurement potential was a pitch pipe, a reel-to-reel tape recorder, and a very slow and smokey spectrograph. Speech–language pathologists had to rely on human perception (i.e., hearing) to indicate what was happening in the client's voice. After years of working in voice with no technology to speak of and then having access to equipment, I have found that the interaction of bits and bytes, sonographs and laryngoscopes, stroboscopes and endoscopes, pneumotachometers and flowmeters enhances my perception but does not replace it.

The perceptual rating of normal and abnormal voices has received considerable attention in the literature on voice disorder (e.g., Gerratt, Till, Rosenbek, Wertz, & Boysen, 1991; Kreiman & Gerratt, 2000). Perceptual judgment of voice is a controversial method. Some authorities find perceptual judgment so invalid and unreliable as to be meaningless and believe that only objective and instrumentally based measurements should be used to discriminate voices. At the opposite extreme is the voice clinician who relies only on perceptual judgment of voice without any objective assessment. In the many voice evaluations that occur daily in clinics, hospitals, private practices, and school systems, however, it is likely that a combination of perceptual judgment and objective assessment is the standard. As Kreiman and Gerratt stated, "Vocal quality is an interaction between an acoustic voice signal and a listener; the acoustic signal itself does not possess quality, it evokes it in the listener. For this reason, acoustic measures are meaningful primarily to the extent that they correspond to what listeners hear" (p. 73). It is also important to remember that when assessing the quality of a client's voice, many of the aspects of judgment are multidimensional. The perception of pitch is typically considered a single-dimensional characteristic; loudness as well. However, when multiple acoustic variables are integrated into voice quality judgment, including pitch, loudness, vibratory patterns of the signal, laryngeal airway resistance, and resonance, judgment becomes a multidimensional task and is extremely more complicated. It therefore becomes even more critical that concerns of validity and reliability of judgment are evaluated.

Readers interested in the question of the value of perceptual ratings should read Kreiman, Gerratt, Kempster, Erman, and Berke (1993). These researchers reviewed 57 articles in which perceptual judgment was a critical aspect of the research and found considerable variance in methodology used and results obtained. Their discussion on the importance of reliability (generally similar ratings) and agreement (same rating) is particularly valuable. Following their extensive review of the literature, they performed two experiments on perceptual judgments of vocal roughness. Generally, listeners varied widely in their level of reliability and agreement but rated normal voices more consistently and appropriately than rough voices. Experience seemed to emerge as a favorable factor in rating, producing higher reliability and agreement. Overall, a rather bleak picture of perceptual voice quality ratings emerged from their findings.

I believe, however, that highly experienced judges are rather good at discriminating parameters of voice with validity and reliability, characteristics that can be taught (see Bassich & Ludlow, 1986), but objective assessment provides highly valuable support for those judgments. Despite the availability of new instruments, I continue to use my ears in the evaluation process.

One concern that occurs when perceptually judging the human voice involves the language of category. Voice literature is filled with terms that confuse, overlap, contradict, or fail to communicate in a valid manner. Boone (1991) compiled a table of 100 word descriptors for voice, including such esoteric terms as *blanched, bleary, burnished, edgy, metallic, painted, silvery, stentorian,* and *whiskey*. Other terms that are more common and perhaps better understood among voice clinicians include *breathy, clear, effeminate, nasal,* and *hoarse*. Between these extremes are terms such as *harsh, rough,* and *strident,* which are commonly found in voice literature but which likely are not used reliably among evaluators. If a scale defines a term and provides an ordinal or interval ranking opportunity for judgment (0 to 4 on an equal-appearing scale), the opportunity for reliable and valid measurement is enhanced. Regardless, the perceptual judgment findings of Kreiman, Gerratt, Precoda, and Berke (1992); Kreiman et al. (1993); and Kreiman and Gerratt (2000) must be considered.

Valuable information can be obtained from critical listening and perceptual ratings of various parameters of voice as part of the overall evaluation process. Several perceptual scales have been developed, but I find simple scales to be the most useful.

Askenfelt–Hammarberg Scale

Askenfelt and Hammarberg (1986) devised an 11-item scale that can be used to perceptually evaluate most of the parameters of voice heard clinically; Kent (1994b) modified their scale (see Table 3.2). Most of the scale items listed are discussed in the following paragraphs.

Breathiness

Most voice disorders involve a factor of increased laryngeal airflow through a compromised glottis during phonation. When perceived, this airflow factor should be objectively measured with a flowmeter such as the Aerophone II Voice Function Analyzer (see Figure 3.7). On the perceptual scale, breathiness is rated on a 0 to 4 (*severe*) scale. If the perceptual rating is 0, it would be unnecessary to submit the client to airflow testing to document breathiness unless such testing is necessary for some other parameter measurement. Breathiness is perceived in patients with all of the vocal abuse pathologies, paralysis, benign and malignant growths, and nonorganic or functional dysphonias. The subtle differences between perceptual ratings of 1, 2, 3, and 4 can often be used diagnostically to guide the evaluation process or as measures of improvement with therapy (see Chapter 4 for indicators of improvement).

TABLE 3.2
Perceptual Scale for Voice Evaluation

Voice Quality	Rating				
1. Breathy (audible escape of air through glottis)	0 none	1	2	3	4 several
2. Vocal fry/creaky (low-frequency periodic vibration)	0 none	1	2	3	4 several
3. Hard glottal attacks (glottal stops at onset of vowels	0 none	1	2	3	4 several
4. Hyperfunctional/tense (strained or pressed quality)	0 none	1	2	3	4 several
5. Hypofunctional/lax (too little tension in vocal folds; weak, lax and breathy quality)	0 none	1	2	3	4 several
6. Diplophonia (two different pitches heard simultaneously)	0 none	1	2	3	4 several
7. Voiced breaks (intermittent register breaks)	0 none	1	2	3	4 several
8. Grating/harsh (high-pitched noise owing to irregular vocal fold vibrations)	0 none	1	2	3	4 several
9. Rough/coarse (low-pitched noise owing to irregular vocal fold vibrations)	0 none	1	2	3	4 several
10. Unstable voice quality or pitch (irregular variation in quality or pitch)	0 none	1	2	3	4 several
11. Register (mode of phonation: modal, middle, or falsetto)		Modal	Middle	Falsetto	
12. Pitch (primary auditory correlate of fundamental frequency)	0 low	1	2	3	4 high

Note. From *Reference Manual for Communicative Sciences and Disorders* (p. 140), by R. D. Kent, 1994, Austin, TX: PRO-ED. Copyright 1994 by PRO-ED, Inc. Reprinted with permission. Based on Tables 2 and 3 of "Speech Waveform Perturbation Analysis: A Perceptual-Acoustical Comparison of Seven Measures," by A. G. Askenfelt and B. Hammarberg, 1986, *Journal of Speech and Hearing Research, 29,* p. 54.

Hard Glottal Attacks

The hard glottal attack is marked by an abrupt onset of vowel production and, in extreme cases, sounds much like a grunt. In ongoing speech, it is more difficult to perceive and would more likely be heard as part of overall vocal tension or hyperfunction. When it occurs in the extreme (rating of 3 or 4), it is a factor of vocal abuse and must be modified, as explained in Chapter 4.

Vocal Hyperfunction or Tension

Vocal hyperfunction or tension is a common characteristic of many voice disorders. In the client with vocal nodules, vocal effort may be caused by an attempt to overcome an inefficient laryngeal mechanism or by some etiological factor. The same is true of the patient with laryngeal paralysis; even though the main quality might be breathiness, both types of patients might also demonstrate vocal tension or hyperfunction in an attempt to increase loudness. In its extreme (rating of 3 or 4), so much resistance to airflow occurs that phonation is stopped intermittently. The characteristic voice profile of the patient with adductor spasmodic dysphonia (see Chapter 5) is typical of this pattern of voice stoppage.

Vocal Hypofunction

Vocal hypofunction is highly correlated with laryngeal breathiness or increased airflow. When breathiness and overall hypofunction occur in voice, loudness is compromised. Some patients, such as those with personality characteristics of shyness and vocal reticence, might have vocal characteristics of hypofunction without breathiness. These patients have the physical traits needed for vocal projection but psychogenically do not use them. The weak voice of a patient with parkinsonism is another example of vocal hypofunction.

Diplophonia

It is often difficult to distinguish perceptually between true diplophonia, or double pitch of the voice, and typical dysphonia, which contains combinations of factors. True diplophonia, which is rather rare, occurs most often in patients with laryngeal paralysis in which one vocal fold has lost significant mass from deinnervation. Two distinct pitches occurring simultaneously must be perceived to justify the perceptual judgment of diplophonia. Often this perception, when it occurs, can be seen on the Visi-Pitch or other pitch extraction device. Cavalli and Hirson (1999) examined diplophonia from perceptual and acoustic analyses and concluded that trained listeners were able to distinguish diplophonia reliably from other aspects of voice, but not as easily as they could identify whisper, voice breaks, or harshness. Their acoustic analysis of samples judged to be diplophonic revealed a significant relationship between subharmonics in the spectrum and measures of frequency and amplitude perturbation. One summary statement indicated that as the perception of diplophonia was judged with greater inter-listener reliability, the number of subharmonics between the primary harmonics increased. These relationships were only correlative, and examples of voices judged to be diplophonic that did not demonstrate subharmonics were presented.

Voice Breaks

In many voice disorders, vocal instability is manifested in the form of voice breaks. These are sudden changes in pitch and have been described as register breaks or changes from chest voice to loft, falsetto. Sometimes the breaks are not so dramatic that the pitch slips into a different register, but when they occur, however dramatically, they indicate vocal instability from structural or functional abnormalities. Voice breaks are heard in patients with vocal abuse disorder; mass changes on the vocal folds, such as polyps or cysts; and psychogenic voice disorder, such as puberphonia (Chapter 5). They should be noted when perceived as part of the voice evaluation process.

Grating/Harsh Voice

Askenfelt and Hammarberg (1986) described a grating/harsh voice as a high-pitched noisy voice resulting from irregular vocal fold vibration. It is likely a combination voice demonstrating high pitch, excessive laryngeal tension, and perhaps a slight nasal resonance quality. Perhaps the easiest aspect of this voice to judge is the grating nature because *grating* is a term commonly used to describe any irritating or annoying noise that causes humans to react strongly, such as the sound of fingernails on a blackboard.

Rough or Coarse Voice

The person with a rough or coarse voice likely has abnormalities on the vocal folds that cause aperiodic vibration, excessive turbulence, increased airflow, and perhaps some degree of hyperfunction. The term *hoarseness* is often used as a correlate to *roughness* or *coarseness* in the voice. This voice consists of many voice components that together result in this unique voice quality. Vocal roughness is heard in patients with any mass change on the vocal folds or any stiffness factor that limits the smooth vibration necessary for normal voice. Many of the disorders covered in this book involve the voice symptom complex of vocal roughness.

Pitch

In perceptual rating of vocal frequency or pitch, the listener must judge whether the person's pitch is age and sex appropriate or whether some aspect of pitch attracts unwanted attention. Judgment involves whether the person's pitch is too low (rating of 0) or too high (rating of 3 to 4) for his or her age and sex. This is an important judgment because, regardless of what the numbers indicate from objective assessment using the Visi-Pitch or similar instrument, if a person's voice pitch draws negative attention, a voice disorder exists. It is also important to assess perceptually whether pitch inflections are extreme in an upward or downward direction. Although the majority of vocal pitch may be in an appropriate range, extreme fluctuations upward in a male might generate sex confusion over the phone, and extreme fluctuations downward in either sex might constitute a factor of vocal hyperfunction and misuse.

Resonance

One aspect of voice not considered in Askenfelt and Hammarberg's (1986) scale is resonance, particularly the oral–nasal coupling resonance that is part of many voice disorders. As indicated in Chapter 5 (on neurogenics) and Chapter 8 (on resonance), many clinical conditions affect the velopharyngeal mechanism and produce hypernasality. Under normal conditions of velopharyngeal closure, there is complete separation of the oral and nasal cavities during speech except in the production of the nasal consonants /m/, /n/, and /ng/. When a client's voice indicates this normal balance of velopharyngeal functioning, a normal judgment of resonance is given, meaning the velopharyngeal port is closed except during the production of these nasal consonants. Although this parameter is not judged in the Askenfelt and Hammarberg scale, it must be evaluated as part of every voice evaluation.

Individuals often display resonance characteristics in which the presence of nasal consonants causes an assimilation of nasality to surrounding consonants and vowels, in which case assimilation nasality is heard. This is a relatively insignificant deviation from normal. When nasality is heard in all vowel sounds, a significant factor of nasal resonance is added to the voice, and this must be noted and managed by the speech–language pathologist. This nasality, which indicates significant velopharyngeal dysfunction, is heard in many of the dysarthric voices discussed in Chapter 5 and in patients with orofacial clefting and additional syndromes of the craniofacial complex discussed in Chapter 8.

Zraick, Liss, et al. (2000) reported nasal voice quality as having multidimensional perceptual qualities. Although synthetic vowels were generated and used in this study, the dimensions of nasality perceived were probably typical of those seen clinically. Three dimensions interacted and accounted for 83% of the total variance in listeners' judgments: nasalization, vocal intensity, and fundamental frequency. Thus it is clear that perceptions of nasality are affected by the intensity and frequency of the voice. It is also common for nasality and other voice dimensions to be evaluated on scales that appear equal in scaling differences, a process known as equal-appearing interval scaling, with parameters similar to those on the Askenfelt and Hammarberg scale. However, Zraick and Liss (2000) reported evidence that scaling involving direct magnitude estimates results in nasality ratings that are more consistent and reliable. In direct magnitude estimates, listeners scale individual voice samples relative to one another or to a standard stimulus usually obtained from the middle of the range stimuli.

Several organic conditions in the nasal cavity can affect normal functioning in resonation in the direction of hyponasality, a condition in which there is too little participation of the nasal cavity in resonance. For example, if a client has a severe cold or nasal allergy, during the production of the nasal consonants the velopharyngeal port opens normally but nasal resonance is restricted because of congestion in the cavity. This dampening of nasal resonance is called hyponasality. The main effect of such a resonance change is that the nasal consonant /m/ sounds more like /b/, the /n/ like /d/, and the /ŋ/ like /g/.

Gelfer Rating Scale

Another useful rating scale includes a set of bipolar perceptual rating items that can be used to relate listener perceptions to physiological and acoustic measures. Through use of measures of confidence, several parameters of voice were eliminated until the aspects shown in Figure 3.11 remained for evaluation by speech–language pathologists.

High Pitch	__1__2__3__4__5__6__7__8__9__	Low Pitch
Loud	__1__2__3__4__5__6__7__8__9__	Soft
Strong	__1__2__3__4__5__6__7__8__9__	Weak
Smooth	__1__2__3__4__5__6__7__8__9__	Rough
Pleasant	__1__2__3__4__5__6__7__8__9__	Unpleasant
Resonant	__1__2__3__4__5__6__7__8__9__	Shrill
Clear	__1__2__3__4__5__6__7__8__9__	Hoarse
Unforced	__1__2__3__4__5__6__7__8__9__	Strained
Soothing	__1__2__3__4__5__6__7__8__9__	Harsh
Melodious	__1__2__3__4__5__6__7__8__9__	Raspy
Breathy Voice	__1__2__3__4__5__6__7__8__9__	Full Voice
Excessive Nasal	__1__2__3__4__5__6__7__8__9__	Insufficient Nasal
Animated	__1__2__3__4__5__6__7__8__9__	Monotonous
Steady	__1__2__3__4__5__6__7__8__9__	Shaky
Young	__1__2__3__4__5__6__7__8__9__	Old
Slow Rate	__1__2__3__4__5__6__7__8__9__	Rapid Rate
I Like Voice	__1__2__3__4__5__6__7__8__9__	Don't

Figure 3.11. Gelfer Rating Scale. *Note.* Adapted from Gelfer (1988).

The scale in Figure 3.11 has many parameters to judge. Some appear redundant, and one point of confusion is apparent: Most of the parameters judged are arranged so that low-number judgments (i.e., 1 to 3) indicate normalcy of voice and high-number judgments (i.e., 7 to 9) indicate abnormalcy. However, this is not always the case. Low-number judgments on the parameters of "high pitch," "breathy voice," "excessive nasal," and "slow rate" do not indicate normal aspects of voice. Thus, each parameter requires individual analysis rather than relying on an overall profile to discriminate normal from abnormal voice characteristics. Gelfer (1988) provided extensive information regarding the development and testing of this scale.

If one were to read the evaluation chapters of the majority of books on clinical management of voice disorders, the disparity of approaches presented by the various authors would be obvious. Each author approaches the perceptual process differently, some with scales, some with elaborate and helpful descriptions of qualities to be evaluated, and others with combinations of scales and descriptions (Andrews, 1999; Awan, 2001; Boone & McFarlane, 2000; Colton & Casper, 1996; Deem & Miller, 2000; Stemple et al., 2000). It is important that the speech–language pathologist who uses perceptual rating scales recognize the inherent weaknesses of perception and the need for extensive experience in voice judgment (Bassich & Ludlow, 1986). Speech–language pathologists should also use objective assessment to complement and enhance the validity of perceptual voice judgments.

ENDOSCOPY AND STROBOSCOPY

In Chapter 2, the rationale and general procedures for using endoscopy and videostroboscopy in voice evaluation were discussed. Here attention is given to clinical interpretation use and of stroboscopic results.

In endoscopy light is emitted in an alternating current pulse of light or direct current of continuous light, and laryngeal tissues and movements are viewed in real time. Vocal fold vibration is sufficiently rapid that the human eye cannot resolve individual vibrations, so movements are blurred. In stroboscopy light is emitted in rapid pulses at the same frequency as or slightly varied from the frequency of vocal fold vibration, providing an illusion of stopped motion (same frequency) or slow motion (1- to 2-Hz difference from the fundamental).

If the speech–language pathologist is using a stroboscope in a nonhospital setting such as a university clinic or private practice, the procedure must be done without anesthesia. I have performed hundreds of such examinations, with approximately a 90% success rate even with strong gaggers. Before I begin the examination, I hand the sterilized rigid endoscope to the patient or client and give these instructions:

> Think of this instrument as a spoon that you are going to place in your mouth. Go ahead and put it into your mouth under your own control. Move it around and continue to breathe through your mouth as you normally do. Keep it in the middle of your tongue. Bring your tongue forward. Now say "ah" with it in your mouth. If you gag a little, that is okay. Now say "ee," and it won't sound much like "ee" with the scope in your mouth. Go ahead and touch the back of your throat gently. That is all I am going to do, only I will have a camera attached.

I have found that this simple procedure helps desensitize patients and eliminate some fear of the examination process.

A proper examination with the stroboscope must involve, when possible, a range of pitch and loudness functions. In this manner the full dynamics of vocal fold activity can be assessed. It is best to have a specific protocol that is memorized or posted by the stroboscope. Some interpretation is possible during the procedure, but it is best to delay detailed interpretation until the video can be analyzed with repeated viewings. Obviously, many examinations result in immediate manifestations of the bases of a client's dysphonia, which must be discussed as the client views the video. I usually mention that the written report may contain some additional details that become apparent with repeated viewings.

Two rigid scopes are commonly available for stroboscopic examination: 90° and 70°. The latter provides a somewhat better view of the larynx without epiglottal obstruction and is the one with which I have the most experience. When the 70° scope is used, the head should be somewhat extended. I ask the client to sit straight, bend forward slightly as though tying a shoe, and then look up at me. This movement should be slight, not exaggerated.

When stroboscopy is being done, a contact microphone (similar to a stethoscope) is placed on the client's neck just lateral to the thyroid cartilage and is usually held in place by Velcro. The examiner asks the client to phonate the "ee" sound and determines the frequency of vibration that is displayed in hertz on the front panel of the stroboscope. Next, while holding the client's tongue with a 4-by-4-inch gauze, the examiner inserts the endoscope slowly without touching tissues as the client continues to phonate "ee". If fogging occurs, the scope must be warmed to body temperature, which can be done by placing it against the client's cheeks or tongue. Care must be taken to prevent mucus from getting on the scope itself. I usually wipe the scope quickly with the gauze after placement on the tissues to warm it.

When the larynx is clearly displayed on the screen, the testing protocol is initiated. The examination should begin with the client's phonating using the speaking pitch. I usually obtain several samples by having the client prolong an "ee" sound for 2 or 3 seconds, stop and breathe, and then prolong another "ee" sound. This is done under nonstrobe lighting. This initial procedure allows the examiner to evaluate general aspects of laryngeal anatomy and physiology. Abnormalities in arytenoid movement during abduction and adduction can be detected, and general tissue char-acteristics of the true and ventricular cords can be evaluated. I ask the client to phonate this normal pitch in different loudness levels (starting softly and moving to a loud voice) as well as different pitches, sometimes leading to a falsetto voice sample. I then evaluate these same samples under stroboscopic lighting.

Many of the foregoing procedures will not be possible with patients who do not tolerate the procedure well and have strong gagging reflexes. If the examination results only in some quickly viewed samples of anatomy and physiology, only limited descriptions are possible.

Interpretation is made easier if the speech–language pathologist follows a chart of items that need to be evaluated. Several such evaluation protocols are available (Hirano & Bless, 1993; Poburka, 1999a). By using an evaluation form such as that in Figure 3.12, the speech–language pathologist can identify and describe the salient concerns of laryngeal anatomy, physiology, and pathology. Pathological identifica-tions made by the speech–language pathologist must be nondiagnostic in a medical sense. This becomes a difficult situation for speech–language pathologists who are examining patients without a physician present. Following an examination, it is appropriate to review the video recording with the patient, who is likely to press for an opinion regarding pathology. I am cautious about stating strong opinions and indi-cate that a copy of the video will be supplied to the referring physician who can inter-pret the pathology. Speech–language pathologists who have examined many patients may have a strong idea about the pathology. Depending on the nature of my relation-ship with the patient, I often express some possibilities. In the case of paralysis, for instance, I may say, "Your right vocal fold is not moving properly. You could see that when we compared it with the left vocal fold. Your physician will have to help us understand exactly why your right vocal fold is not moving."

Although the speech–language pathologist cannot make medical diagnoses, it is within the scope of practice to diagnose the effect of various pathologies on the voice. It is appropriate to state that a patient's voice quality, loudness, or pitch is affected by specific abnormalities noted on the stroboscopic examination. For example, one patient with a significant dysphonia was referred for a stroboscopic examination by an otorhinolaryngologist, who stated that the left vocal fold was red and inflamed. He was not sure why and wanted the increased diagnostic potential of stroboscopy to help with the diagnosis and treatment. This patient had a long history of cigarette smoking but had quit within the past year.

My examination showed the left vocal fold to be truly red and inflamed, as the physician had noted, but stroboscopic examination showed that the left vocal fold was also stiff and not vibrating. I explained to the patient that stroboscopy showed that one of his vocal folds was not vibrating to any degree, which is a likely cause of his dysphonia, but I was not sure what pathology was causing the stiffness. He pressed me for an explanation. Because of his history of smoking and the appearance of the

STROBOSCOPIC ASSESSMENT

Name _____

Address _____

Date_____ Phone_____ Referred by: _____

Arytenoid Approximation

_____ Equal and symmetrical

_____ Right normal; left with little to no movement

_____ Left normal; right with little to no movement

_____ Both do not fully approximate but do have some medial-lateral
movement

Describe:_____

Vocal Fold Approximation

_____ Total and equal bilateral approximation

_____ Bowing: R; L; Both

_____ Chink: Anterior; Posterior; Midfold

_____ Irregular

_____ Hourglass

_____ Incomplete without bowing

_____ Hyperfunctional

Describe:_____

Vocal Fold Edge

_____ Both smooth and regular

_____ Irregular edge: R; L; Both

_____ Pathology apparent: R; L; Both

Describe:_____

Vocal Fold Surface

_____ Normal: Whitish gray with light yellow ends

_____ Size: R>L; L>R; both enlarged

_____ Edema/Inflamed: R; L; Both

_____ Hemorrhagic: R; L; Both

_____ Pathology apparent: R; L; Both

Describe:_____

Figure 3.12. Stroboscopic assessment form.

STROBOSCOPIC ASSESSMENT *Continued.*

Vibratory Behavior

_____ Regularity/Phase (periodicity)

_____ Both vocal folds open and close equally (on time) per cycle

_____ Irregular movement (timing is off): Sometimes; Always

Describe:_____

Amplitude (lateral excursion)

_____ Both move laterally equal distance (~ *1/3 the width of the visible vocal fold*)

_____ R>L; L>R

_____ Both reduced

_____ No lateral movement with attempted vibration

Describe:_____

Mucosal Wave (loose tissue) Function

_____ Equally present and fluid bilaterally (~ _ *the width of the visible vocal fold*)

_____ Reduced (slightly stiff): R; L; both

_____ Absent (very stiff): R: L; both

_____ Adynamic segment: R; L; both

Ventricular Behavior

_____ Normal: both in the lateral position during phonation

_____ Adduction occurs during phonation: TVFs adducted

_____ Complete adduction during attempted phonation; TVFs not visible
(Plica Ventricularis)

Describe:_____

Other

Describe:_____

Summary and Recommendations

_____

_____

_____

Evaluated by:

_____

Figure 3.12. *Continued.*

left vocal fold, I was suspicious that the final diagnosis would be unfortunate, but I was unwilling to speculate with him. I reported my findings and provided a copy of the video to the physician, who indicated that a biopsy would be needed. The patient was found to have a squamous cell carcinoma (my suspicion).

Videostroboscopy has revolutionized the world of voice evaluation and treatment and increased knowledge about normal anatomy and physiology. As a professor teaching normal anatomy and physiology, I have found the stroboscope invaluable in teaching about the subtle aspects of vocal fold anatomy and physiology. In a clinical sense, I cannot imagine voice evaluations being done without this procedure. I recommend the books by Hirano and Bless (1993) and Karnell (1994), who provide comprehensive coverage of all aspects of the technology, procedure, interpretation, clinical management, and clinical utility of videostroboscopy in managing various dysphonias. Even though the technology has changed somewhat since these books were written, the general background and processes involved in the evaluation and reporting of stroboscopic findings remain helpful. Additional references on stroboscopy that are helpful include Stemple et al. (2000), Woodson (1998), and Karnell and Langmore (1998). As reviewed by Sataloff (1999), two excellent video resources on the use of videostroboscopy have been provided by Cornut and Bouchayer (*Assessing Dysphonia: The Role of Videostroboscopy*) and by Stasney (*Atlas of Dynamic Laryngeal Pathology*). These videos cover numerous pathological conditions of the larynx and explain how to interpret video imaging findings. Bless and Poburka (2001) have also provided a video tutorial on this subject.

CASE EXAMPLE OF VOICE EVALUATION

This evaluation was conducted at the Arizona State University Speech and Hearing Clinic (Case, 1994). It is presented here in abstract form.

Background and Case History

J. B., a 62-year-old woman and former nurse, was evaluated at the Arizona State University Speech and Hearing Clinic. She had a long history of vocal hoarseness and low pitch, with gender confusion over the phone, which she attributed to 43 years of cigarette smoking. She had quit smoking approximately 1 year prior to this evaluation. She described herself as a strong-willed and aggressive individual who supervised her nursing staff with authority. She was referred by a local otolaryngologist who thought her dysphonia might be related to vocal fold dryness, vocal strain, esophageal reflux, and depression. He did not indicate in his report any pathological basis for her dysphonia but wanted a stroboscopic examination to clarify her disorder.

J. B. reported that, although she had always noticed a raspy quality and low pitch in her voice, her voice significantly deteriorated approximately 9 months prior to this evaluation. She attributed this sudden voice change to asthma and esophageal reflux. She was medically treated for both conditions without voice improvement. J. B. also reported a feeling of constant pain in her throat.

A vocal history was taken, and the following factor of vocal abuse/usage was identified: constant conversation on the phone and in person in a noisy work environment. Perceptual judgment of her voice was reported as follows: J. B. presents with a raspy and consistently dysphonic voice characterized by low pitch (near the bottom of her range), vocal tension that can be heard and seen in her neck area, reduced loudness potential in which increased vocal effort only increases the tension in her neck without significantly increasing vocal loudness, and some combination of breathiness and overpressure in her voice.

The Kay Elemetrics Visi-Pitch was used to obtain specific pitch or frequency measurements. J. B.'s habitual pitch (or speaking fundamental frequency), obtained by having her count from 1 to 20 in a normal voice, was 124.5 Hz. This is typical of a man's speaking frequency and clarified why she was experiencing gender confusion over the phone. Her basal frequency was 115.7 Hz, and her ceiling frequency was 258.6 Hz. This vocal range of 13.9 semitones is significantly below the average of 24 to 36.

Exploring and measuring her vocal pitches resulted in finding an improved voice, nearly normal in quality, which was shaped into simple conversation. The habitual pitch of this improved voice, again determined during counting, was 190.7 Hz. Her two voices were acoustically compared using the Kay Elemetrics Digital 5500 Sono-Graph interfaced with a laryngograph. The following measurements were obtained:

Voice	Jitter	Shimmer	Harmonic/ Noise Ratio	F_0
Low/dysphonic	1.55%	1.24 dB	2.73 dB	145.5 Hz
More normal	0.80%	0.63 dB	14.83 dB	190.1 Hz

These values matched the perceptual judgments of both her dysphonic and more normal voices. The reduced jitter and shimmer values and increased harmonic-to-noise ratio for her more normal voice indicated improved laryngeal physiology. The next step was to view her larynx under both voice conditions.

Videostroboscopic examination revealed that, when the patient used her dysphonic voice, her ventricular folds nearly obliterated the view of her true vocal folds. Clearly, her primary dysphonia was caused by ventricular dysphonia. When she produced her more normal voice, however, ventricular involvement was eliminated and true vocal fold vibration was observed. Her true vocal folds appeared somewhat swollen and slightly erythemic, particularly in the middle portion of intermembranous tissue on the right side. The swelling was likely due to vocal hyperfunction, as part of her ventricular dysphonia, and is expected to improve as she habitually uses her improved voice. She was referred to a speech–language pathologist to stabilize her newly found voice.

The sudden change in J. B.'s voice approximately 9 months prior to evaluation also needed explanation. My suspicion was that perhaps ventricular dysphonia began about that time, which closely paralleled the cessation of smoking. Perhaps her years of being aware of a slightly raspy and low-pitched voice began to change when she quit smoking, and the improved vocal quality did not match her self-perception of a strong-willed person with an aggressive and authoritative personality. She perhaps attempted to maintain her old vocal quality as her larynx improved following smoking cessation, and vocal hyperfunction was introduced gradually into her vocal self-image.

This evaluation covers many of the topics discussed in this chapter regarding the importance of a good case history, acoustic measurement, visual documentation, and an attempt to provide some measure of vocal modification as part of the evaluation. Although much of the discussion is speculation and perhaps a little too far-reaching into the psychogenic realm, J. B. presents with an interesting profile of vocal dysphonia.

SUMMARY

Several evaluation procedures have been described, including voice screening; medical referral; taking case histories; and vocal parameter evaluation of pitch, loudness, quality, resonance, and vocal efficiency using perceptual scales and instrumentation. Specific measurement of vocal parameters and the technology needed were covered, as were techniques of acoustic measurement and visual documentation, particularly videostroboscopy. Not all of these processes and procedures must be followed in the evaluation of every client; however, the speech–language pathologist should be familiar with each of these procedures so as to select the proper ones for each case.

Clinical Management of Vocal Abuse

One of the most dramatic examples of how the delicate tissues of the larynx can be abused or misused was captured on film by Moore and von Leden (1958). During one segment, a person's cough was filmed in high-speed cinematography (5,000 frames per second) but projected at the normal rate of 16 frames per second. The ultraslow motion shows what happens to the vocal folds and surrounding laryngeal tissues during a brief cough.

For the several seconds of the film (1 second in real time), the tissues of the larynx are tossed about as though caught in a hurricane. The arytenoid cartilages are in chaotic and frenzied motion, matched by the turbulent actions of the vocal folds. The entire larynx is adversely affected by this aerodynamic turmoil. It is impossible to watch this coughing episode without realizing how laryngeal tissues are affected by even common occurrences such as a cough. With this perspective, consider how vulnerable these tissues are to continuous forms of vocal abuse behavior such as yelling and screaming.

Considering that during normal phonation the vocal folds are vibrating from one hundred to several hundred times each second (depending on the pitch of the voice), it is surprising that tissue trauma from all of this action does not occur more commonly. Furthermore, considering the great number of fans heard screaming at sporting events, it is even more surprising that thousands of people have not damaged their vocal folds by abnormal vocal behavior.

Although the total is not great, some individuals have developed voice disorder from vocal abuse, which is found at all ages and in most segments of society. Children yell and scream on the playground, and adults yell and scream at sporting events. Children enjoy making strange and loud toy and animal noises during play, and adults enjoy singing in styles and environments that foster vocal abuse. Loud and aggressive children verbally intimidate and bully other children, and these same verbal characteristics can be found in many adults. The general designator *vocal abuse* as a label for such behavior has been increasingly replaced *phonotrauma* because it is the nature of vocal behavior that causes the changes in voice quality and laryngeal status (Verdolini, 1999). Here the designators *vocal abuse*, *vocal misuse*, and *phonotrauma* are used interchangeably.

When children grow into adulthood, many enter professions with highly demanding verbal requirements: teaching, law, professional singing and acting, auctioneering, sales, and the ministry. Many of the verbal activities in these professions are incompatible with good vocal hygiene and can damage the delicate tissues of the larynx, producing a voice disorder caused by vocal abuse or misuse. This chapter provides speech–language pathologists with information for evaluating and remediating voice disorder cases resulting from various types of vocal abuse. The two most common and significant voice disorders that result directly from vocal abuse or misuse are vocal nodules and contact ulcers.

Many strategies can be employed to treat the client with vocal abuse that causes vocal and tissue changes. The most important goals are to identify all abuse forms, gain the client's cooperation or compliance in eliminating or reducing them, and encourage the client to maintain these changes. Murry and Woodson (1992) provided documentation that various approaches, including surgery, can be effective in the treatment of such patients, but the most important factor is compliance to vocal abuse reduction through voice therapy. Such therapy can be difficult to accomplish in the case of the professional voice user and some children, and the speech–language pathologist must be resourceful and energetic. The rewards, however, can be great when vocal quality, durability, and career stability are accomplished through these efforts.

VOCAL NODULES

The most common voice disorder resulting from vocal abuse or misuse, and the most common cause of hoarseness in children and adults, is a condition of vocal nodules or vocal nodes (Benninger & Gardner, 1998; Meyerhoff & Rice, 1992). Vocal nodules are also called "singer's nodules," "screamer's nodules," "cheerleader's nodules," "parson's nodules," and "teacher's nodules" (Lancer, Syder, Jones, & LeBoutillier, 1988), markers that identify the etiology of this voice disorder.

Vocal nodules are benign growths that develop at the margin or junction of the anterior and middle thirds of the glottal length, including intermembranous and intercartilaginous portions (see Figure 4.1). Nodules are typically found bilaterally, but a few cases of unilateral nodules have been reported (Lancer et al., 1988; McFarlane & Watterson, 1990). Because vocal abuse and various forms of phonotrauma are the primary etiologies of vocal nodule pathogenesis, it is difficult to explain how vocal abuse could cause only one vocal fold to develop a nodule while the other fold remains uninvolved, but this appears to be the case in instances of unilateral vocal nodules.

The nodules I have seen have all been bilateral but usually asymmetrical in severity. It is rare to see perfectly symmetrical bilateral vocal nodules. I have seen many cases of vocal nodules in which the nodule is remarkable on one side and only slightly

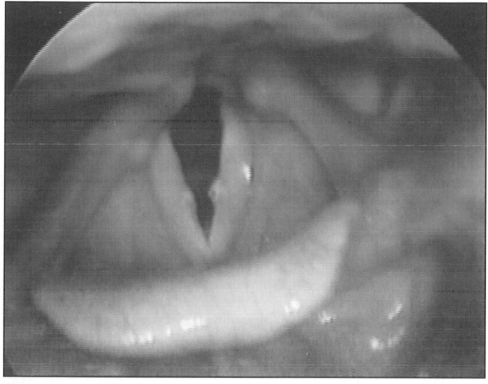

Figure 4.1. Vocal folds with nodules

developed contralaterally. One must be careful not to incorrectly identify a cyst or some other type of growth as a vocal nodule when using mirror examination. Without the careful documentation of stroboscopy, however, it would be easy to make such a mistake. McFarlane and Watterson (1990) reported significant variation in the size and location of vocal nodules in both children and adults, including an instance of quadruple vocal nodules (two nodules on each fold) in a 38-year-old woman. The majority of their adult cases were women, both singers and nonsingers.

The reason nodules develop at the junction of the anterior and middle thirds of the intermembranous glottis can be understood by reviewing the nature of vocal fold vibration. The anterior two thirds of the glottal opening is composed of muscular tissue that vibrates during phonation. The posterior third is composed of cartilaginous tissues (arytenoids) that do not vibrate during phonation. Therefore, the junction of the anterior and middle thirds, where nodules develop, represents the midpoint of vocal fold vibration. During the vibratory cycle, it is at this junction that the excursion from midline is widest and the vocal folds contact with greatest energy during normal or abnormal phonation. It is logical and consistent with known principles of voice science that vocal nodules should develop at this location when phonation is abusive over time. As the vocal folds begin to change dimensions due to phonotrauma, such as generalized edema, the entire configuration of vocal fold vibration can be affected. Alipour and Scherer (2000) provided an elegant biophysical computer model to determine how various bulging (edema) effects change phonation patterns. They determined that vocal fold bulging increases glottal flow resistance, changes in lung pressure values, reductions in glottal width area, and decreased values of mean volume velocity during phonation.

The pathogenesis of vocal nodules occurs in two stages, acute and chronic. The acute nodules are soft, reddish, vascular, and edematous, and they resemble laryngeal hematomas. They often are surrounded by generalized edema of the entire vocal fold tissues, and the entire glottis appears erythemic (reddish). The surrounding edema and erythema usually appear only in the acute stage of development. In the chronic stage, the nodules can be hard, white, thickened, and fibrotic, but little evidence of significant edema in the nodule or in the surrounding tissue can be noted. This is particularly true when past history of vocal misuse has caused the nodules to be well established but current behavior is only sufficient to maintain the nodules. When nodules are present and instances of current significant phonotrauma are present, generalized edema, focal evidence of hemorrhage, and general erythema can often be seen.

Kleinsasser (1986) reported that microlaryngoscopy reveals vocal nodules to be hyperplastic, acanthotic (thickened), squamous epithelial growths with markedly thickened basal membrane. The submucosal connective tissue of Reinke's space does not show any fibers connecting or fixing the epithelium to the vocalis muscle. Hirano and Bless (1993) reported that vocal nodules are always located in the superficial layer of the lamina propria. They cautioned that any surgical attempt to remove them should be strictly limited to this layer.

Arnold (1980) reported that in chronic vocal nodules the thickened epithelium becomes altered by acanthosis (hypertrophy), keratosis (horny growth or calluses), pachydermia (abnormal thickening), and metaplasia (change in the type of cell), and advanced lesions may show precancerous changes, including leukoplakia (white patches). I have seen one patient in whom vocal nodules removed during one surgery were found to be benign, but those removed during a second surgery were found to contain malignant cells that were extensive enough to later require a laryngectomy. Typically, however, vocal nodules remain benign growths, and no remarkable evidence exists to concern the person with vocal nodules that they may become malignant. Any person who develops laryngeal cancer in the presence of vocal nodules is likely experiencing coexisting conditions with separate etiologies.

When their delicate tissues are irritated by abusive voice production, vocal folds may worsen from the beginning stage of generalized vocal fold swelling (edema) and redness (erythema) to the final stage of full nodular development. Thus, the tissue reacts to vocal abuse by developing tiny growths of extra tissue that form the nodule. Nodules have been compared with corns or calluses on toes and hands, which develop from excessive rubbing and physical abuse. Vocal nodules develop in children as well as adults, and a gender ratio of 2:1 to 3:1 (male to female) is typically seen.

EFFECTS OF NODULES ON VOICE CHARACTERISTICS

The voice is affected in several ways when nodules develop. Voice quality is altered slightly in the early stages and dramatically when the nodules are well developed. The most common complaint is that the voice is raspy, hoarse, breathy, and less durable. Speech–language pathologists use these same terms to describe the voice characteristics, although these descriptive terms are usually accompanied by objective measurements to clarify the meaning of the language used.

The main factors involved in producing these perceptible characteristics are increased laryngeal airflow or breathiness; increased respiratory effort; overpressure (medical compression) of the vocal folds, perceived as voice tension; and asymmetrical vocal fold vibration (Sapienza & Stathopoulos, 1994). Two reasons can account for the breathiness factor:

1. The nodular mass on the vibrating edge of each vocal fold prevents complete approximation from occurring. This allows excessive air to escape during phonation through the glottal chinks anterior and posterior to the contact between the nodules.

2. Constant abuse of the voice structures produces irritation in the tissue, particularly in the posterior area around the arytenoid cartilages. This irritation can add a slight pain factor in phonation, causing the client to avoid hard approximation of the arytenoid cartilages at the onset of and during phonation, which also allows excessive air to escape and further causes the voice to be breathy.

The excessive overpressure (tension) factor usually is caused by the client's attempt to exert increased effort to overcome the incomplete approximation of the vocal folds. This increased effort is the basis of the tension. Because a nodule on one fold rarely matches the mass size of the nodule on the opposite fold, each vocal fold vibrates in a slightly different phase, resulting in aperiodicity. All of these factors contribute to the voice quality heard in clients with vocal nodules.

Objective measurement of the hoarseness found in patients with vocal nodules is part of clinical procedure, and I recommend the documentation discussed in this book for all dysphonias. However, P. Schneider (1993) reported lack of correlation between acoustic measures and laryngeal status in a single patient evaluated several times over a 2-year period using acoustic and visual tracking.

Voice characteristics of persons with vocal nodules usually include increased jitter, shimmer, and lower harmonic-to-noise ratios. A narrow-band spectrogram (see Figure 1.13) shows the obliteration of upper harmonics in a patient with hoarseness, such as would occur with vocal nodules, compared with a matched normal phonation pattern. As the upper harmonics are affected by the nodule, the spectrogram displays significantly increased spectral noise compared to the intensity of the harmonics. Thus, the filtering of the spectrographic instrumentation is unable to distinguish vocal harmonics from spectral noise.

Further voice characteristics of persons with vocal nodules include reduced maximum phonation durations and abnormal s/z ratios (Eckel & Boone, 1981; Rastatter & Hyman, 1982; Tait et al., 1980). Although the results of these studies reveal some inconsistencies, Rastatter and Hyman are less enthusiastic about the s/z ratio as an indicator of vocal nodules and other laryngeal pathology than are Eckel and Boone. The maximum phonation durations for /z/ typically are shorter than those for /s/, and the ratios of persons with nodules are greater than 1.40. The speech–language pathologist should at least consider short maximum phonation durations and s/z ratios greater than 1.40 as an indication of laryngeal inefficiency, without making a statement about diagnosis of vocal nodules based on these measurements.

The pitch of individuals with vocal nodules usually is too low, considering their age and sex. Early literature in speech and language pathology suggested lowering the habitual pitch level clinically because one factor of causation was a high pitch (Van Riper & Irwin, 1958). However, it is now recognized that vocal nodules lower the voice because of extra mass of the folds, which reduces the fundamental frequency vibration. In some individuals, an attempt to maintain a low voice pitch is an etiological factor in the development of the nodules. Thus, the speech–language pathologist must decide whether the lower-sounding pitch is etiologically related to the development of the nodules or a by-product of their presence.

Some persons may attempt to compensate for the vocal nodules and the increased breathiness of the voice by increasing the tension in the folds, thus possibly causing an increase in pitch, but typically the pitch is found to be too low. The person with nodules may not be attempting consciously to lower the pitch, so it probably is occurring because of the mass factor, but this must be determined clinically. Clinically raising the pitch should be done only when an etiological factor is involved (discussed in the next section).

Pitch control and stability also are problems for persons with vocal nodules. Upward or downward pitch breaks can occur regularly at the onset of phonation. They reflect a highly unstable laryngeal mechanism. Mattson (1980), in a study of the pitch changes over 10 months of a single subject (a cheerleader) with vocal nodules, found significant fluctuation of habitual pitch. These changes occurred between morning and night voice, before and after cheerleading, and particularly the day following extensive cheerleading. On one occasion, the cheerleader's pitch changed from a habitual level of 220 Hz to 174 Hz overnight as a result of cheer-leading the previous night. Many similar pitch fluctuations were revealed during the 10-month span. This same client experienced significantly reduced vocal durability from morning to night, another common characteristic of persons with vocal nodules.

ETIOLOGY OF VOCAL NODULES

Although there are some exceptions (Kay, 1982), the etiology of vocal nodules is thought to be vocal abuse or misuse (Andrews, 1999; Boone & McFarlane, 2000). Several specific forms of vocal abuse and associated causal factors must be considered, including the following:

- Yelling and screaming
- Voicing with a hard glottal attack
- Singing in an abusive manner (as a professional or an amateur)
- Inadequate hydration
- Speaking in a noisy environment
- Coughing and excessive throat clearing
- Grunting when exercising and lifting
- Calling others from a distance
- Inappropriate pitch in speaking or singing
- Speaking excessively during allergy episodes and upper respiratory infections
- Vocalizing under conditions of excessive muscular tension
- Smoking or speaking in a smoky environment
- Speaking or performing excessively during premenstrual or menstrual periods
- Vocalizing excessively
- Speaking with inadequate breath support
- Laughing hard and abusively
- Vocalizing excessively while taking excessive amounts of aspirin or aspirin-based products
- Cheerleading, aerobic instruction, or pep club activities
- Vocalizing toy and animal noises

- Engaging in athletic activity involving yelling, such as coaching or serving as a football quarterback

- Aggressive personality factor

- Arguing with others

- Excessive use of alcohol

- Medications

- Classroom teaching

- Miscellaneous factors such as religious chanting

This compendium seems comprehensive, yet the speech–language pathologist will find unique and individual forms of vocal abuse that do not appear on any traditional list. For example, Murry and Rosen (2000) reported on three patients whose primary phonotrauma was crying, causing vocal fold hemorrhage. Preparing a checklist such as that shown in Figure 4.2 can assist the speech–language pathologist in determining possible causes of a client's vocal abuse and misuse. Most of the types listed are discussed in this chapter.

Yelling and Screaming

Yelling and screaming are so common that they appear almost normal in many circumstances. Children of all ages seem to yell and scream regularly in both organized playground activities, such as sporting events, or in unorganized play in the backyard or street. During school recess, as most teachers can attest, children seem to release their contained emotions through their voices as much as by running and jumping. Some children are more vocal than others and become the "generals" of the playground, continually yelling instructions to the others in an attempt to establish and maintain a leadership role. Verbal arguments develop over trivial matters and end in a yelling match that involves no verbal logic, only loudness of voice. One wonders why nearly all such children do not hurt their voices and develop vocal nodules.

Adults also yell and scream. Both men and women can become emotionally involved in sporting events and cheer or boo with gusto. Parents of children in organized games scream at kids on the field, umpires, referees, coaches of opposing teams, and anyone else considered a threat to victory. Many adults who become coaches of youth teams find themselves yelling continually at the players. This is particularly noticeable in youth football, in which the players' ears are partially covered by helmets, making it difficult for coaches to communicate without yelling. Again, one wonders why every coach of a youth team does not have vocal nodules, particularly those with losing records.

Name _____

Date _____

VOCAL ABUSE AND MISUSE	EXPLANATION
_____ Yelling and screaming	_____
_____ Hard glottal attack	_____
_____ Abusive singing	_____
_____ Inadequate hydration	_____
_____ Speaking in noise	_____
_____ Coughing/throat clearing	_____
_____ Grunting in exercise	_____
_____ Calling at a distance	_____
_____ Inappropriate pitch	_____
_____ Excessive talk with allergy or upper respiratory infection	_____
_____ Muscular tension	_____
_____ Smoking factor	_____
_____ Alcohol factor	_____
_____ Speaking in menstrual cycle	_____
_____ Excessive speaking	_____
_____ Inadequate breath support	_____
_____ Laughing hard	_____
_____ Excessive aspirin (drugs)	_____
_____ Cheerleading, aerobics instruction, pep clubs	_____
_____ Toy/animal noises	_____
_____ Athletic activity (coaching, etc.)	_____
_____ Aggressive personality	_____
_____ Arguing	_____
_____ Miscellaneous factors	_____

Figure 4.2. Vocal abuse and misuse checklist.

When a child or adult is referred or screened out for voice therapy because of vocal nodules, the speech–language pathologist must take care to explore all possibilities of yelling and screaming as causal factors. Yelling episodes that occur frequently might be significant but easily overlooked.

Hard Glottal Attack

Even though vocal nodules develop at the junction of the anterior and middle thirds of the glottis, swelling and inflammation in the posterior region around the arytenoid cartilages are not uncommon. One factor that could explain this is the tendency for some people to begin phonation abruptly, a process called hard glottal attack or *coup de glotte* (attack of the glottis). Andrade et al. (1999) found that patients with various dysphonias presented with more significant numbers of hard glottal attacks than a control group. If a client presents with dysphonia and has a tendency to initiate voice with abrupt vocal behavior, specific management and clinical attention to eliminate this behavior might be required.

In hard glottal attack, phonation is begun with a forceful closure of the arytenoid cartilages. Such slamming together does not cause vocal nodules but can account for generalized swelling in the entire glottal region. Clients should be made aware of this tendency and should be helped to modify such behavior. Several recent studies have investigated contact pressures in the endolarynx during phonatory and non-phonatory behaviors (Jiang & Titze, 1994; Verdolini, Hess, Titze, Bierhals, & Gross, 1999). The methodology involves placing pressure transducers in the larynx under conditions of videoendoscopy and topical anesthesia. Using these procedures, contact pressures at various points along the glottis can be measured. Hess, Verdolini, Bierhals, Mansmann, and Gross (1998) reported interarytenoid pressures were greater than intraglottic pressures, interarytenoid pressures were greater for lower pitches than higher pitches, and both interarytenoid and intraglottic pressures were remarkably large during observed hard glottal attacks. These studies confirm the significance of the hard glottal attack and general-impact stress in the larynx as forms of phonotrauma.

Singing in an Abusive Manner

One of the most vocally demanding professions is that of a professional singer. Regardless of the style of music—the classical music of the opera, in which the performer is well trained in vocal usage, or the more popular style involving the big-time business of recording and touring, or the small-time nightclub circuit, in which performers may have little or no vocal training—the demands for vocal effort are great. A growing body of literature addresses the issue of singing and laryngeal concerns (Cleveland, 1994; Mishra, Rosen, & Murry, 2000; Sataloff, 1998c). Much of the literature on professional voice concerns comes from the Voice Foundation and its publication, the *Journal of Voice*. Articles from this journal cover such topics as country and western singers (Burns, 1991; Stone, Cleveland, & Sundberg, 1999; Sundberg, Cleveland, Stone, & Iwarsson, 1999), the effects of vocal fatigue and attrition (Kitch & Oates, 1994; Mann et al., 1999; Sapir, 1993), phonational profiles of singers and nonsingers (Brown, Morris, Hicks, & Howell, 1993; Rosen & Murry, 2000), the suggested requirements in training for those working with the professional voice user (Gregg, 1997; Titze, 1992), perceptual aspects of singing (Sundberg, 1994), and respiration concerns in singing (Sataloff, 1988; Thomasson & Sundberg, 1999).

Care of the professional singer's voice must be approached with great caution and expertise. A team approach is valuable in identifying concerns a professional singer might have about his or her vocal instrument and its care. As Titze (1992) suggested, there is a growing need for including the performance techniques of theater and the musical arts in the traditional speech–language pathology curriculum. Although I have some performance background in singing and acting, I am cautious about giving advice regarding performance technique. A team concept allows for ideas to be presented to the professional voice user from the scientific view (the measurement of voice acoustics and visualization) and from the artistic view (musical or theatrical pedagogy). Monthly at Arizona State University, I meet with a professor of theater arts, a professor of opera, and, when possible, the otolaryngologist involved when medical consultation is needed to evaluate students in the performing arts. I can provide the acoustic and visual documentation of vocal concerns, add advice and direction about nonperformance vocal usage, and support the instructions given by my colleagues in the art of vocalization on the stage. I try to understand the borders of my knowledge and stay within them. This philosophy is compatible with the advice given by Wilder (1998) regarding speech pathology and the professional voice user.

I recently participated in the voice evaluation of a professional singer whose art is exceptional and performances are demanding. Each night, this man performed on the stage in singing demands that tolerated little variation because of the familiarity of the musical score. The acoustic and visual documentation I provided as part of this evaluation identified essentially normal vocal folds and acoustic range and accuracy. He had been evaluated by some of the finest otolaryngologists and speech–language pathologists in the nation as he toured with the show. His routine, which I certainly approved but had not directed, is an excellent one for any professional voice user involved in demanding performance. Following are the salient aspects of his own professional voice care, based on the advice given to him by many professionals (many of these items are discussed in more detail later in this chapter):

• *Vocal rest.* To conserve his voice for performance, he spends little time engaged in frivolous conversation when it can be avoided. After his performance, he avoids as much as possible the mingling and autograph-seeking crowds. Although he feels it would be nice to mingle and hear their comments about his performance, he knows it would be at the expense of vocal hygiene. Such mingling might be nice for the ego but deleterious to already overworked vocal tissues.

• *Irritants.* Each breath involves moving air past his instrument, the larynx, and he is cautious about the quality of that air. I am sure he feels that if he owned a Stradivarius violin, he would protect it from any element that might harm its surface. His larynx is his Stradivarius, and it is just as priceless. He never smokes and avoids smoky areas; he uses humidifiers to maintain a high moisture content of the air he breathes; he avoids extremes of hot, cold, or dry temperatures as much as possible. Although he is not a hermit, he is very cautious.

• *Hydration*. He follows the advice often given to professional voice users to "sing wet and pee pale." He continually consumes large amounts of water and monitors his intake by observing the color of his urine. He also avoids the intake of substances that have a diuretic effect, such as caffeine.

• *Diet and acid reflux*. He is aware that performers tend to work at night, avoid too much eating before a performance, and then are starved after the show. He plans his mealtimes to avoid eating before bedtime, because of the increased probability of gastric reflux that would harm his laryngeal tissues.

• *Vocal warm-up and cooldown*. When be awakens after a restful night's sleep, he tests his voice very carefully by humming a midrange tone at a low intensity. Throughout the day he lightly vocalizes to keep his voice somewhat active. As he approaches his performance, he begins his warm-up with easy vocalizations accompanied by relaxation techniques he has learned from his vocal coaches. He expands his vocal pitch and loudness ranges cautiously. By showtime, he has increased the usage of his vocal instrument to a performance level. After his performance, he goes through a cooldown process, ending with easy vocalizations in his shower before retiring for the night.

As I listened to this artist's descriptions of vocal preparations prior to performance, I mentally compared him with a great athlete. An excellent amateur or professional athlete would never consider performance without many minutes of stretching and tuning the muscles prior to the first pitch, first dribble, first huddle, or first serve. The performer, a vocal athlete, must approach the performance with the same gradual warming process. Only in the past decade have speech–language pathologists spoken of the importance of a cooldown process at the end of a vocal performance (Saxon & Schneider, 1994; Schneider, Saxon, & Dennehy, 1998).

Care of the professional singer or performer requires effort with few degrees of freedom. The demands for vocal control are greater with this population than with any other clinical population. Even singers who are well trained in musical pedagogy can develop laryngeal tissue changes as a result of their singing. Singers of the great arias and choral selections face the most challenging of musical scores. Not only are the high and low tones often near the upper and lower limits of a singer's range, but the notes must be hit precisely. A singer must have precise and rapid control over laryngeal adjustments because experienced listeners notice when the singer is off by just a few hertz. The singer must be well trained, and the larynx must be in superlative shape. Any swelling or abnormal change in the vocal fold tissues would make such singing essentially impossible.

Vocal productions that are near to or that exceed the vocal capabilities of a performer can be presumed to be deleterious to the performer's laryngeal tissues. Coleman (1987) provided a method that a singer can use to determine whether a given musical score falls within his or her performance limits. This phonetogram method can help a performer avoid scores with damage potential.

In working with, for example, a nightclub singer who has vocal nodules, the speech–language pathologist's analysis must involve viewing the performer in action on- and offstage. Modification or elimination of behaviors that are not related directly to the performance can make a difference in the singer's durability. Abuses that are not part of the act are the only ones over which the singer has much control without taking away the means of employment. It is highly unlikely that the typical nightclub performer will have the talent or means to become a trained singer and advance to a better performance situation. It is also unlikely that this singer will be willing to modify the singing to be less abusive if it means changing what the person perceives as a truly individual vocal style. By observing the singer in the work setting, the speech–language pathologist can discover abuses that can be modified rather easily but can make a significant difference in vocal durability.

The speech–language pathologist is more likely to work with a nontrained singer who has developed vocal nodules than with a classically trained one. Rosen and Murry (2000) found that classically and well-trained singers reported less difficulty on the Voice Handicap Index than other singers and nonsingers. The less trained singer will often choose music that challenges the vocal range and potential of his or her voice, and all of the concerns of the well-trained singer apply. When an untrained singer is successful and popular, even with a singing style and vocal quality that are unacceptable to the well-trained singer, the speech–language pathologist will likely have little success if an attempt is made to change the style and vocal quality that foster such success. Rather, the speech–language pathologist must be prepared to help the nontrained successful singer modify those aspects of vocal behavior that can be modified without sacrificing the successful singing style.

The typical nightclub crowd is noisy, with constant chatter, laughter, clinking glasses, and jukebox music during breaks. Singers must compete with this noise as they mingle and are forced to almost yell simply to communicate, when what they need most is vocal rest. The larynx is not given time to recuperate before another intense musical set begins. These between-set conversations can be as abusive to the voice as the actual singing, because amplifiers can reduce vocal strain during singing.

Even a client who engages in amateur singing must be evaluated to determine whether this is a contributing factor to the development of nodules. People often sing with the radio while doing housework or other activities around the home, while in the shower, or while driving. These all bring joy to the heart but trauma to the vocal folds when done in an abusive manner. Many people are members of church, youth, or community choirs, and those activities also can contribute to vocal abuse.

Amateur singing that occurs only occasionally seldom constitutes a significant factor in the pathogenesis of vocal nodules; however, when a person has developed nodules from other causes, even amateur singing can constitute a sufficient abuse factor to maintain the nodules. Therefore, speech–language pathologists should recommend that most amateur singing be halted temporarily during the weeks of therapy.

One rather important laryngeal concern for all singers, regardless of extent of training or singing style, is the general position in the neck of the larynx during singing. Shipp (1987) provided extensive information showing that singers with classical vocal training maintain a vertical laryngeal position at or below the resting level of the larynx, whereas untrained singers typically position the larynx higher, well above the resting position, particularly as vocal pitch is raised. Shipp reported that maintaining a low position during singing results in (a) facilitating a vocal fold vibratory pattern that produces substantial energy in the higher portion of the resonance spectrum; (b) a greater opening of the vocal tract, enhancing vocal resonation; (c) a greater easing of transitions of voice from one vocal register to another; and (d) a reduction of vocal fold contact or closure forces that might be considered a vocal abuse factor.

Inadequate Hydration

Most speech–language pathologists encourage increased hydration in patients with voice disorders, especially those in dry climates. I advise patients to establish a baseline of water consumption and try to at least double it. If they report little water consumption, or indicate that fluid intake comes from the coffee machine or the soda machine, there is a critical concern for voice management.

Verdolini-Marston, Sandage, and Titze (1994) and Verdolini, Titze, and Fennell (1994) have documented what seems intuitive. In the former study, the investigators used a double-blind, placebo-controlled treatment protocol and found that increased hydration benefited patients with nodules and polyps. This evidence of improvement was supported by the second study (Verdolini, Titze, & Fennell), another double-blind, placebo-controlled study investigating phonatory control under three hydration levels: tropical treatment (high humidity, administration of 2 teaspoons of a mucolytic drug, and lots of water consumption); control treatment (normal humidity, no drug, and no instructions on water consumption); and the Arizona treatment, which consisted of a drying process (low humidity, administration of 2 teaspoons of a decongestant drug, and no water intake for the 4 hours of the experiment). The results favored the phonatory control obtained under conditions of increased hydration. The assumption was that heightened hydration would increase laryngeal tissue viscosity (stickiness vs. dryness), which was not measured directly, and this likely happened, as evidenced by improved laboratory performance and subjective self-assessment of patients in the tropical treatment group. Additional researchers have confirmed the importance of maintaining adequate hydration when doing voice performance (Solomon & DiMattia, 2000).

These studies add documentation to the clinical view that it is wise to encourage patients experiencing voice disturbance to maintain significant water intake. Additionally, physicians can administer synthetic saliva products, such as Salivart, as an oral spray.

Speaking in a Noisy Environment

When a person speaks in a noisy environment, several things happen to the larynx and speech system. First, the high ambient noise level makes it difficult to monitor how loud the conversation is, so the individual is unlikely to eliminate excessive vocal effort. Second, to be heard above the noise, the person generates greater lung airflow, to which the vocal folds respond with greater resistance equivalent to what is perceived as laryngeal tension. Although the resistance is quantifiable and measurable, the instrumentation necessary to do so does not work well in a noisy environment such as a nightclub or a factory.

An easy way I have found to demonstrate the effect of a high ambient noise level on conversation involves making a tape recording of the noise in a nightclub (the quality of the recording is not important). I then play back the recording at a noise level typical of a nightclub and engage the client in conversation. The widely known Lombard effect will cause the client's voice to become more intense (loud), usually in direct proportion to the loudness level of the tape. I can then demonstrate what is happening to the client's voice by suddenly turning off the tape recorder in the middle of the client's speech. The client usually will notice that he or she has been nearly shouting and generating considerable tension to compete with the noise. The impact of this demonstration can be helpful in convincing a client with vocal nodules how important it is not to compete with a noisy environment.

Coughing and Excessive Throat Clearing

The speech–language pathologist can use the example of the cough photographed and shown in ultraslow motion discussed earlier to communicate the deleterious effect of coughing and excessive throat clearing on the larynx. An endoscopic view under normal lighting conditions of a person coughing is just as effective. Coughing occurs when the protective valving mechanisms of the larynx are stimulated by a foreign irritation. It is a reflex act and hard to control or eliminate when caused by an upper respiratory infection or allergy. Antihistamine–decongestant medicines are often helpful in reducing this reflex act, and clients with vocal nodules should be encouraged to solicit the help of a physician when an upper respiratory infection or allergy is present.

As in the case of a hard glottal attack, coughing and excessive throat clearing are unlikely to cause vocal nodules, but then can act as generalized irritants to the larynx and add a vulnerability factor to other forms of vocal abuse. Therefore, it is important that the speech–language pathologist discuss the effect of coughing and excessive throat clearing and provide modification support. This can include physician referral as well as instruction on cough and throat-clearing modification.

The manner of coughing and throat clearing can be modified when a person is taught to do them with less intensity and glottal explosion. Zwitman and Calcaterra (1973) discussed the "silent cough" method of eliminating the abusive aspects by teaching the client to push air from the lungs in blasts, being careful not to produce sound whenever the urge to cough or clear the throat occurs. Even reflex coughing during upper respiratory infection can be modified in this manner. Most throat clearing is not reflexive, and behavior modification can help eliminate it. The speech–language pathologist should point out that most throat clearing is unproductive in terms of actually removing the stimulating mucus from the glottis and that swallowing quickly after a small air blast is more likely to clear the area of the mucus than is a loud, phonated grunt.

Grunting When Exercising and Lifting

Grunting is a significant but often overlooked form of vocal abuse. Anyone who has been on the sidelines of a football game can attest to the grunting that goes on during blocking and tackling. Fortunately, those engaged in this strenuous vocal activity usually are large and strong, so their larynges are frequently strong enough to resist the abuse involved. However, I recently worked with a 345-pound offensive lineman for a professional football team who had developed vocal nodules and was having a difficult time using his voice at the line of scrimmage to let his fellow players know what he was going to do. He said, "If I can't get my voice back, I am out of a job." I was intrigued that this giant of a human being was being sidelined by two tiny muscles in his larynx.

Many of the general public's activities, however, involve the same kind of laryngeal trauma. Daily exercise and lifting involve glottal closure under pressure in order to contain air in the lungs to stabilize the chest cavity so that skeletal muscles can function efficiently. Push-ups, pull-ups, weight lifting, hard tennis serves or volleys, and jumping usually involve hard closure of the glottis. Clients should be informed of this potential form of vocal abuse so that they can analyze their behavior with regard to it. Figure 4.3 shows the larynx of a patient with a well-developed body who spent 2 to 3 hours each day in vigorous weight lifting accompanied by loud grunting and laryngeal overpressure.

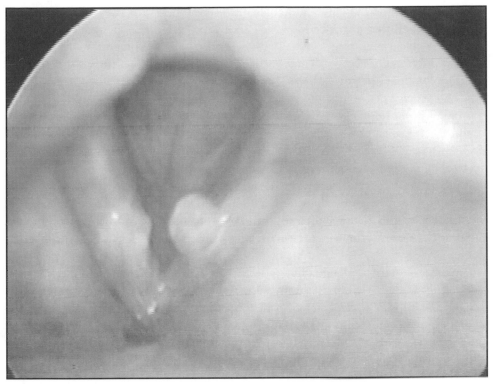

Figure 4.3. Cyst and generalized edema on larynx of patient who was a weight lifter and bartender in a noisy nightclub.

Calling Others from a Distance

Men, women, and children who develop vocal nodules often are surprised to discover how often they yell from room to room or yard to yard to communicate with other people or pets. It seems easier to yell than to walk closer for communication. However, walking—a simple activity—can help both the cardiovascular system and the vocal folds and can eliminate significant abuse to laryngeal tissues. The speech–language pathologist should encourage clients to make the extra effort to decrease the distance before communicating verbally, especially when there is noise in the environment, such as in a house with the radio or television playing.

Using Inappropriate Pitch Levels

Pitch characteristics of vocal abuse clients merit considerable attention. The speech–language pathologist must evaluate the basal, habitual, and optimal pitch levels in such individuals and modify any significant disparity found between habitual pitch and pitch levels that might be too low. This low pitch must be viewed in the overall context of vocal physiology, including laryngeal tension. As mentioned previously, the low pitch might also be a consequence of increased mass on the vocal folds, and the pitch will naturally elevate as improvement occurs.

The average person usually speaks at a fundamental frequency average above the bottom of his or her range. Any tendency for a person to speak at a pitch level lower than this typical pattern will place the habitual pitch very close to the basal level. At or near the basal level, the larynx does not function efficiently in phonation, so considerable tension and effort must be expended to initiate voice. For a high pitch to be abusive, it would have to approach the upper limits of the vocal range, a level rarely approached by most people. However, a high-pitched and tense voice is also abusive.

In singing, it is common for untrained but professional vocalists to attempt to use tones at the extreme limits of their range, either too high or too low. Falsetto singing does not need to be abusive, but in pop music, where it is common, it often is. Falsetto singing that is abusive is more often falsetto screaming and has affected many professional singers adversely. One of the first signs that a singer's larynx has been damaged by vocal abuse is loss of control on high tones, including falsetto. However, singers usually do not try to transpose the pitch or range requirements of certain songs to fit their voice range but rather work harder to achieve the target pitch as written. In the long run this is counterproductive to good vocal performance and is abusive to laryngeal tissues.

Speaking During Allergy Episode or Upper Respiratory Infection

When the delicate tissues of the larynx are inflamed by allergy or upper respiratory infection, they are more vulnerable to vocal abuse. Even normal communication during these episodes can harm the tissues, but when verbal abuse is intense, prolonged, at inappropriate pitch levels, or in any other way abusive, the negative effect is compounded. Therefore, it is important to determine whether such inflammations exist when the individual is evaluated.

A medical examination is required to distinguish between inflamed tissues that are caused by an allergy or by an upper respiratory infection, but the adult client's impression as to whether either is present can be helpful. In any case medical attention is necessary, and the client should be encouraged to seek such service. Cohn, Spiegel, Hawkshaw, and Sataloff (1998) provided an excellent account of the effect of allergies on the voice, particularly on the voice of performers. Jackson-Menaldi, Dzul, and Holland (1999) suggested using screening tests for performers who have a history of allergies, such as a screening radioallergosorbent test or a screening panel of scratch/intradermal skin tests. Most of the allergies discussed affect the mucous membranes of the nose and throat, including the delicate tissues of the larynx, caus-ing inflammation and often swelling of laryngeal tissues. The fundamental frequency and vibratory characteristics of the voice are therefore affected negatively by such tis-sue change. These changes constitute a factor of concern beyond the vulnerability to vocal usage caused by allergy.

Allergies to molds and dust affect some professional voice users performing in concert halls due to the curtains, backdrops, and stage equipment that are rarely cleaned. The musty theater smell might produce nostalgic sensations, but at the same time it can stuff up the nose and swell the vocal folds.

An extension of the concern for allergic reactions is the possibility of tissue reac-tion to toxic substances such as asbestos, silicone, alcohol, caffeine, and many pre-scribed drugs. Sataloff (1994, 1998c) discussed the general concerns of tissue reaction to the presence of these toxic substances in the environment.

Vocalizing Under Musculoskeletal Tension

The speech–language pathologist must give considerable attention to the evaluation of excessive muscular tension in the laryngeal area during phonation as a vocal abuse factor. A. E. Aronson (1990) advocated physical manipulation of the larynx and surrounding tissues when excessive musculoskeletal tension or vocal hyperfunction is present. Aronson suggested the following steps to physically manage such tension:

1. Encircle the hyoid bone with the thumb and middle finger, working them poste-riorly until the tips of the major horns are felt.

2. Exert light pressure with the fingers in a circularmotion over the tips of the hyoid bone and ask if the patient feels pain, not merely pressure. It is important to watch the facial expression for signs of discomfort or pain.

3. Repeat this procedure, with the fingers working into the thyrohyoid space, begin-ning from the thyroid notch and working posteriorly.

4. Find the posterior borders of the thyroid cartilage just medial to the sternocleido-mastoid muscles and repeat the procedure.

5. With the fingers over the superior borders of the thyroid cartilage, begin to work the larynx gently downward, also moving it laterally at times. Check for a lower laryngeal position by estimating the increased size of the thyrohyoid space.

6. Ask the patient to prolong vowels during these procedures, noting changes in quality or pitch. Clearer voice quality and lower pitch indicate relief of tension. Because these procedures are fatiguing, rest periods should be provided.

7. Once a voice change has taken place, the patient should be allowed to experi-ment with the voice, repeating vowels, words, and sentences.

Generally using the procedures outlined by A. E. Aronson (1990), Roy and Leeper (1993) documented the change in voice of 17 patients. Voice recordings and acoustic and perceptual baseline data were obtained prior to a single treatment session of physical laryngeal manipulation using the steps suggested by Aronson. The majority of patients experienced considerable voice improvement following the treatment. These patients were not being seen because of vocal abuse and had no laryngeal pathology (vocal nodules, etc.), but the primary vocal symptom was one of vocal hyperfunction, a characteristic that is common in patients with vocal nodules. The techniques suggested by Aronson (1990) and confirmed by Roy and Leeper (1993; Roy, Ryker, & Bless, 2000) might well apply to patients with vocal nodules and generalized vocal abuse or misuse, particularly those with professional voice demands, such as actors, who must often perfom vocally challenging and violent behaviors.

Subjectively, the speech–language pathologist can monitor excessive tension by palpating the extrinsic laryngeal muscles (sternocleidomastoid, mylohyoid, sternohyoid, masseter, etc.) even if the strict protocols of A. E. Aronson (1990) and Roy, Ryker, et al. (2000) are not used. If tension is found in the extrinsic musculature during pho-nation, it also is likely to be present in a hyperfunctional manner in the intrinsic musculature responsible for voice. Such hyperfunctional effort contributes to the overall pattern of vocal abuse and should be modified as part of the therapeutic process.

Smoking or Speaking in a Smoky Environment

Smoking tobacco is well documented as a significant health hazard generally, and its effect on laryngeal tissue is likewise well known. Meyerhoff and Rice (1992), Sataloff (1991, 1998c), and Stone, Chagnon, and Ossoff (1994) have reported on the abusive effects of smoking on the larynx. Sataloff stated the concern in unambiguous terms: "The deleterious effects of tobacco smoke on mucosa are indisputable. It causes erythema, mild edema, and generalized inflammation throughout the vocal tract. Both smoke itself and the heat of the cigarette appear to be important" (Sataloff, 1991, p. 80). Tobacco smoke is also often an allergen and can be an irritant to respiratory tract tissue. Nicotine constricts the peripheral blood vessels, reducing blood flow. The usual effect of excessive smoking is a lowering of the fundamental frequency of the voice, particularly in women (Gilbert & Weismer, 1974).

The irritating effects of smoking on the vocal folds are so substantial that it is not unreasonable for the speech–language pathologist to expect the client with vocal nodules or other abuse conditions to significantly cut down or eliminate smoking to establish a good prognosis for therapy. As with many factors, smoking—even excessively—does not cause vocal nodules but does add a significant vulnerability factor.

Fritzell and Hertegard (1986) reported data from a retrospective study investigating the deleterious effects of cigarette smoking on laryngeal tissues with chronic vocal fold edema. A questionnaire was sent to 140 patients previously treated for this condition. One of the most significant bits of data was that 123 of the 126 patients (98%) who responded to the questionnaire were smokers at the time of initial treatment. Of these patients 94% were women. Many of these patients had undergone surgery or voice therapy. A follow-up clinical examination was performed on 95 of the responding patients, and only 16 had stopped smoking. When the results of this retrospective clinical examination study were complete, the authors stated that stopping smoking yielded significant improvement in all tested dimensions, whereas failure to stop smoking yielded long-term results indicating that surgery, therapy, or a combination of both treatments failed to result in a favorable outcome.

Smoking marijuana is also a significant hazard in many cases. Although marijuana (cannabis) is an ancient drug, its use by a significant part of society has occurred only since the early 1960s. Many smokers report dry mouth and throat, raspiness in the voice, and difficulty with pitch change (Sataloff, 1991, 1998c). Professional singers, particularly those who tour extensively and sing traditional rock and roll, often use marijuana, which has a deleterious effect on singing control, especially in reaching high notes at low intensities. The singer who has vocal nodules experiences an even more significant effect from tobacco and marijuana smoke. Therefore, even casual marijuana use should be discouraged in clients with vocal nodules.

Excessive Vocalization During Menstrual Cycle

Several authors have reported on the effect of menstrual cycles on vocal changes in women (Davis & Davis, 1993; Golub, 1992; Sataloff, 1998a). Although these changes may be subtle and not experienced by all women, the speech–language pathologist should alert female clients to be cautious about excessive vocalization during premenstrual and menstrual periods. It may be necessary to document in a specific client whether voice quality and pitch seem to change just before menstruation. If so, it would indicate that tissue edema is sufficient to establish a vulnerability factor on the effects of abuse on the vocal folds.

Abitbol et al. (1989) studied 38 women during the ovulation and premenstrual phases of two monthly cycles. They found that alterations in estrogen and progesterone levels associated with these cycles caused laryngeal water retention, edema of the interstitial tissue, and venous dilatation, causing vocal hoarseness and vocal fatigue in 22 of the 38 women. All of these women were vocal performers (classical, jazz, vocal teachers, or actors). Only 5 of the women smoked cigarettes. These women were studied with acoustic measurement, videostroboscopy, and glottographic instrumentation. Davis and Davis (1993) found abdominal bloating to be the most common complaint of female singers and difficulty singing high notes as the most common vocal finding. These studies, along with others (Higgins & Saxman, 1989; Newman, Butler, Hammond, & Gray, 2000; Rubin, 1987), provide significant documentation that hormonal changes in women can affect the larynx and the voice, particularly in those who perform vocally.

Excessive Vocalizing

It is not necessarily the amount of vocalization that becomes abusive but the nature of it. When a person has vocal nodules, however, it can be helpful to suggest the elimination of nonessential communication during the early weeks of therapy. The speech–language pathologist must judge whether such a suggestion would add so much stress to the client as to be counterproductive, but eliminating superfluous talking should at least be considered.

Inadequate Breath Support

The volumes of respiration necessary for phonation support were discussed in Chapter 3, along with a description of instrumentation needed for objective evaluation of the human respiration system. Here a more clinical description of the breath support necessary for the phonation and articulation processes of speech is provided. Boone (1988) provided practical steps for improving breath support for speech by explaining to the client that inspiratory–expiratory respiration is a continuous movement and by providing drills that maximize those processes in speech and singing. He emphasized speaking in simple terms (e.g., bigger breath, smaller breath, renewed breath, expiratory control) rather than in the complex terms of respiratory measurement (e.g., vital capacity, inspiratory capacity, expiratory reserve volume). His four-step approach provides a practical solution to many respiratory problems encountered in voice therapy.

One benefit of formal singing or acting training is the realization of how important breath support is for proper laryngeal function, including specific instructions for proper breathing. When the larynx is supported well by proper breathing, it is as though vibration is occurring with little effort. Without such support, the larynx must be tense and must work hard to produce the vibration. It is important for the speech–language pathologist to evaluate clients with vocal nodules to determine whether breath support is adequate. This is not a major etiological consideration in vocal nodule therapy, unlike the case for some neurologically based speech disorders, but evaluation of the utilization of the respiration system may be an important consideration in some patients.

Good breath support for phonation requires sufficient inhalation of air but rarely requires a maximum effort, as it would, for example, in measuring vital capacity. A deep inhalation beyond tidal inhalation is all that is required. This occurs with the abdominal muscles essentially relaxed so as to facilitate contraction of the diaphragm.

The diaphragm is a dome-shaped muscle surrounding a central tendon that separates the abdominal cavity, which contains the stomach, intestines, and visceral organs, from the thoracic cavity, which contains the lungs, heart, and mediastinum. When the diaphragm contracts, by virtue of its shape and skeletal attachments, it pulls itself downward and forward, expanding the vertical dimensions of the thoracic or pulmonary cavities and therefore enlarging the lungs in that direction. This expansion draws air into the lungs and inhalation (inspiration) occurs.

For inhalation sufficient to support running phonation and speech adequately, the diaphragm must be able to contract without excessive resistance. Resistance is less when the abdominal muscles have decreased tonicity. As the diaphragm contracts, its movements displace the visceral organs in a forward and lateral direction, distending the abdominal wall.

The functions of the diaphragm during inhalation are complemented by musculature that lifts the rib cage to produce lung expansion in an anterior direction. In other words, deep inhalation requires that the stomach and visceral organs be displaced in a forward direction at the same time that the chest wall is expanding. If the client puts a hand on the stomach during proper inhalation, the inspiration should push the hand forward slightly. The deeper the inhalation, the farther the hand should move forward.

Following the inhalation cycle, the air is exhaled by essentially a reversal of that process. The diaphragm relaxes and pulls itself back to its precontraction position, and the muscles that lifted the rib cage relax, allowing the rib cage to be lowered. These relaxation processes have the effect of decreasing the dimensions of the lungs, squeezing out their air through the open glottis. If phonation is to occur during this exhalation cycle, the glottis is closed, generating subglottic pressure, and the exhaled air vibrates the vocal folds.

The early stage of exhalation is essentially passive, with tissues (diaphragm and rib cage) merely returning to their precontracted state. Air inhaled into the inspiratory reserve volume and tidal air are exhaled by this passive process. Beyond tidal exhalation, the process of exhalation becomes active, involving contraction of the abdominal muscles to compress the abdominal cavity by displacing the visceral organs up against the diaphragm, which in turn compresses the lungs to force exhalation.

This lung compression is aided by the compression of the rib cage by muscles antagonistic to rib elevation (intercostals, transversus thoraces, serratus posterior inferior, and abdominal muscles). These compression forces have the effect of decreasing the vertical and anterior dimensions of the chest wall cavity to complete the exhalation involved in the expiratory reserve volume. The abdominal muscles also facilitate rapid and efficient contractions of the diaphragm for quick inhalation without significant interruptions in speech flow during running conversation.

The following are indicators that the client with vocal nodules has inadequate breath support for phonation:

- Phonation is attempted before adequate inhalation.

- Phonation is started after considerable exhalation has occurred, forcing voice and speech with little respiratory reserve.

- Poor reciprocity is exhibited between the muscles of inhalation (inspiration) and exhalation (expiration).

This information on breathing for speech is important in treating the typical client with vocal nodules or some similar vocal abuse disorder, such as contact ulcers. It is based on the assumption that breathing is essentially normal and devoid of pathology and merely needs to be maximized to support better the phonation and articulation processes of speech.

Laughing Hard and Abusively

The speech–language pathologist never wants to be accused of suggesting that a client eliminate the joy of a good laugh, but laughing is an altered form of phonation, and some of its forms can involve considerable abusive stroking of the vocal folds. This concern for laughing patterns usually is not a very significant item in the treatment of vocal abuse, but some attention may need to be directed to modifying abusive laughter during the early weeks of therapy or following surgical removal of vocal nodules.

Cheerleading, Aerobics Instruction, and Pep Club Activities

Perhaps the classic example of vocal abuse in school-age children is organized cheerleading and pep club activities. In most junior and senior high schools, students are encouraged to abuse their vocal folds physically to improve school spirit and support the team. It is almost as though the chosen cheerleaders have been elected to sacrifice their voices on the altar of team victory. Organized cheerleading also is found in Little League baseball and Pop Warner football programs.

For several years some of my graduate students in speech–language pathology studied the effects of cheerleading on the voice and vocal folds. Several high school and university cheerleaders were investigated longitudinally through basketball and football seasons. One study involved 10 varsity basketball cheerleaders. Before the beginning of the basketball season, 8 female and 2 male cheerleaders were examined medically by an otolaryngologist and found to have normal larynges. Baseline voice recordings were obtained on each. Before and after home basketball games during the season, voice recordings were made of each participant.

At the end of the season, each person was medically evaluated by the same otolaryngologist. Both male cheerleaders had developed vocal nodules. One significant finding was that the voice recordings, which were judged by three independent experts and also were used to obtain spectrographic measurements, were not specific in identifying the presence of the vocal nodules; only the medical inspection identified them. This study was significant in that subjects with identified normal larynges were involved in a vocally abusive activity that resulted in a 20% incidence of developed vocal nodules. Observation of the cheering styles of the 2 males revealed an abusive pattern that was significantly different from that of the 8 females, who did not develop vocal nodules (Case, Beaver, & Nenaber, 1978).

A further study involved voice and laryngeal characteristics of high school cheerleaders and an additional group of university students. These groups were followed longitudinally through a football season. Each cheerleader was evaluated by an otolaryngologist at the beginning and the end of the football season, as well as periodically throughout the season. Each participant's voice also was recorded at the time of each medical examination. The voice recordings also were used for listener judgments and spectrographic analyses.

In the high school group, initial medical examinations revealed that none of the 9 participants (all female) had laryngeal pathology. After this initial examination, the 9 participated in a weeklong cheer camp, then were examined medically again. Four of the 9 subjects had laryngeal pathology (i.e., early vocal nodules and laryngeal edema), which the otolaryngologist attributed directly to vocal abuse. The cheerleaders reported that the cheer camp was an intense and vocally abusive experience that involved continual yelling in both formal and informal cheering sessions.

The listener judgments and spectrographic analyses were in agreement with the medically diagnosed status of the cheerleaders' larynges: 100% when no pathology was present and from 68% to 79% when pathology was present. These findings indicating the presence of pathology among many of the subjects made it more difficult to obtain agreement. Both false positives and false negatives were obtained; that is, medical inspection revealed pathology when listener judgment or spectrographic analysis indicated a normal larynx, or vice versa. By the end of the football season, even with some counseling from the authors of the study, 2 of the participants continued to have vocal nodules, as confirmed by medical inspection.

The 12 university football cheerleaders studied presented a different pattern. They were evaluated medically the day before the first football game. An otolaryngologist examined each cheerleader's larynx and took a medical case history. Voice recordings for listener judgments and spectrographic analyses also were obtained. Surprisingly, 9 (5 males, 4 females) of the 12 were found to have laryngeal pathology related to vocal abuse—a 75% prevalence. It had been hoped that examining the cheerleaders prior to the first game would reveal normal larynges. As it turned out, however, the members of the squad had been practicing their yells intensely for several weeks, and this was obviously responsible for the high prevalence of laryngeal pathology.

The research team felt obliged to inform the team members of the condition of their larynges and the probable causes of the pathology. This was done with slides and discussion about the development of vocal nodules. By the end of the football season, only 7 (4 males, 3 females) of the 12 cheerleaders (58%) continued to have laryngeal pathology from vocal abuse. In this study, probably because of the high prevalence of preexisting laryngeal pathology, agreement between spectrographic analyses and medical inspections and between listener judgment of voice quality and medical inspections was lower than in the previous studies (56% and 64%, respectively; Case, Thome, & Kohler, 1979).

Because many of the cheerleaders in these studies developed pathology but others did not, it was important that the distinguishing causal factors be determined. From observation and subjective judgment, the following behaviors seemed to be excessive in the cheerleaders who developed the nodules and other laryngeal pathologies:

- Cheering without good abdominal breath support
- Cheering with an energy focus in the larynx
- Cheering with excessive tension in the laryngeal area
- Using hard and abrupt onset of voice (hard glottal attack)
- Cheering during colds, infections, or allergy attacks
- Cheering at an inappropriate pitch level (too high or too low)
- Excessive individual cheering in addition to the group yells
- Cheering without amplification when it could be used

In addition to the preceding factors, researchers have identified others that must be considered when working with cheerleaders to prevent vocal difficulty. Perhaps one of the most important factors is screening out those cheerleading applicants who predictably will have vocal difficulty. Campbell, Reich, Klockars, and McHenry (1988) developed a screening protocol that can easily be incorporated into the selection process. Many factors were found to be important considerations, even when not statistically significant:

- Frequency of sore throats or tired voices at day's end
- Severity of progressive aphonia and dysphonia on noncheering days
- Severity of acute vocal problems at cheerleading camp or during tryout periods
- Frequency of coughing and throat clearing
- Amount of loud talking when not cheerleading
- Aggressive personalities (as determined by a personality scale)

Through use of this list and consideration of additional factors that would be obvious to one who understands the vocal demands of cheerleading, the speech–language pathologist can help improve selection of cheerleaders and reduce the high prevalence of laryngeal and vocal difficulties experienced by this high-risk group. The speech–language pathologist who might consult in the selection and care of these youth can refer to Reich and McHenry (1987) and Reich, McHenry, and Keaton (1986) for additional help. Considering the high prevalence of laryngeal pathology in cheerleaders, it seems important that the speech–language pathologist evaluate cheerleaders to determine whether vocal abuse is affecting their voice quality and laryngeal structures. It also is suggested that before practices cheerleaders and pep squad members be advised of cheering techniques that are less abusive, in accordance with the principles outlined.

Whereas cheerleaders have been abusing their larynges for decades, only recently have patients presented vocal abuse symptoms from aerobics instruction. Heidel and Torgerson (1993) and Long, Williford, Olson, and Wolfe (1998) provided documentation from self-reporting of aerobics instructors and participants that such activity can be harmful to the larynx. In another case I documented on audiotape and videotape the effect of only one session of aerobics instruction done without the benefit of amplification. I performed a series of visual examinations of the larynx of a professional aerobics instructor who developed vocal nodules, including one taken 1 hour before she had to teach a class without a microphone, although she usually had one available. I documented her voice, she then taught the class, and the next morning I saw her for a replication of the visual and acoustic documentation. The results were dramatic. Her hoarseness was dramatically worsened, and her pitch was lowered from a speaking fundamental frequency of 186 Hz to 145 Hz. She also reported losing her voice by the end of the night, and she experienced some soreness. The visual documentation was also dramatic, with her larynx showing increased edema along the entire phonating edge and her vocal folds being considerably more erythemic.

Schwan, Case, and LaPointe (1996) reported evidence of phonotrauma among aerobics instructors when 20 instructors were medically and stroboscopically evaluated. Eighty-two percent of the vocal folds of these instructors were found to have laryngeal pathology attributed to the extensive vocalization involved in directing classes in aerobics.

Vocalizing Toy and Animal Noises

Verbal dramatics is often an important part of children's play. Bears growl, lions roar, monsters make weird noises, airplanes scream as they dive in combat, machine guns and rifles make sharp bangs, and bicycles become motorcycles—all in the children's voices. Numerous play activities seem to require children to mimic sounds, thus abusing the larynx. The speech–language pathologist who works with a child with vocal nodules should explore these verbal activities thoroughly. Some children engage in many such activities, others in only one or two but often and routinely.

For example, the child who merely makes motorcycle sounds when riding a bicycle, but does so often, can abuse the larynx sufficiently to produce nodules even when good vocal hygiene is practiced in all other circumstances (T. S. Johnson, 1983).

Athletic Activity Involving Yelling

The high school athletic coach, particularly in football, basketball, and wrestling, is in a high-risk profession for vocal abuse and the development of vocal nodules. The wrestling coach, for example, continually yells instructions during a match in an atmosphere of extreme noise and emotional tension. A typical wrestling match involves three rounds of 2 minutes each, and it is not unusual for the coach to be yelling throughout each round, telling the wrestler to execute one move or another to gain points or avoid being pinned. Hand signals or gestures will not work because the wrestler's eyes usually are buried in his opponent's armpit. Only the voice can be used to communicate. This occurs match after match until often, by the end of the meet, the coach is voiceless, and the next morning it is worse.

It is a great challenge for the speech–language pathologist to help the athletic coach solve the dilemma of preventing vocal abuse while still functioning effectively as a coach. To accomplish this, the speech–language pathologist must carefully consider with the client ways of modifying the communication process to eliminate as much of the abuse as possible.

Aggressive Personality Factor

A. E. Aronson (1990) classified vocal nodules as a psychogenic voice disorder because abuse or misuse most often is not the primary etiology. Rather, abuse is an intermediate link in the chain of causes that begins with an emotionally determined tendency to vocalize in an aggressive manner. This attitude was shared by Toohill (1975), who reported that 62 of 77 children with vocal nodules were described by their parents as screamers, incessant talkers, or loud talkers who were aggressive, hyperactive, nervous, tense, frustrated, or emotionally disturbed. Throughout the literature children with vocal nodules have been described as having these aggressive personality characteristics, as well as greater feelings of inadequacy, poorer relationships with parents and siblings, and greater difficulty controlling themselves in verbal relationships.

Some of these factors have been corroborated in my clinical experience but not to the degree reported by A. E. Aronson (1990) and Toohill (1975). The possibility that a client with vocal nodules has a significant personality disturbance as a contributing factor in the etiology of the disorder certainly must be considered; in such cases, referral to a psychologist or psychiatrist is in order as an adjunct to vocal abuse therapy.

McHugh-Munier, Scherer, Lehmann, and Scherer (1997) reported on personality and coping strategies of female patients with vocal nodules or polyps and found that these patients tended to use more emotional than cognitive coping strategies. Roy, Bless, and Heisey (2000) studied a group of patients with vocal nodules as one part of a larger study involving other dysphonias, focusing on personality traits that might have a bearing on the development of their nodules. They reported that patients with vocal nodules registered as socially dominant, stress reactive, aggressive, and impulsive on the Multidimensional Personality Questionnaire. This article is an excellent one to read when considering the personality traits of patients with various dysphonias.

Arguing with Others

The aggressive personality factor often manifests itself in frequent arguments with other people, including peers and siblings. To a certain degree, this is a normal part of social and family life, unless it occurs in the extreme. The client with vocal nodules (or, if a child, family members also) must be interviewed about the prevalence of such behavior. In children, this often is such a meaningful factor in voice abuse that it is wise to include peers and significant others in the early therapy sessions to enlist their help in avoiding such confrontations. If a sibling or significant peer is not willing to cooperate in avoiding verbal arguments, it is hard to convince the client to become verbally passive when conflict arises.

Alcohol Intake

The interaction between alcohol intake and cigarette smoking as a factor in the development of laryngeal cancer is discussed in Chapter 7. In this section I discuss alcohol as it relates to vocal abuse. I see many university students in whom one factor of vocal abuse is the tendency to socialize with friends while drinking alcohol in a smoky environment. The degree of vocalization and its intensity often relate proportionately to the degree of alcohol intake. After such an episode of pleasure, the next morning the voice is usually significantly altered. Was it the talk? The competing noise? The smoky environment? The alcohol? The answer is likely all of these factors.

Some evidence exists documenting negative changes in the mucosa of laryngeal tissues and in voice performance under conditions of alcohol intake. Watanabe et al. (1994) studied 48 subjects who consumed alcohol under laboratory testing conditions. Among the extensive findings was that vocal range and mean laryngeal airflow decreased as voice roughness increased. Vocal efficiency deteriorated in almost all of the subjects. Within 1 hour of alcohol intake, changes observed included engorgement and tissue changes in the subglottal, false fold, and arytenoid regions. These findings lend support for the concern about the effects of alcohol intake on voice function.

Medications

In Chapters 2 and 3, I generally discussed the importance of considering medications in the development and maintenance of a dysphonia. Those general considerations apply here in a discussion of vocal abuse and the development of vocal nodules and other related dysphonias. A growing body of literature exists regarding these considerations, particularly studies of professional voice users such as singers and actors. Sataloff et al. (1998) discussed many of these medications and warned of the possible positive and deleterious effects of antihistamines, mucolytic agents, corticosteroids, edema medications, sprays, mists, inhalants, antibiotics, antiviral agents, antitussive medications, antihypertensive agents, gastroenterologic medications, vitamins, sleeping pills, analgesics, hormone replacement medications, bronchoactive medications, beta-blockers, psychoactive medications, and medications to treat various neurological disorders. Because each of these medications can have positive as well as significant deleterious consequences on the voice, it is the responsibility of the patient's physician to monitor all medication usage, but the speech–language pathologist working with a client with dysphonia must be aware of possible effects of medications. Sataloff et al., along with the *PDR* references in Chapter 2, is an excellent general reference guide to the effects and side effects of medications on professional voice users. Sataloff (1998b) also provided guidance on medication usage for the traveling performer who must adjust to capricious performance milieu. He stated that it is particularly challenging for a performer who travels outside the United States to obtain necessary medications, and it is common for such performers to carry with them a "bag of goodies" that past experience has indicated might be needed.

Neely and Rosen (2000) reported on an opera-singing patient who had been placed on Coumadin to treat atrial fibrillation. This 59-year-old voice professor and elite professional opera singer presented with red vascular lesion of the midportion of his right vocal fold consistent with a hemorrhagic vocal fold polyp. After microlaryngoscopy the patient underwent excision of the vocal fold polyp and carbon dioxide laser ablation of the vascular ectasia feeding the polyp. Coumadin was stopped perioperatively for 3 weeks. Surgery was successful and the patient resumed singing until 8 weeks postoperative, when he developed recurrent dysphonia. The authors found that he had been restarted on Coumadin. Coumadin anticoagulation therapy was found to be etiologically related to the development of the patient's polyp because it thins the blood and generates increased potential for hemorrhage to abused tissues. In this case, laryngeal tissues used in singing were most vulnerable. Neely and

Rosen cautioned against performers' using aspirin, nonsteroidal anti-inflammatories, and hormonal replacement therapies without strict physician monitoring of voice factors.

Professional Teachers

Schoolteachers seem to be particularly vulnerable to the development of dysphonia related to phonotrauma. A growing body of professional literature supports this concern (Kostyk & Rochet, 1998; Rantala & Vilkman, 1999; Russell, Oates, & Greenwood, 1998). E. Smith, Gray, Dove, Kirchner, and Heras (1997) stated that teachers were more likely than a nonteaching control group (15% vs. 6%) to report having a voice problem. E. Smith, Kirchner, Taylor, Hoffman, and Lemke (1998) reported that female teachers were more likely to experience voice difficulty (38%) than male teachers (26%). More than 38% of both female teachers and male teachers believed that teaching had an adverse impact on their voice status. Simberg, Laine, Sala, and Ronnemaa (2000) stated that this concern about dysphonia among teachers needs to be extended and evaluated in those training to become teachers. They reported that 19% of 226 students had organic voice disorder, reinforcing the notion that teachers and prospective teachers should be monitored carefully for voice difficulty, which could significantly hamper their careers.

Miscellaneous Factors

The list of possible forms of vocal abuse is so extensive as to preclude an inclusive list. For example, I evaluated a man who was referred after surgery for contact ulcers. He presented with many of the vocal abuse forms discussed previously, and I thought that we had compiled a comprehensive list of target behaviors. At the end of the evaluation, he mentioned that he loved to perform Buddhist chanting and wondered whether it was vocally abusive. I had no experience with such chanting, but he presented an audiotape of the behavior. I was immediately taken by how vocally intense and potentially abusive the chanting was as presented in the audio recording. I asked him to demonstrate how he chanted.

Regardless of whether he chanted appropriately from a religious point of view, it was obvious that he chanted in such a way that, although his soul might benefit, his larynx could not be saved. His breathing was nonsupportive and prolonged, his pitch was at the bottom of his range, and vocal and laryngeal tension were obvious. He would attempt to stretch his vocalizations on one breath to the maximum and then take a quick inhalation and resume. He mentioned that often he would do this chanting several hours each day. Clearly, his chanting would have to be modified or it would lead to further surgery.

The story of this individual illustrates the important clinical interview technique of ending a vocal abuse interview with a general question about additional forms of abuse not covered. I usually state, "We have been talking about various forms of vocal abuse or misuse activity. Can you think of anything you do, even if it does not occur often, that might also be a concern to us?" In this manner, miscellaneous concerns can be identified.

EVALUATION AND THERAPY
PROCEDURES FOR VOCAL NODULES

Persons with vocal nodules receive the services of speech–language pathologists either by screening or teacher referral in school or by physician referrals in clinics, centers, and private practice. When a student is screened or referred by a teacher, the speech–language pathologist first must determine the nature of the problem and the possible causes and effects. The only information available initially is that the student has a hoarse or raspy voice. The etiology of the vocal symptoms is not known until a medical inspection is conducted, which should begin as soon as it has been established that persistent voice disorder exists.

Once the medical confirmation of vocal nodules is obtained, formal evaluation of the client can proceed. The evaluation session is done first, but therapy emerges in the final stage of the evaluation session. There is no clear distinction between evaluation and therapy processes in cases of vocal nodules. The following management protocol is designed to help the speech–language pathologist working with clients with vocal nodules.

Evaluation Session

The evaluation session involves completing the case history and vocal abuse checklist, performing acoustic and visual assessments, and outlining the therapy process and the initiation of vocal abuse reduction. The case history must explore general background aspects related to the development of the nodules (refer to "The Case History" section in Chapter 3 for procedural suggestions). After this case history, the speech–language pathologist should have a good understanding of the pathogenesis of the client's dysphonia. As part of the case history, the speech–language pathologist should work with the client to complete the Vocal Abuse and Misuse Checklist (see Figure 4.2). This checklist provides an opportunity to determine which forms of vocal abuse apply. Once all forms of vocal abuse have been identified, strategies can be employed to reduce or eliminate them.

Acoustic and visual assessments depend on the instrumentation available. I typically do the following (the specific processes are outlined in Chapter 3):

- Obtain digital recording (or high-quality analogue recording) of the client's voice, documenting the date, time, speech sample (e.g., the "Rainbow" passage; Fairbanks, 1960), and a vowel prolongation sample in the natural voice.

- Measure pitch using the Kay Elemetrics Visi-Pitch II or similar device to obtain measures of speaking fundamental frequency, basal frequency, ceiling frequency, and vocal range in semitones.

- Measure vocal parameters using the Computer Speech Laboratory, digital spectrograph, or laryngograph to obtain jitter, shimmer, and harmonic-to-noise ratio.

- View the larynx through endoscope and stroboscope and video-record the results.

- Measure laryngeal airflow.

Once the acoustic and visual assessments are complete, the evaluation session becomes one of instruction to the client. The speech–language pathologist explains the findings and relates them to the vocal abuse forms identified. If available, visual documentation makes the explanation process much easier. After freezing an image of the client's nodules on the computer screen, the speech–language pathologist can orient the client to the view and structures shown, compare the view of the nodules to a photo or video of normal structures, and begin the explanation of pathogenesis. Some patients require only a simple explanation, whereas others require a detailed explanation of tissue changes and vocal consequences.

At the end of this part of the evaluation session, the patient or client should understand vocal abuse and its consequences. Then the speech–language pathologist can explain the therapy process. My philosophy of therapy is based on two general principles:

1. All forms of vocal abuse identified must be significantly reduced or eliminated.

2. Speech and voice must become vocally hygienic, with proper respiratory support, laryngeal involvement in phonation, and resonatory control.

To help patients significantly reduce or eliminate vocal abuse, I have developed a protocol of awareness by which progress can be measured. It is based on the notion that abusive vocal behavior will be eliminated immediately in some cases and progressively in others, depending on the difficulty of changing the behavior. I explain that, as a result of the instruction received during the evaluation about the nature and consequences of vocal abuse, change will occur in progressive steps, as follows:

1. *After-the-fact awareness.* Most of the abuse forms identified in the evaluation will continue for a while; however, if the client is interested and compliant in therapy, there will be an increase in after-the-fact awareness of abuse forms. The client will think, "Uh oh, I shouldn't have done that!" Even though the abuse form has occurred

and the harm has been done, the awareness level has increased and after-the-fact recognition has occurred. This is the beginning of change.

2. *Concurrent awareness.* When the client becomes more aware of vocal abuse, he or she will think, as the abusive vocal behavior is occurring, "Uh oh, I shouldn't be doing this!" Again, even though the behavior is occurring and the damage is being done, therapy progress is being made because of heightened awareness of the negative behavior.

3. *Before-the-fact (a priori) awareness.* This stage represents the best sign of therapy progress. The client is about to do some form of vocally abusive behavior but thinks, "No, I am not going to do that." When this stage is reached and maintained on a given form of vocal abuse, positive results will occur to the degree that the abuse form was contributing to the development of vocal nodules.

These stages of vocal abuse awareness and reduction can be charted for each behavior listed in Figure 4.2 that applies to a client. As the various forms of vocal abuse are being modified and eliminated, therapy must also be directed toward making vocalizations more hygienic through proper respiratory support, laryngeal involvement in phonation, and resonatory control. This process is begun at the first therapy session.

At the conclusion of the evaluation session, the client with vocal nodules should (a) understand the pathogenesis of vocal nodules, (b) understand how nodules affect the voice, (c) know the specific behaviors that must be modified for improvement to occur, (d) understand the therapy process ahead, and (e) have no remaining questions. I recommend also that, assuming the client wants therapy and is ready to begin, he or she be put on a modified form of vocal rest, a hypofunctional voice, which Colton and Casper (1996) called the confidential voice. This voice is just above a whisper in the middle of the speaking range, low in intensity and relaxed in effort. It is the sort of voice one might use speaking about a confidential matter, in church, in the library, or for pillow talk. I spend time at the end of the evaluation session instructing the client on this voice and, when I am convinced it can be used properly, ask the client to use this voice as much as possible until the next visit.

The rationale for using this confidential voice is twofold. First, it puts the brakes on a tendency to drive the voice as though competing in the Grand Prix. It is incompatible with most forms of vocal abuse and places the client on vocal "crutches." I explain this analogy as follows: "If a physician has placed you on crutches for a twisted knee, you cannot leave your crutches for even a short game of volleyball without damaging your knee. It is also true of vocal crutches. You cannot expect to use a hypofunctional voice and then abandon this control to yell, scream, or otherwise abuse your voice even for a short moment without undoing the good accomplished by hours of good control." Second, the hypofunctional or confidential voice allows abused and swollen tissues to somewhat heal, and often voice quality and acoustic measures, perhaps even visual measures, show improvement after a few days. This can inspire the client to realize that the body can heal itself when proper vocal care is engaged. (This is also a good reason to use audio documentation of the baseline voice so that comparison can be made.)

First Therapy Session After Evaluation

The first therapy session, the follow-up to the evaluation session, should follow within a week of the evaluation. At this therapy session, the speech–language pathologist should be prepared to (a) record the client's voice after a few days of hypofunctional voice usage to compare with the baseline recording; (b) present a list of abuse forms, in some order of severity (see hierarchical analysis later in chapter), that will require attention; and (c) instruct the client on principles of good vocal hygiene. The speech–language pathologist can begin the session by asking how well the client did in using the hypofunctional voice. If this went well and the client was able to decrease vocalizations by using it, a favorable prognosis is established for therapy. If the client states that he or she was unable to change to any significant degree, the therapy process will be a long one.

Assuming a favorable response to the hypofunctional assignment, the therapy proceeds with instruction on principles of good vocal hygiene, which has three main components: (a) proper respiratory support for speech, (b) efficient phonation, and (c) tone-focus away from the larynx into the mask of the face. The speech–language pathologist may find it helpful to show the client a model of the human torso while explaining good vocal hygiene as follows:

The lungs are housed in the chest, or thoracic cavity, as you see here, and this lower cavity, the abdominal cavity, houses several organs, including the stomach and intestines. These two cavities, the thoracic cavity for the lungs and the abdominal cavity for these other organs, are separated by an important breathing muscle, the diaphragm. The diaphragm is the floor of the thoracic cavity and the roof of the abdominal cavity. The diaphragm is a major breathing muscle. When it contracts in breathing, the diaphragm moves essentially downward and the chest cavity is increased vertically; thus air is drawn into the lungs. You can also expand the chest cavity by lifting your chest upward at the same time, like this [demonstrate]. Doing that, however, creates muscular effort and tension in the neck and larynx areas, and we don't want that. Let's teach a breathing pattern that does not involve the upper chest as much.

For the diaphragm to move downward easily, the abdominal muscles must be fairly relaxed. So I want you to relax your stomach muscles and breathe so that you feel much movement in the stomach area. I want you to breathe so that movement occurs from the breast level down and little movement is occurring in the chest area above the breast level. Can you feel that? As you breathe in, you should have the feeling that air is going into your stomach. It is not, of course, but the downward movement of the diaphragm and the movement of the organs gives that impression. Now breathe a few cycles and notice that feeling of expansion in the stomach or abdominal area as you inhale.

When you breathe for speech, you should have this sensation of expansion from the breast level down on inhalation and a reduction of that expansion when you exhale. Practice a few cycles of that breathing.

Now I want you to add voice to this process. Place your tongue in the bottom of your mouth, open your teeth as far as you can, and still have your lips lightly together. Now I would like you to take a fairly deep breath, expanding from the breast level down. Exhale and hum an easy tone, like this [demonstrate]. Good. Now do it again, and this time see if you can feel your lips tingle with the vibration of the voice. Did you feel it? If you did, repeat that process several times and produce this easy voice, while humming, and feel the vibration around your lips. Now repeat it once again and see if you can expand the facial vibration around your nose and eyes, what we can call the mask of your face.

Continue to produce voice and feel the facial vibration. Keep the tone very light and effortless. Now on exhalation produce the consonant–vowel combination of /mi . . . mi . . . / mi/. [Move from the repetition of /mi/ to /mai/ and so on.] Now that you are producing these simple vocalizations with good breath support and facial resonance, notice that there is no focus of effort in the area of your larynx or vocal folds. It is almost as if nothing is happening there. That is because the voice is being used efficiently and most of the vocal energy is resonating in the upper vocal tract and is felt mainly in the mask of the face.

Now that you feel your voice resonating in the mask of the face, notice once again that little tension is present in your neck area around your vocal folds. Next I would like you to count from 1 to 10 in this easy voice. You will not feel vibration in the mask of the face as clearly, but what you should feel is the absence of tension in the larynx area. Keep the breathing support deep and full from the breast level down and count easily without driving the voice.

I want you to practice these drills to help you better understand how to produce voice with good breath support, relaxation in the neck area, and resonance in the mask of the face. Your assignment is to practice these drills three or four times each day for about 10 minutes. Each time you do it, it should be easier for you to produce voice this way. In the next therapy sessions, we will move from these drills to normal reading and conversation using these principles.

At the same time we are teaching you to speak with better vocal control (vocal hygiene), we need to progressively eliminate forms of vocal abuse until they are essentially out of your life. We will use the Vocal Abuse Reduction Protocol [Figure 4.4] to target the behaviors we need to eliminate first. On this page we will identify all of the abuse forms that need to be eliminated, starting with the first priority, the next priority, and so on down the list. We will target the first two [or one, or three] to work on this week.

As you move each abuse form from after-the-fact to concurrent to before-the-fact awareness, we will mark the date of accomplishment. This will help you to understand where you are on mastering this control.

VOCAL ABUSE REDUCTION PROTOCOL

Client Name_____   Date of Initial Therapy _____

VOCAL ABUSE FORMS	AFTER-THE-FACT DATE	CONCURRENT DATE	BEFORE-THE-FACT DATE
1.			
2.			
3.			
4.			
5.			
6.			
7.			
8.			
9.			
10.			

Vocal Abuse Forms: List all forms of vocal abuse that require modification in hierarchical order. Number 1 is the first priority.

After-the-Fact: The vocal abuse is recognized by the client, but after it has occurred. Mark the therapy date in which the client indicates to you that this awareness level has been achieved for this abuse form.

Concurrent: The vocal abuse is recognized by the client as he or she is doing it. Mark the therapy date in which the client indicates to you that this awareness level has been achieved for this abuse form.

Before-the-Fact: The vocal abuse is recognized before it occurs. Mark the therapy date in which the client indicates to you that this awareness level has been achieved for this abuse form.

Figure 4.4. Vocal Abuse Reduction Protocol.

Additional Sessions

Additional therapy sessions will follow the same general routine as the first therapy session. First, the speech–language pathologist determines how well the client accomplished the task of practicing the drill activities for good vocal hygiene. Second, the therapist determines how well the client was able to move the chosen vocal abuse forms from after-the-fact awareness to before-the-fact control. Client judgment on the particular stage of abuse modification is critical, but confirmation from a parent may be needed for youngsters. Each therapy session should also involve a short audio sampling of the client's voice for serial comparison. I have found a nice correlation between the quality of the voice and the accomplishments recorded on the Vocal Abuse Reduction Protocol.

Typically, the first therapy session is scheduled a few days after the evaluation, and subsequent sessions occur twice weekly for the initial weeks, moving to once a week as control is established. However, this schedule may be adjusted by the speech–language pathologist, who can sense how often a client needs to be seen and make that judgment on an individual basis.

Hierarchy Approach to Abuse Elimination

Because some forms of vocal abuse are more difficult than others to eliminate, attention must be directed toward a systematic approach to therapy. A hierarchical approach to abuse elimination has been widely used. The speech–language pathologist must help the client eliminate the easier levels of abuse first and move systematically toward the harder levels. This concept is depicted in Figure 4.5.

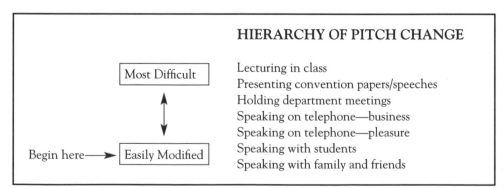

Figure 4.5. Pitch change hierarchy in vocal nodules cases. *Note*. From *Clinical Management of Speech Disorders* (p. 206), by D. E. Mowrer and J. L. Case, 1982, Austin, TX: PRO-ED. Copyright 1982 by PRO-ED, Inc. Reprinted with permission.

When therapy has produced the desired results, including the elimination or significant reduction of vocal abuse forms and the establishment of good vocal hygiene in general communication, therapy should move into a maintenance schedule. The speech–language pathologist might schedule the client once every 2 weeks, then 3, then 4, as long as control is maintained. The criteria for dismissal include the following considerations:

- The client feels that sufficient change has occurred and no longer feels the need for therapy.

- The referring physician reports that vocal pathology is no longer present.

- Vocal parameters (jitter, shimmer, harmonic-to-noise ratio, spectrographic analysis, vocal range, and quality judgments) are within normal limits.

- Vocal durability (maintaining parameter improvement) is significantly improved or normal.

- The speech–language pathologist senses that improvement has plateaued and feels that no further benefit can occur from continuation.

At the conclusion of therapy, both acoustic and visual replications of baseline documentation should be done. The accountability provided by such documentation should be part of every therapy dismissal.

Several authors have reported various treatment methods for the clinical management of patients with vocal nodules. Some of these methods involve strict counting of each instance of vocal abuse and are structured in an operant methodology involving reinforcement when significant reduction of instances occurs. Many of these principles of counting and reinforcement can be applied to any therapy technique. The use of reinforcement in modifying behaviors generally and speech in particular has been well documented in the literature (e.g., Mowrer, 1982). Mowrer described principles of reinforcement in detail to help the speech–language pathologist use them in programming the therapeutic process. Mowrer and Case (1982) explained how these principles can be part of the therapy process in a vocal nodules case. Toward the end of the evaluation–therapy process with a child, the speech–language pathologist should discuss with the parents the concept of reinforcement and determine what type should be used. This might involve short-term reinforcement as well as more significant reinforcement after a medical examination has confirmed that the vocal nodules are gone.

Principles of behavior modification using techniques of operant conditioning have been used in the treatment of vocal nodules by a number of authorities, including Drudge and Philips (1976), T. S. Johnson (1985) in the *Vocal Abuse Reduction Program*, and Boone in *The Boone Voice Program for Children* (1993) and *The Boone Voice Program for Adults* (1982). These various programs include procedures for identifying and reducing abuses, with tight reinforcement schedules either for eliminating the abuse or counting the target behaviors accurately. When the proper reinforcement is chosen—whether it is money, verbal praise, the opportunity to carry out enjoyable activities, or whatever—the client is motivated to count and eliminate abusive verbal behaviors. The precision with which behaviors are counted, charted, and reinforced distinguishes programs that are based on truly operant conditioning from those that merely involve reward or reinforcement. In either case, with chidren it is a good idea to include the concept of reinforcement for following therapy suggestions, however precisely this is done. Before the end of the first therapy session, the speech–language pathologist should determine the role of reinforcements, select specific ones toward which the client will work, and establish criteria for attaining them.

Less structured approaches to the clinical management of patients with vocal nodules have been presented by Morrison and Rammage (1998), Boone and McFarlane (2000), and several authors in Stemple (2000) in the section titled "Treatment of Hyperfunctional Voice." In Stemple's book, experts provide direction on objective documentation and the use of the confidential voice (Janina Casper), psychosocial aspects of children's behavior (Moya Andrews), family education (Leslie Glaze), soft whisper approach (John Hufnagle), and tone focus (Linda Lee) and use of an auditory feedback device to facilitate voice therapy (Stephen McFarlane and Shelley Von Berg). These and other authors provide excellent case studies of management for vocal hyperfunction.

There are many approaches to therapy for vocal abuse and misuse, phonotrauma, and hyperfunction of the larynx, and they have been called by many names. A recent trend in therapy is to describe approaches that are not specific to any disorder as holistic approaches to voice management. Holistic voice therapy programs integrate all of the voice subsystems, such as respiration, phonation, and resonation, into the rehabilitation process (Stemple, 2000). Stemple's Case Study Patient B is an excellent outline of comprehensive voice therapy, which includes attention to the physical environment of the patient and a methodology to strengthen the voice with vocal function exercises.

CONTACT ULCERS AND GRANULOMAS

Much of what has been discussed about the nature of vocal nodules and their pathogenesis, evaluation, and treatment applies to contact ulcers and their sequelae. Some patients with contact ulcers have significant vocal abuse or misuse as a clinical concern. In other patients, clinical conditions or medical procedures generate the ulceration process, and vocal abuse or misuse exacerbates the process. The speech–language pathologist must be prepared to evaluate all aspects of this disorder.

Whereas vocal nodules develop on the tissues involved in phonatory vibration, contact ulcers generally develop in the region around the arytenoid cartilages. The ulceration process, when vocal abuse or usage is concerned, begins with contact forces between the cartilages. Forceful adduction of the arytenoid cartilages at the onset of phonation (Hess et al., 1998) generates a force on the soft tissues covering the cartilages and causes a necrosis of tissue in the contact area. This process of change typically begins with tenderness or inflammation, followed by necrosis as the abuse continues. The body may then attempt to heal the injury with layers of tissue described by Hirano (1996) as proliferated capillaries, fibroblasts, collagenous fibers, and leukocytes. Soon a mass of extra tissue, called a granuloma, is present unilaterally or bilaterally in the cartilage area. Hirano described three types of granulomas: contact granuloma (from vocal abuse), intubation granuloma (from intubation surgery), and gastroesophageal reflux granuloma (from the acid from reflux pooling in the laryngeal area).

Regardless of the etiology of the granuloma, voice can be affected, depending on the granuloma's size. The voice affected by granuloma is typically described as low in pitch, hyperfunctional in effort, and often breathy. In Figure 4.6 the unilateral granuloma would prevent the vocal folds from completely adducting during phonation. Some of the voice characteristics heard in patients with granuloma are etiologically related to the disorder, and other characteristics result from the tissue buildup that prevents complete adduction.

Although contact ulcer granulomas historically have been described as typically a disorder of adult males who are verbally intense and professionally upwardly bound and aggressive, this finding was refuted by Watterson, Hansen-Magorian, and McFarlane (1990), who reported that 21% of 57 contact ulcer patients were female and 44% were younger than 40 years of age. I have evaluated and treated several women affected by granulomas, including the patient whose vocal folds appear in Figure 4.6. She is a high school physical education teacher who is continually teaching and yelling instructions on the athletic field and who also engages in continual verbalization while jogging each morning and evening with her husband.

Among the clients of granuloma recently seen in the voice clinic at Arizona State University were the female adult physical education teacher and the male Buddhist chanter mentioned previously, as well as a high-level politician and a school superintendent. In each of these cases, voice therapy was responsible for the elimination of the granuloma except in the female teacher, who changed her behavior but required surgery to remove the tissue.

Esophageal reflux, or more specifically gastroesophageal reflux disorder, has been found to have a significant etiological relationship to the development of contact ulcers and granulomas. Emami, Morrison, Rammage, and Bosch (1999) reported on a 12-year retrospective analysis of patients with these disorders and found that 77% of 76 patients had complete resolution of their laryngeal pathology with an essentially

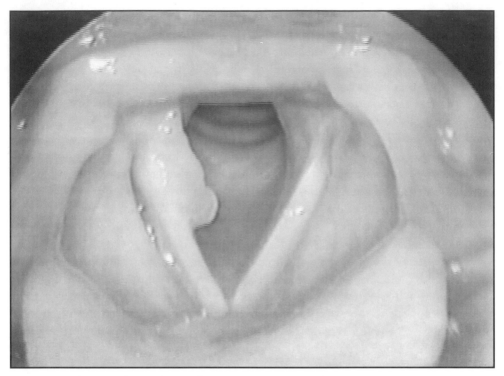

Figure 4.6. Contact ulcer with granuloma.

nonsurgical approach that involved significant management of gastroesophageal reflux disorder. Ylitalo and Hammarberg (2000) reported similar success with the nonsurgical management of contact granuloma patients with therapy that focused on reducing vocal hyperfunctions.

GASTROESOPHAGEAL REFLUX DISORDER

Symptoms of gastroesophageal reflux disorder can range from near subclinical (minor) to life threatening (airway obstruction due to laryngeal stenosis or laryngospasm). Between these extremes most patients complain of hoarseness, globus pharyngeus (a sensation of a lump in the throat), dysphagia (difficulty swallowing), and chronic throat clearing and coughing (Koufman, 1995; Sataloff, 1998c). The importance of investigating reflux as an etiological consideration in patients with dysphonia cannot be overstated. When a patient complains of heartburn and the need for antacid usage, reflux should always be suspected.

Patients who experience moderate amounts of esophageal reflux complain of awakening with an acid taste in the mouth and a burning larynx. Coughing is commonly associated with such an incidence. However, many patients with reflux deny ever having a symptom. The laryngologist can identify the tissue changes and recommend diagnostic and therapeutic intervention. Often the symptoms can be relieved by diet change, less nighttime eating, lifestyle changes to alleviate stress, antacid usage, and medications when symptoms persist. The treatment for reflux is entirely medical, and the speech–language pathologist should merely support diagnostic and therapeutic efforts of the physicians involved. Knowledge about this condition, however, is critical to understanding many dysphonias, particularly those involving contact ulceration and granuloma development (Emami et al., 1999).

Patients with dysphonia from contact ulcers and granuloma should be evaluated and treated using the same general procedures described for the patient with vocal abuse. Even when the etiology of the granuloma is intubation trauma or esophageal reflux, a voice component likely needs to be addressed. Sataloff, Castell, Katz, and Sataloff (1999) produced a complete reference on reflux laryngitis and related disorders, and it is recommended for those working with patients who have reflux disorder.

VOCAL NODULE AND GRANULOMA SURGERY

General principles of phonosurgery were discussed in Chapter 2. The speech–language pathologist should also be aware of special considerations for managing patients with vocal nodules who may be facing surgery, one of the most controversial areas of voice management. Sataloff (1991) provided considerable guidance regarding surgery for patients with vocal nodules: "Surgery for vocal nodules should be avoided whenever possible and should virtually never be performed without an adequate trial of expert voice therapy including patient compliance with therapeutic suggestions" (p. 269). He also suggested that silence is not necessary but proper voice usage, under the direction of a speech–language pathologist (or singing teacher for the performer), should be followed prior to the surgery. In this way the patient can learn the techniques that will be necessary to use after surgery. This philosophy was restated years later (Sataloff, 1998c; Sataloff, Spiegel, Heuer, & Rosen, 1995).

The greatest threat from surgery for vocal nodules is the possibility of submucosal scarring, which causes adynamic segments. This can happen even under conditions of expert surgery. I have evaluated many patients who after surgery have had residual dysphonia even though the physician reported that the vocal folds appeared normal and healthy. The key is the method of examination used to determine "normal and healthy." If an indirect method of inspection is used under normal lighting, or even flexible endoscopy, adynamic segments cannot be seen during vibration. Stroboscopy is needed to observe such segments. When adynamic segments are noted using stroboscopic analysis, the prognosis for a return of normal vibratory function is rather poor. There is a strong possibility that the patient might have a slight residual dysphonia and restricted high range usage.

Sataloff (1991) also stated that surgery on nodule areas should be strictly confined to the lesion area and that "no vocal stripping" should occur (p. 270) on professional voice users with benign disease. As mentioned earlier, surgeons should also stay superficial to the intermediate layer of the lamina propria and preserve the mucosal tissue along the leading edge of the vocal fold (Benninger & Gardner, 1998). The laser is useful, according to Sataloff (1998c), when surgery is needed for ulcer granulomas.

CHANGING THE PITCH IN VOCAL ABUSE THERAPY

There seems to be a movement away from the notion that pitch levels should be changed independent of general factors of phonation physiology. As discussed in Chapter 3, the concept of optimal pitch is controversial (Colton & Casper, 1996). There are, however, instances in which changing the pitch will eliminate a contributing factor of vocal abuse. If a person is attempting to sound more authoritative or masculine, or feels that by lowering the pitch the voice will project better, the person might be deliberately lowering the pitch toward the bottom of the range. When this is done, strain occurs and the pitch should be changed in an upward direction. When vocal hyperfunction is present in the voice, eliminating the tension will often result in an automatic raising of the pitch. However, when pitch is deliberately lowered for some effect, therapy should include trying to raise it.

Instrumentation can be helpful in changing the pitch of the voice. The Visi-Pitch, for example, has a horizontal cursor that provides real-time feedback on pitch usage. The horizontal cursor can be used as follows to change the pitch:

1. Have the client hum, and the vocal pitch will appear on the screen in some relation to the horizontal cursor that is set at the target level; it will likely be somewhat below the target cursor.

2. Direct the client to continue to hum, while raising the pitch until it is close to the horizontal cursor level.

3. When the pitch is close to the horizontal cursor level, have the client produce a hum with various vowels in a monotone level.

4. When the match is close, have the client say simple words or count in a monotone, keeping the voice near the horizontal cursor setting.

5. Have the client say simple phrases, such as "My name is Jim," and encourage an upward inflection above the cursor level at the end of the phrase.

6. Set two horizontal cursors for a range of pitch usage, and instruct the client to say phrases and keep the voice within the upper and lower cursors; pitch variety should now be encouraged instead of monotone usage.

7. Use reading to establish normal pitch usage while the client maintains pitch between the cursors.

8. Then use conversation to establish normal pitch usage; the client can hold the microphone near his or her face and occasionally open it with the key switch to measure whether the voice pitch is being maintained at the appropriate level.

9. Once pitch is controlled in a clinical setting with the feedback of the Visi-Pitch, carryover can be approached using a hierarchical approach, as outlined in Figure 4.5.

10. If the hierarchical approach is not needed, the change in vocal pitch can be monitored by asking the client whether pitch control is in the after-the-fact, concurrent, or before-the-fact stage.

VOCAL ABUSE TREATMENT IN CHILDREN

Slight vocal hoarseness is common in children. When hoarseness is a stable part of the voice profile in the presence of heightened vocal activity, the child and family members will likely show little concern. When more moderate hoarseness is present, however, the parents, teachers, family physician, and speech–language pathologist—everybody but the child—will likely become concerned.

When vocal screening occurs in the schools and a child's vocal hoarseness is heard and found to be persistent, a medical diagnosis is necessary to eliminate significant medical concerns such as papillomatosis, webbing, or other laryngeal pathologies. Slight vocal nodules from typical childhood yelling and screaming might not change the voice enough to warrant this medical attention. However, should the professional and family seek (a) medical inspection of the larynx, which confirms nodules, and (b) voice therapy, then the therapy process is the same as with adults but with a changed orientation. The explanation of vocal abuse and its consequences on the voice must be reduced to a child's level of understanding. Boone (1993) developed a kit with photos and directions to help the speech–language pathologist work with a child. Andrews (1986, 1999) also provided excellent directions for working with children who have vocal nodules. The primary differences compared with the adult approach are the level of photos (drawings rather than actual laryngeal structures), the language used to describe vocal abuse, the documentation of abuse instances (more-specific counting and charting), and the notion of specific reinforcement for behavior change.

SUMMARY

This chapter has identified the common forms of vocal abuse and the consequences of such abuse to tissues. The primary focus is on the commonly observed disorders of vocal nodules and contact ulcers with granuloma. The tissue changes initial to these forms of vocal pathology were also discussed. A methodology that can be used by the speech–language pathologist in treating patients with vocal abuse is also outlined. Surgical considerations as part of patient management were also discussed.

Neurogenic Voice Disorders

This chapter reviews abnormal neurological functions in the motor speech system, with particular emphasis on laryngeal neurological dysfunctions. Some of the disorders covered result from central disruption of motor speech functions, but the primary emphasis is on disruptions of the peripheral nervous system causing vocal fold paralysis.

The neurological bases of human laryngeal functions are complex yet remarkably stable in both biological and phonatory aspects. For example, the larynx functions well in its valving processes during swallowing to keep food, liquids, saliva, and other substances from entering the delicate respiratory system. However, should some foreign substance enter the larynx and stimulate the sensory end organs, it is forcefully expelled by the motor cough reflex. Thus, laryngeal sensory and motor integration of function protects the delicate tissues of the respiratory system from foreign matter.

As a sentinel and protector of the respiratory tract, the larynx senses that which approaches from above and determines whether it is appropriate to enter. If clean air approaches, the larynx opens the valve and allows entrance into the respiratory tract. When it senses food or liquid, the laryngeal sentinel tightly closes to stop it from entering the respiratory tract; the substance bypasses the larynx and enters into the esophagus and stomach. These biological functions—the larynx is open for breathing and closed for swallowing—sound rather simple, but the performance of these simple biological maneuvers requires sophisticated sensory and motor innervation (Cooper & Lawson, 1992; Matthews, 2000; Sanders, 1995; Webster, 1999).

This same laryngeal structure can be so delicately controlled by the nervous system as to allow a great singer, for example, to set the vocal folds with the perfect amount of longitudinal tension and medial compression to vibrate at a frequency perfectly matched to the orchestra at an exact loudness level with few trial-and-error adjustments (Lovetri, Lesh, & Woo, 1999). Thus, laryngeal sensory and motor integration of laryngeal function, once again, acts to perform, only this time in phonation during communication.

INNERVATION OF LARYNGEAL STRUCTURES

To understand the complexities of neurogenic dysphonias, it is necessary for speech–language pathologists to have a thorough appreciation of the innervation of the larynx from central and peripheral nervous system structures. The following section is designed to accomplish that goal.

Central Nervous System

The central nervous system innervation to the larynx is extensive from both left and right cortical hemispheres (Bear, Connors, & Paradiso, 1996; Netter, 1983; Webster, 1999). The motor cortex for laryngeal control is in the inferior and lateral aspects of the motor cortex and primary motor strip. When this area of the cortex is stimulated using microstimulation techniques, a bilateral laryngeal response is observed, indicating bilaterality of innervation from the cortex. This projection from the cortex is likely polysynaptic, passing to the midbrain and then to the nucleus ambiguous in the brain stem. This pathway is considered an upper motor neuron tract (Bear et al., 1996; Gacek & Malmgren, 1992; Zemlin, 1998).

The cortical tracts that innervate the larynx likely junction, as indicated, in the midbrain area. From the midbrain, additional upper motor neuron tracts pass to the nucleus ambiguous in the brain stem at the level of the medulla oblongata. The midbrain to nucleus ambiguous tracts show rather ipsilateral (same side) predominance. Some fibers cross to the nucleus ambiguous on the contralateral side of the brain stem, but most remain ipsilateral. Thus, the upper motor innervation to the larynx begins in the cortex as described and passes to the nucleus ambiguous after connections in the midbrain.

Peripheral Nervous System

The lower motor neuron innervation to the larynx and pharynx begins at the nucleus ambiguous, which initiates the vagus nerve system, the final common pathway to the larynx. The vagus nerve system provides sensory and motor innervation to the larynx and is part of the peripheral nervous system. The peripheral nerves involved in laryngeal and pharyngeal innervation include the vagus (cranial nerve X) and the accessory (cranial nerve XI), which integrate outside the brain stem at the nodose (inferior) ganglion. From this nodose ganglion, the innervation is essentially considered the vagus nerve system.

The peripheral nervous system innervation to the larynx is ipsilateral, with the right and left halves of the larynx (including vocal folds) innervated by the right and left sensory and motor peripheral nerves, respectively. The bilateral control to the larynx stops at the peripheral nerves. Therefore, the right and left halves of the larynx are innervated centrally by both cortical hemispheres directed through the right and left peripheral nerves, respectively (Benninger & Schwimmer, 1996; Netter, 1983; Webster, 1999). Because of this bilateral contribution to each peripheral nerve, under normal circumstances laryngeal functions are completely symmetrical with regard to right and left vocal fold function. The peripheral nerve nuclei that serve the sensory and motor functions of the larynx, as well as related structures such as the velopharynx, are located in the nucleus ambiguous of the medulla oblongata in the brain stem. The nucleus ambiguous constitutes the connection between the central and the peripheral nervous systems.

It is essentially impossible for the right and left vocal folds to function out of phase with each other in adduction and abduction. Therefore, when the structures of the larynx are devoid of pathology, only a lesion or some form of disorder in the nervous system can disrupt normal symmetrical laryngeal functions.

Figure 5.1 shows the sensory and motor innervation of the larynx provided by the central and the peripheral nervous systems. The first branch off the vagus is the pharyngeal nerve, which innervates the muscles of the pharynx and all soft palate (velum) muscles except the tensor veli palatini, which is innervated by the motor division of the trigeminal nerve (cranial nerve V). Pharyngeal innervation is accomplished with the help of motor innervation from the glossopharyngeal nerve (cranial nerve IX).

Two additional branches off the vagus are important for laryngeal innervation: the superior laryngeal nerve and the recurrent laryngeal nerve. Upon exiting the vagus, the superior laryngeal nerve divides into internal and external branches. The internal branch is essentially sensory and is responsible for touch and pain innervation to the laryngeal mucosa in the ipsilateral supraglottal section of the larynx. The external branch is motor to the ipsilateral cricothyroid muscle (major pitch control muscle). Therefore, if superior laryngeal nerve innervation is normal, the sensory functions of the upper larynx (vocal folds and above) and motor control of the cricothyroid muscles are property maintained. Figure 5.2 shows the larynx and epiglottis as innervated by the superior and inferior (recurrent) laryngeal nerves. The nerve supply as shown is the result of Sihler's stain.

If the recurrent laryngeal nerve innervation is normal, the sensory functions of the lower larynx (infraglottal region) and motor functions of abduction, adduction, and partial vocal fold tension (vocalis contraction) are properly controlled. Much information about laryngeal innervation comes from research done on animals to experimentally determine the exact nature of laryngeal innervation, with findings then extrapolated to humans. The details of such investigation are complex and somewhat equivocal, but considerable documentation has been provided. The details of animal studies, which possibly help clarify human laryngeal central and peripheral innervation, can be found in Blitzer, Brin, Sasaki, Fahn, and Harris (1992).

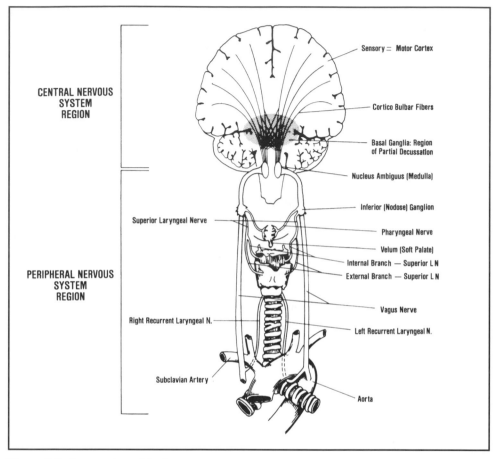

Figure 5.1. Innervation of the larynx.

NEUROLOGICAL DISORDERS IN CHILDREN AND ADULTS

Several possible disruptions can occur along the sensory and motor tracts of the central and the peripheral nervous systems to affect laryngeal function and produce a neurogenic voice disorder. Traumatic, infectious, vascular, neoplastic, chemical, or degenerative disruptions produce voice disorder. The voice symptomatology depends on the level of disruption and can occur as an isolated dysphonia or as a more broadly involved disorder of the entire motor speech system.

The term *dysarthria* refers to neurogenic speech disorders that involve disruption of the respiration, phonation, resonation, and articulation sensory–motor speech systems to some degree. *Anarthria* refers to the complete stoppage of speech because of

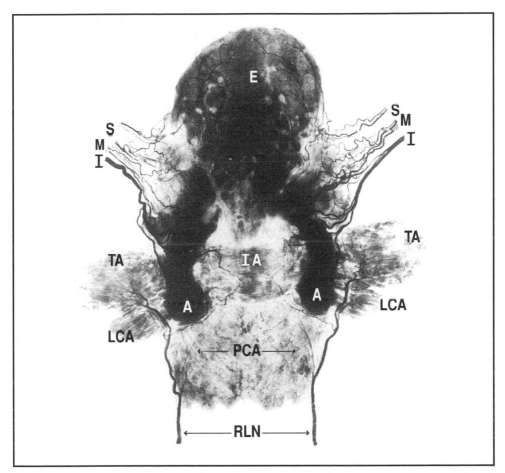

Figure 5.2. The nerve supply of the human larynx. An entire human larynx was processed with Sihler's stain, a technique that renders soft tissue translucent while counterstaining nerves. The larynx was then dissected to isolate the superior (*SMI*) and recurrent laryngeal nerves (*RLN*) as well as all laryngeal muscles and the arytenoid (*A*) and epiglottic (*E*) cartilages.

The RLNs are seen entering the larynx from the inferior direction. The first muscle to be innervated by the RLN is the posterior cricoarytenoid muscle (*PCA*). The second RLN branch travels beneath the PCA to innervate the interarytenoid muscle (*IA*). Finally, the RLN gives off a branch to innervate the lateral cricoarytenoid muscle (*LCA*) before terminating in the thyroarytenoid muscle (*TA*).

The superior laryngeal nerves enter the larynx from the superior direction. They travel down the lateral sides of the larynx and give off branches that pass medially to supply sensory innervation to the laryngeal mucosa. The superior laryngeal nerve usually divides into three main branches: a superior branch (*S*) innervates the epiglottis (*E*), a middle branch (*M*) innervates the false vocal cord, and an inferior branch (*I*) innervates the arytenoid (*A*) and postcricoid area.

Note. From "The Microanatomy of the Vocal Folds," by I. Sanders, 1995, in *Diagnosis and Treatment of Voice Disorders*, edited by J. S. Rubin, R. T. Sataloff, G. S. Korovin, and W. J. Gould, New York: IGAKU-SHOIN. Copyright 1995 by Lippincott. Reprinted with permission.

disruption in these systems (Duffy, 1995; McNeil, 1997). This chapter discusses the symptomatic, etiologic, evaluative, and treatment considerations of common neurogenic dysphonias, including the dysarthrias that involve dysphonia.

VAGUS NERVE LESIONS

Lesions can occur at any point along the vagus nerve from the nucleus ambiguous in the brain stem medulla to its peripheral ending where it enters the larynx. The symptoms involved depend on the level of the lesion.

If some lesion or disease process disrupts the vagus nerve at the nucleus or any point before the pharyngeal nerve exits, the sensory and motor innervation to the pharynx and larynx are affected and a flaccid paralysis is present on the ipsilateral half of both the velopharynx and the larynx. Velopharyngeal closure is disrupted on that side, as are vocal fold abduction, adduction, tension, and relaxation on the affected vocal fold. The paralyzed side of the velum does not lift upward and backward in velopharyngeal closure, and the paralyzed vocal fold cannot adduct, abduct, or lengthen. The sensory aspects of laryngeal control also are lost on the ipsilateral side of nerve damage.

The nuclei of both vagus nerves can be affected by a brainstem lesion, in which case bilateral symptoms of the pharynx and larynx are likely evident. A lesion outside the brainstem less commonly produces bilateral damage except in the case of widespread trauma or disease that damages both vagus trunks. The most common condition is some sort of unilateral lesion.

The speech symptoms of unilateral vagus damage above the pharyngeal nerve include hypernasal resonance on vowels, nasal air emission on pressure consonants, breathiness in the voice, reduced loudness, and lowered pitch. Diplophonia (double pitch) can also occur when longevity of damage produces tissue atrophy and mass differences of the two vocal folds (Cavalli & Hirson, 1999).

Nonspeech symptoms include a weakened coughing mechanism that does not have a sharp coup at the onset of the cough. Aspiration of food or liquid into the larynx is common during swallowing, causing choking and coughing. Because of reduced pharyngeal activity, swallowing is labored and slow. If a person swallows liquids in a bent-over position, such as at a water fountain, regurgitation of the liquid through the nose because of inadequate velopharyngeal closure often occurs.

If the lesion is in the brainstem and the nuclei of both vagus nerves are damaged, these symptoms in speech and nonspeech areas are present in increased severity. For example, if the vocal folds are paralyzed in a fairly intermediate position, the voice usually is so breathy as to approach whispered speech. Even though both vocal folds are in an abducted position, however, there is enough closure potential during speech effort to produce a slight amount of voicing, although the overwhelming quality characteristic is severe breathiness. Loudness is compromised and the pitch of the very weak voice is lowered. The biological protection afforded the respiratory tract by the larynx is so severely damaged from such a bilateral lesion as to produce a life-threatening condition because all sensory and motor functions are affected. Respiratory difficulties are expected and tracheostomy is likely when bilateral paralysis occurs.

A lesion can occur on the vagus nerve below the point of exit for the pharyngeal nerve but above the exit of the superior laryngeal nerve. In such cases, all of the laryngeal symptoms described are present, with no pharyngeal involvement. Therefore, although the voice is breathy, with reduced loudness and lowered pitch, no hypernasality or nasal air emission on consonants occurs. The vocal fold affected still is paralyzed in the abducted position, from which it cannot adduct. Although rare, this same condition could occur bilaterally.

A common occurrence in neurogenic voice disorder is some condition that damages the vagus nerve below the exit of the superior laryngeal nerve or injures only the recurrent laryngeal nerve after it exits the main trunk of the vagus. This can happen unilaterally or bilaterally. In the case of a unilateral occurrence, the ipsilateral vocal fold is paralyzed in the paramedian position, from which it cannot adduct or abduct. Some slight adduction might be observed due to the bilateral innervation of the interarytenoid muscles. The voice is slightly breathy, is slightly reduced in loudness and pitch, and has some possibility of diplophonia, particularly after a prolonged paralysis and subsequent atrophy of the involved vocal fold. The most common nonspeech complaint is dyspnea (difficulty in breathing). This is particularly noticeable under conditions of extreme effort, such as running or similar activity. The dyspnea occurs because the paralyzed vocal fold is in a position near midline (paramedian) and does not abduct during inhalation. Therefore, all air must pass through the glottis, which is decreased in openness by nearly 50%. Under labored breathing, voice can be heard on inhalation, a condition called laryngeal stridor. Swallowing functions are essentially normal, and little aspiration occurs.

When the recurrent laryngeal nerve is damaged bilaterally, a much more serious condition exists (see Figure 5.3). Airway obstruction is sufficient to require emergency tracheostomy in most cases. Although the voice is near normal, this is of little comfort because of the dyspnea. Bilateral recurrent laryngeal nerve damage can happen to children as well as adults. The long-term treatment consists of surgery to improve the airway (specific procedures involved are discussed later).

It is important that the speech–language pathologist understand why the vocal folds are paralyzed in varied positions, depending on the site of the lesion. As indicated earlier, a lesion that prevents innervation to the larynx from both the superior and the recurrent laryngeal nerves causes the vocal fold to be paralyzed in a somewhat abducted (intermediate) position, whereas recurrent nerve damage paralyzes the vocal fold closer to the adducted midline position. The key to understanding this difference lies in

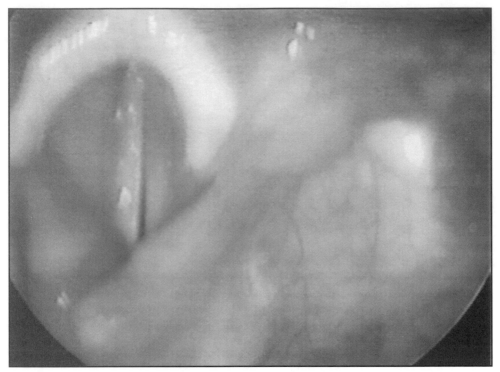

Figure 5.3. Bilateral vocal fold paralysis. (Photo taken as patient attempted inhalation.)

the function of the external branch of the superior laryngeal nerve that provides motor control to the cricothyroid muscle. That muscle elongates the vocalis muscle to provide much of the longitudinal tension involved in increasing pitch. When this muscle functions properly, it pulls the vocal fold closer to midline by increasing the longitudinal tension. The following case study explains how an intact superior laryngeal nerve can influence the degree to which a paralyzed vocal fold can be moved toward midline.

CASE EXAMPLE OF LARYNGEAL NERVE PARALYSIS

This case illustrates the voice disorder resulting from unilateral lesion of the recurrent laryngeal nerve and demonstrates that cricothyroid contractions can mask the severity of the disorder.

M.S., a 29-year-old man, was referred by his fellow employee, who was a speech–language pathologist. M.S.'s main vocal concern was his vocal pitch, which he felt was too high. His case history revealed that 6 years earlier he had had cancer of the thyroid gland, which required surgical removal of much of the gland. During the surgery, his left recurrent laryngeal nerve had been severed, after which he "hardly had a voice at all." In the ensuing years, M.S. experienced gradual improvement in the strength and quality of his voice. His only concern was that his pitch seemed too high and that he often was mistaken for a female on the telephone.

An evaluation of M.S.'s voice revealed essentially normal voice quality, indicating essentially adequate approximation of his vocal folds at midline. However, his habitual pitch was found to be around 174 Hz, typical of the pitch of a mature female. He also experienced pitch breaks into the falsetto range. M.S. complained of some dyspnea as well, particularly when he ran or exercised.

Indirect laryngoscopy revealed a paralyzed left vocal fold, as expected from the case history, but with near-normal midline approximation of the vocal folds during phonation at his habitual pitch level of 174 Hz. It was hypothesized that the midline approximation occurred because the extensive contraction of his cricothyroid muscles was sufficient to raise his pitch to the 174-Hz level. It was hypothesized further that, by lowering his pitch to a normal male level, the compensation mechanisms would be eliminated and the paralytic dysphonia that normally would be expected from recurrent laryngeal nerve damage would be unmasked.

Therapy during the next 3 weeks was directed at lowering M.S.'s pitch from around 174 Hz to around 123 Hz. When this had been accomplished, his voice quality became breathy and significantly reduced in loudness. Indirect laryngoscopy confirmed that a significantly altered positioning of the left vocal fold had occurred during phonation and that the fold was paralyzed in a more abducted position, producing a significant chink between the folds during phonation at the lower level. His true paralytic dysphonia had been unmasked by eliminating the compensatory involvement of cricothyroid contraction.

Although this case illustrates the relationship that exists when the recurrent laryngeal nerve is deinnervated without damage to the superior laryngeal nerve, this concept of vocal fold position is not always seen clinically, nor has it been verified completely by research (Smith & Ramig, 1995). In my clinical experience I have found that the position of the paralyzed vocal fold can be quite variable regardless of suspected etiology, and I have seen several examples of paralysis in which the vocal fold is significantly fixed away from midline when a known recurrent laryngeal nerve etiology has been established.

LESIONS OF THE SUPERIOR LARYNGEAL NERVE

A unilateral lesion of the superior laryngeal nerve, which is rare, primarily affects the elongation potential of the vocal fold on that side (external branch dysfunction). A sensory disorder also is manifested in the larynx above the vocal folds on the same side (internal branch), but this does not contribute to the dysphonia. Normal adduction and abduction of the vocal folds remain, although a rotational effect on the larynx toward the normal side occurs during phonation, caused by the intact cricothyroid contraction on the uninvolved side. There also can be a slight bowing of the vocal fold on the side of damage, resulting in a slight breathiness of the voice. The quality of the voice might appear somewhat hoarse because of the rotational effect and the bowed paralytic vocal fold, which cause asymmetrical (aperiodic) vibration of the vocal folds (Tucker & Lavertu, 1992). Unilateral superior laryngeal nerve paresis, weakness, or paralysis will produce a "twisted larynx" as described by Nasseri and Maragos (2000). (Their treatment strategy for such a condition is discussed in a later section.)

When a bilateral lesion of the superior laryngeal nerve occurs, these same characteristics are present on both sides. The one significant difference is that the larynx does not rotate during phonation, because of equal noninvolvement of the cricothyroid muscles. The anterior commissure of the larynx is masked by the overhanging epiglottis, and the vocal folds are bowed symmetrically in the middle portion of the glottis. The voice is breathy and reduced in loudness, with significantly reduced pitch variability. Increased aspiration and choking result from reduced sensory function in the upper larynx. Tucker and Lavertu (1992) reported that most cases of superior laryngeal nerve dysfunction are caused by viral neuropathy.

Bevan, Griffiths, and Morgan (1989) reported three cases of cricothyroid paralysis from disruption of the superior laryngeal nerve, which required careful diagnoses using videostroboscopy and EMG analyses. Only when these objective assessment techniques were used was the etiology of each patient's dysphonia identified. Hartman, Daily, and Morin (1989) also reported an interesting case of coexisting superior laryngeal nerve dysfunction (unilateral) from an idiopathic (of unknown cause) inflammatory process and psychogenic dysphonia manifesting as a vocal conversion reaction. Voice therapy proved effective for alleviating the psychogenic component, and time eradicated the neuropathy. An additional concern is Reye's syndrome, a severe acute encephalopathy seen in children. Thompson, Rosenthal, and Camilon (1990) reported on four cases of Reye's syndrome in which superior laryngeal nerve paralysis caused absent laryngeal sensitivity. These children also had paralysis of the recurrent laryngeal nerves bilaterally.

Eckley, Sataloff, Hawkshaw, Spiegel, and Mandel (1998) reported on 56 adults presenting with superior laryngeal nerve paresis or paralysis confirmed by laryngeal electromyography. The most common etiology was neuritis (67.7%), followed by iatrogenic and unknown etiologies. Trauma represented nearly 9% of the etiologies. Many of these patients were singers trained at various levels. Eckley et al. reported that those singers with classical singing training, particularly the female singers, had less effect in vocal performance as measured by physiological frequency range and musical frequency range of phonation. The most common presenting symptoms of voice, particularly of the nonsingers, was hoarseness, loss of high range, and vocal fatigue. Breathiness was also reported among the patients. Those who were singers generally were able to continue to perform but with increased difficulty.

ETIOLOGIES OF VAGUS NERVE LESIONS

Several studies of the etiologies of vocal fold paralysis of the unilateral and bilateral varieties have been reported. Tucker and Lavertu (1992) reviewed many of these studies and reported on the selection, diagnosis, etiologic factors, and management of many patients with unilateral or bilateral vocal fold paralysis. Their analysis showed that vocal fold paralysis can be caused by trauma, thyroid surgery in which the recurrent laryngeal nerve is severed, surgery to manage malignancies, and a large category of idiopathic paralyses and pareses, including viral infections. Many patients with idiopathic etiology recover function within 1 year.

Laryngeal paralysis is often seen in infants, as reported by Andrews (1986, 1999). She listed many of the laryngeal dysfunctions in children, including congenital conditions affecting respiration, swallowing, and phonation. Many of the conditions she reported include nonneurological factors of airway obstruction (mucosal edema and hyperemia, granulated tissue formation, cricoid cartilage destruction, subglottal stenosis) and others involving neurological status (dislocation of arytenoids, inter-arytenoid fixation, and other forms of laryngeal paralysis). When the paralysis is bi-lateral, symptoms include severe respiratory distress, stridor (voice on inhalation), cyanosis (skin color change from inadequate oxygenation), and sometimes aspiration. Many of these children undergo tracheostomy. Often the tracheostomy is long term. Rosin, Handler, Potsic, Wetmore, and Tom (1990) reported that with medical management 16% of such children had spontaneous recovery and were decannulated (tracheostomy tube was removed). Andrews (1999) provided extensive information regarding management when tracheostomy is required:

- Be aware that long-term tracheostomy in children might affect expressive language and speech development, even when receptive language remains typical.

- If a child has a tracheostomy tube and has a viable laryngeal mechanism for voice, the speech–language pathologist can assist the child in learning to occlude the tube with a finger to produce voice. Also, assistance can be given to increase the duration of prosthesis usage, improve voice onset timing with speech, increase length of exhalation, learn to phonate at the top of the inhalation cycle, and improve phrasing and prosody.

- Even with a "talking trach" or Passy-Muir valve, which closes automatically on exhalation to divert the airstream into the larynx for phonation, children will require help on timing issues.

Cohen, Geller, Birns, and Thompson (1982), who reported on many cases of laryngeal paralysis involving children, identified the following factors: sex of the patient, etiology, disease onset, mother's type of pregnancy and delivery, disease-related symptoms, type of paralysis, vocal fold(s) position, need for tracheostomy, age of decannulation, preoperative diagnosis and neurological status, congenital and associated anomalies, course and progress of the disease, and statistics on recovery and resolution of the problem. It is significant that central nervous system diseases occurred in 18% of the patients, birth trauma accounted for 19% of the cases, surgical and blunt trauma to the neck accounted for 11%, and the etiology of 36% of the paralyses was unknown. A tumor (neuroblastoma) of the neck was the cause in one case.

Fifty-eight percent of the paralyses occurred within the first 12 hours of life. Bilateral abductor vocal fold paralysis occurred in 62% of the children studied, 45 of whom (73%) required a tracheostomy. Several neurological abnormalities, including hypotonia (floppy child), cerebral palsy, and various syndromes, were found in 33%. Cohen et al. (1982) underscored the prevalence and nature of laryngeal paralysis in children.

The significance of laryngeal paralysis or other abnormalities requiring prolonged tracheostomy and other forms of medical management as they relate to speech and language development was reported by Narcy, Contencin, and Viala (1990). An excellent study on 319 children with airway obstruction, including paralysis requiring tracheotomy, was described by Crysdale, Feldman, and Naito (1988), who reported that the average duration of tracheostomy is almost 1 year. Of the 319 children in this study, 222 had tracheostomies because of airway obstruction of various etiologies. In adults recurrent laryngeal nerve disruption occurs because of trauma, surgical sectioning of the nerve in thyroid and chest area cancer treatment, viral infections, and idiopathic etiologies. When known sectioning has occurred and the innervation is damaged, medical management of the paralysis can proceed as soon as it is identified. With idiopathic or viral etiologies, a waiting period of 6 months to 1 year is required because of the common occurrence of spontaneous recovery.

Altman and Benninger (1997) reported on an algorithm to identify patients presenting with unilateral vocal fold immobility. They investigated the charts of 169 such patients. In most cases the etiology of the weakness was revealed by case history and physical examination. When such history and physical examination did not identify the etiology, it was suggested that the following protocol should be used: If history and examination fail to determine the etiology or to further direct the evaluation, chest radiography should be done. A negative radiography is followed by computed tomography.

Victoria, Graham, Karnell, and Hoffman (1999) presented an interesting case of laryngeal paralysis following the application of electrical energy to the heart in the treatment of dysrhythmia. An 81-year-old woman was referred for dysphonia following the cardiac countershock (cardioversion) procedure. Her voice was high-pitched and dysphonic, and she had no history of such voice prior to the incident.

MEDICAL TREATMENT
OF LARYNGEAL PARALYSIS

The medical management of patients with various forms of laryngeal paralysis depends on several factors. Of primary importance is the status of the larynx in biological protection of the airway. Cannon and McLean (1982) reported on four patients with laryngeal paralysis who required laryngectomy because of chronic aspiration of food, liquids, and saliva into the tracheobronchial tree. An unsuccessful attempt was made to manage these patients medically with less radical procedures.

When the vocal folds are paralyzed in an abducted position and cannot close, aspiration is the primary difficulty. Although voice is weak and breathy, it is of secondary consideration. If, however, the vocal folds are paralyzed in an adducted position and cannot open, voice is not significantly dysphonic and aspiration does not occur to any unusual degree, but the patient struggles for breath (dyspnea). Medical management should be directed toward improvement of laryngeal dilatory functions and is often an emergency procedure requiring tracheostomy. This is a well-understood rule between abduction and adduction forms of laryngeal paralysis.

Management of Abduction Paralysis

The most widely used procedure for treating bilateral vocal fold paralysis when the folds are fixed in a midline or near-midline position is tracheostomy to maintain an adequate airway. This can be followed by surgery in the form of arytenoidectomy. The procedure involves unilateral removal of one arytenoid cartilage and cauterization of the muscular attachments to stimulate fibrosis and contracture and thereby provide improved dilation of the glottal space. The success of the procedure depends on whether the patient is able to breathe freely without needing a tracheostomy, has some degree of phonation, and does not aspirate food and liquid (Tucker & Lavertu, 1992). The degree to which a patient is managed with significant procedures such as tracheostomy and surgical opening of the airway depends on how well the patient is able to maintain an adequate lifestyle. Many patients with bilateral paralysis in which the vocal folds are fairly medialized are able to get along quite well even with reduced airway capacity (Benninger & Gardner, 1998).

Nerve–Muscle Pedicle Reinnervation

Attempts to reestablish innervation to the larynx using techniques of nerve attachment (anastomosis) have met with mixed results. Two fine references on the potential of the process are those by Crumley (1994) and Gordon (1994). Crumley explained various possibilities for recovery of the recurrent laryngeal nerve after trauma. One is neural regeneration with synkinesis, meaning a scrambling of innervation to abductor and adductor muscles. A second possibility is partial regeneration with synkinesis, in which either abduction or adduction is relatively intact but not both. Another possibility is total paralysis without any recovery.

An extension of nerve reestablishment involves taking a pedicle of some neck strap muscle with innervation and suturing it into the posterior cricoarytenoid muscle for reinnervation when abduction is needed. A variation is to suture the muscle into the adductors when medialization is needed. The rationale for this procedure is based on the notion that neck muscles are involved in various breathing activities and firing the nerve in that process can stimulate firing of the denervated muscle of the larynx.

Tucker (1997) reported on 52 patients with unilateral vocal fold paralysis who were managed by a combination of surgical medialization (discussed later) and nerve–muscle reinnervation. This combined procedure provided the added benefit of reduced muscle atrophy in 92% of the patients. Tucker (1999) followed his 1997 report by stating that "combining nerve-pedicle reinnervation with surgical medialization of the paralyzed vocal fold would appear to meet most of the short- and long-term needs of the patients with unilateral paralysis" (p. 255). He uses this combined procedure when there is no electromyographic evidence that innervation is present.

Management of Adduction Paralysis

Several medical procedures can aid in the management of disorders involving difficulty in laryngeal adduction. Historically, Polytef (Teflon) mixed with a 50% glycerine base was injected into the lateral margins of the paralyzed vocal fold to displace it toward a more midline position. Although voice improved, the development of granulomas that are difficult to remove have led to reduction in the use of this procedure (Watterson, McFarlane, & Menicucci, 1990). Benninger and Gardner (1998) used Teflon paste in patients who had a paralyzed vocal fold and whose life expectancy was short or whose general health made them a poor risk for more significant surgery.

Teflon laryngoplasty appears to have been replaced as a treatment choice by surgical techniques involving a less permanent material such as Gelfoam, fat, or collagen, which are typically absorbed in 2 to 3 months, with reinjections necessary to maintain results. Medialization (thyroplasty) has also replaced Teflon use significantly. However, the use of Teflon remains an option, and some physicians continue to recommend it. The criticisms against the use of Teflon relate to the obliteration of the mucosal wave, migration of the Teflon into regions of the vocal fold not intended, and the difficulty of removing it once injected should it become problematic. Dedo and Izdebski (1999) reported on more than 500 cases of injected Teflon for unilateral paralysis or vocal fold bowing using mainly an indirect technique under topical anesthesia. The indirect and topical approach allows the patient to phonate during the procedure so that fine-tuning of the voice can be accomplished as the injections occur. One of primary purposes of Dedo and Izdebski was to respond to the criticisms of colleagues who no longer advocated Teflon usage. They documented procedures that, if done properly, would eliminate many of the difficulties associated with Teflon use. They concluded with the recommendations that Teflon be used in patients (a) who require immediate injection after lung cancer, have known section of the recurrent laryngeal nerve, have serious aspiration, or have significant interference with work ability because of dysphonia, particularly breathiness; (b) for whom injection is delayed for 6 months because of the possibility of nerve function return (e.g., after thyroid or other neck surgeries when there is a suspicion that the nerve has not been sectioned, merely traumatized); and (c) for whom injection is delayed for 1 year (e.g., after spontaneous recurrent laryngeal nerve paralysis or carotid thromboendarterectomy). Under these criteria, only 2 patients of 500 had return of recurrent laryngeal nerve function that required removal of the Teflon, which was easily accomplished. Dedo and Izdebski also discussed the criticism that Teflon is often related to the development of granulomas and provided evidence that this seldom occurs with their patients.

The injection of Gelfoam, fat, and collagen provides temporary improvement when it is not known whether spontaneous recovery of nerve function is possible. This is a common method, particularly when the larynx is affected unilaterally. The procedure may be done by indirect or direct laryngoscopy, but Tucker and Lavertu (1992) recommended the indirect approach because vocal fold tension is not altered by the laryngoscope and anesthesia. Therefore, topical anesthesia permits the patient to phonate during the procedure so that vocal quality can be used as the guide to the placement and quantity of Gelfoam injected to provide maximum improved vocalization. These indirect procedures have also been advocated by Bastian and Delsupehe (1998) and Thumfart, Platzer, Gunkel, Maurer, and Brenner (1999).

Thyroplasty I (Medialization)

The foregoing procedures for medializing a paralyzed vocal fold by injecting a substance (Teflon) lateral to the fold to displace it more toward midline, or into the fold (Gelfoam, collagen, or fat) to improve the voice, form the foundation from which laryngeal framework surgeries were developed. These surgical techniques have been described by Isshiki (1998) as thyroplasty procedures. He classified them into four types: Type I (medialization), Type II (lateralization), Type III (relaxation), and Type IV (stretching or lengthening of the vocal fold). Thyroplasty Type I is the most commonly used procedure and is designed to accomplish the same sort of medialization to eliminate glottal insufficiency that Teflon and Gelfoam are designed to provide.

Many physicians have reported using Thyroplasty I to treat vocal fold paralysis that results in insufficient closure of the glottis for phonation (Isshiki, 1998; Kelchner, Stemple, Gerdeman, Le Borgne, & Adam, 1999; Maragos, 1998; Nasseri &

Maragos, 2000; C. A. Rosen, Murry, & DeMarino, 1999; Tucker, 1999). It involves testing with manual compression—a gentle squeezing of the thyroid lamina—to determine whether such compression results in an improved voice quality. Objective acoustic and stroboscopic documentation should be done to support perceptual judgment. When such documentation reveals that compression improves the voice quality, Thyroplasty I can provide a permanent medialization of the paralyzed vocal fold. Blaugrund, Isshiki, and Taira (1992) provided a step-by-step outline of the surgical procedure involved, and the foregoing references provided slight variations. The basic procedure is summarized as follows:

- The procedure is usually done under a local anesthesia because the patient must be able to phonate during the procedure to obtain optimal results.

- After surgical exposure to the thyroid cartilage, a point midway between the superior notch and the inferior border is identified and marked with methylene blue. This point corresponds to the level of the vocal fold.

- In this region, a rectangular window is drawn measuring 3 to 5 mm × 10 to 12 mm.

- The upper line of this rectangle should correspond to the upper surface of the vocal fold that will be displaced.

- Using a fine, sharply pointed dental bur, the surgeon cuts the rectangular-shaped window, taking care not to damage the inner perichondrium of the thyroid lamina.

- The preceding procedure provides a free-moving cartilage wedge that can be moved inside to put medial pressure on the vocal fold, displacing it toward midline. The degree of medialization can be observed and monitored by endoscopy. During this segment of the procedure, the patient is asked to phonate until the desired voice is obtained.

- The position of the wedge is stabilized using a Silastic wedge that matches the rectangle. It is held in place by nylon sutures. The wedge is flush with the level of the thyroid lamina.

- The approach to the larynx is surgically closed.

Thyroplasty Type I can be done as an isolated procedure or in combination with arytenoid adduction (Isshiki, 1998) or reinnervation (Tucker, 1999). It can also be performed on children (Link et al., 1999). Computerized tomography has also been used to customize the Silastic implant to fit the individual size and shape of the patient's larynx (Safak, Gocmen, Korkmaz, & Kilic, 2000). The general procedure of thyroplasty has resulted in significantly improved voice function, particularly when coupled with voice therapy before and after the surgery (Kelchner et al., 1999). One additional positive aspect of this procedure is its reversibility and modification potential. Although the voice expected by the procedure can typically be assessed during the surgical procedure, should the long-term result be less than anticipated, the procedure can be modified to increase or decrease the medialization. Thyroplasty can also be done without significantly compromising laryngeal airflow for respiration, even with the paralyzed vocal fold statically positioned at or near midline (Janas, Waugh, Swenson, & Hillel, 1999).

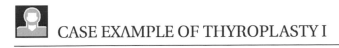

CASE EXAMPLE OF THYROPLASTY I

P. D. is a 26-year-old man whose larynx was injured by a gunshot wound during a robbery. After medical stabilization he was left with a paralyzed right vocal fold in an intermediate position from which no abduction or adduction could occur. His voice was weak in intensity (64 dB SPL at 1 meter), breathy (airflow of 270 ml/sec), low in pitch (fundamental frequency of 89 Hz), and short in vocal durability. He was able to say only a few words before taking a new breath because of the excessive airflow through his incompetent larynx. His maximum phonation duration was 5 seconds. Stroboscopic examination revealed a right vocal fold paralysis and persistent glottal chinking or insufficiency during phonation along the entire phonating edge.

A thyroplasty Type I procedure was done under a local anesthetic. The surgeon monitored the procedure through flexible fiber-optic endoscopy but relied on vocal sounds to determine the fixed position of the rectangular wedge. I was present in the operating room to help with perceptual judgments of the voice. When the expected position had been obtained, the surgeon asked P. D. to phonate and count from 1 to 10 several times as he adjusted the wedge. When the surgeon and I agreed on the best voice quality, stabilization was done and the operation was over.

P. D. was seen for a follow-up evaluation of vocal parameters 2 months after his surgery. A replication of the presurgery voice measurements revealed significant improvement in performance. His speaking intensity for conversation was 72 dB SPL at 1 meter. His airflow was 125 ml/sec for vowel prolongation, and his speaking fundamental frequency was around 122 Hz. His maximum phonation duration was 15 seconds (best of three trials). Stroboscopic examination revealed a paralyzed vocal fold resting near midline, and during phonation there was no glottal chinking or insufficiency. Some vibratory asymmetry was noted, but this was not considered a significant clinical finding. P. D. was very pleased with his new voice and expressed no difficulty in communication.

The case of P. D. illustrates the excellent possibilities of laryngeal framework surgery to improve glottal insufficiency. Several research articles, as mentioned earlier, have documented this improvement potential. Ford, Bless, and Prehn (1992) provided specific details about the Type I thyroplasty procedure and voice results.

They documented in 20 patients that thyroplasty Type I can be used as a primary procedure (8 patients) or as an adjunctive and secondary procedure to other surgical procedures, such as Teflon (3 patients), collagen injections (7 patients), and other microsurgery procedures (2 patients). The etiologies of the glottal insufficiency ranged from paresis or paralysis, sulcus vocalis (see Chapter 8), postcordectomy for cancer (see Chapter 7), and vocal fold bowing. Some patients had vocal fold scarring. Preoperative voice analysis on all 20 patients included perceptual judgment, voice function testing, improvement from self-reporting, and stroboscopic inspection. Only 15 patients completed all posttesting; 19 patients completed some of the posttests. Manual compression testing was done on all patients prior to surgery to determine its value in success prediction. Following are the findings of this well-documented study:

- Seventeen of 19 patients reported subjectively that voice was improved.

- Perceptual judgments of skilled listeners revealed improvement in 9 patients, decrement in 2 patients, and little change or disagreement in 5 patients.

- Transglottal airflow and maximum phonation time increased.

- Signal-to-noise ratios did not change.

- Improvement occurred in intensity range, frequency range, jitter, and shimmer.

- Although many of the preceding measures increased or manifested a positive change, statistical significance was not reached for any tested measure. Mean data were obscured by spurious subjects, which affected statistical significance. Scatterplot analysis provided a better picture of change.

- Patients with neurological disease (paralysis or paresis) seemed to improve more than those with contralateral disease or vocal fold scarring.

- Two patients seemed worse after surgery, one with sulcus vocalis and one with bowing and concomitant abductor spasmodic dysphonia. In the latter case improved glottal closure was offset by increased abductor spasms, and the surgical procedure was reversed.

Although Ford et al.'s (1992) study revealed that the best results occurred for patients with neurological paralysis who received thyroplasty Type I as a primary procedure, previous techniques of vocal fold medialization did not preclude the possibility of improvement in voice. However, their findings do support the notion of caution when vocal fold scarring and bilateral disease are present.

Pushing Exercise Program for Glottal Insufficiency

One technique discussed in the literature to improve glottal insufficiency in cases of laryngeal paralysis is the pushing technique. This procedure is somewhat controversial in that there have been few reports of documented improvement in which one vocal fold is unable to achieve midline status for phonation. Boone and McFarlane (2000) did not discuss this technique in the most recent edition of *The Voice and Voice Therapy* but included it as a facilitating technique in previous editions (Boone & McFarlane, 1988). Basically, the technique involves having the patient push against restraint, as in lifting, to generate reflexive closure of the vocal folds. When the pushing generates closure, phonation is paired with the process to determine whether voice is stronger and less breathy under pushing conditions. If so, the technique is continued and pushing is gradually eliminated while improved phonation continues.

This clinical process may be helpful, however, in some cases of glottal insufficiency. Yamaguchi et al. (1993) provided data indicating that an exercise program of pushing and phonation can produce positive results when careful documentation and visual feedback of performance are provided. In three cases of glottal approximation difficulty, pushing was used as a specific therapy technique, producing improved loudness and glottal waveform function. Yamaguchi et al. suggested using this technique prior to and following thyroplasty (when insufficient improvement requires surgery) but did not recommend the technique when there is vocal fold insufficiency and posterior arytenoid medialization. Colton and Casper (1996) argued against using therapy directed toward effortful closure, as in the pushing technique, but other clinicians continue to use these techniques with varying degrees of success.

Stemple (2000) provided several case studies of therapy approaches to managing various degrees of glottal insufficiency and recommended vocal function exercises to improve voice parameters. Some of these case studies were specific to vocal fold paralysis, including one patient who was an orthodontist experiencing considerable difficulty in his practice. Vocal function exercises improved his voice quality, including decreased breathiness and pitch breaks. McFarlane and Von Berg (2000) provided similar examples of voice improvement using therapy techniques of head turning, lateral digital manipulation of the thyroid cartilage during phonation, and facial tone focus, among others.

It is obvious that laryngeal paralysis can manifest itself in many forms and have various etiologies. Good clinical management involves medical techniques to improve the status of the paralyzed vocal fold(s), either temporarily or more permanently (e.g., thyroplasty), with supportive therapy provided before and after medical management has accomplished maximum results. Many therapy techniques that apply to the management of patients with neurogenic dysphonia are explained later.

DYSTONIA

Dystonia is a term that applies to a variety of central nervous system dysfunctions that produce a variety of abnormal movements in the body. Dystonia is a syndrome of sustained muscle contractions, frequently causing twisting and repetitive movements or abnormal postures (Fahn, 1999). There are generalized dystonias in which major movement functions are abnormal in the entire body and specific dystonias that affect isolated body parts, called focal dystonias. Focal dystonias include movement disorder in the eyelids (blepharospasm), mouth region (oromandibular dystonia), larynx (adductor or abductor spasmodic dysphonia), neck (spasmodic torticollis), and arm (writer's cramp). When two or more focal dystonias exist, the dystonia is referred to as segmental (Brin, Fahn, Blitzer, Ramig, & Stewart, 1992; Fahn, Marsden, & DeLong, 1998).

The diagnosis of dystonia is generally based on information provided by the patient regarding his or her condition coupled with thorough physical and neurological examinations. There is currently no blood test, X ray, or brain scan to aid in diagnosis. Children who experience new-onset dystonia could be tested for the DYT1 gene to rule out or in the hereditary form of dystonia (Comella, 1999). Movement disorder similar to many forms of dystonia is seen in a variety of neurologically based disorders, such as Parkinson's disease, amyotropic lateral sclerosis (ALS), and Huntington's disease, but one significant difference that distinguishes dystonia is the general lack of degeneration. Although often the condition becomes more severe, dystonia does not progress relentlessly in association with degeneration of brain cells, as occurs in many other neurological diseases (Bressman, 1999).

Many focal and generalized dystonias significantly affect speech and voice. For example, oromandibular dystonia causes jaw and lip movements that impede motor speech production. Blitzer, Brin, Green, and Fahn (1989) treated 20 patients with this dystonia using injections of botulinum toxin (BOTOX) and reported an average of 47% improvement in various injected muscle groups (masseters, temporalis, orbicularis oris, etc.). These patients reported improvement in eating and speaking, as well as reduction of pain.

A variation of oromandibular dystonia that involves blepharospasm, or eye twitching, is Meige's syndrome. It is characterized by writhing and undulating movements in the facial region, including the tongue and mandibular structures. In some patients with Meige's syndrome, sustained and fluctuating contractions of the velum, pharynx, esophagus, and respiratory structures are found. Involvement of motor speech processes can vary from mild to severe. Most medical and chemical treatments for dystonia have been successful to some degree in relieving the general movement symptoms of Meige's syndrome patients but without improving the overall dysarthria manifested. Dworkin (1996) used a custom-designed bite-block that was placed between the teeth in a position to stabilize movement of the jaw with as little interference of motor speech functions as possible. Excellent results were obtained in two patients when speech was compared with or without the block. Upon insertion of the bite-block, both patients immediately became intelligible, and many of the hyperkinetic movements of the motor speech structures were neutralized.

Spasmodic torticollis is a focal dystonia that involves mainly the neck. Duane (1988) has evaluated and treated well over 1,500 cases of spasmodic torticollis, many involving voice and speech dysfunction. Case, LaPointe, and Duane (1990, 1993) reported on 70 patients with idiopathic spasmodic torticollis and patients with other forms of dystonia affecting voice and speech characteristics. Patients with IST have significantly reduced levels of pitch range, /s/ and /z/ durations, phonation reaction times, and alternate movement rates for /pʌ/, /tʌ/, and /kʌ/. Additional data on voice differences were provided by Zraick et al. (1993), who found that patients with spasmodic torticollis have higher jitter and shimmer values and lower than normal harmonic-to-noise ratios in voice production. These differences are not from the abnormal head postures that are part of torticollis, because nondysphonic persons do not have the same difficulties when placed in the typical postures of these patients (LaPointe, Case, Duane, & Date, 1994). Apparently, the torquelike focal dystonic contractions that create the neck postural and movement abnormalities characteristic of idiopathic spasmodic torticollis have a considerable impact on the voice and speech characteristics of these patients, independent of head positions.

Spasmodic Dysphonia

Perhaps no voice disorder has received more attention from the medical and speech–language pathology communities in the past few years than spasmodic dysphonia (SD). Since the first edition of this book in 1984, significant changes have occurred in the classification of this disorder, knowledge of its etiological bases, documentation of its neurological aberrations, understanding of its relationships with other neurological and psychological disorders, and treatment methodologies employed. It is an exciting time for patients who have suffered with this puzzling voice disorder.

SD is classified as a focal dystonia in the larynx and is subdivided into adductor and abductor forms. Adductor SD is the more common form (Blitzer & Brin, 1992a; Salvatore, Cannito, & Gutierrez, 1999). A. E. Aronson (1990) categorized varieties of adductor SD into those of conversion reaction, those of musculoskeletal tension, and those of organic (essential) voice tremor. Adductor forms of SD generally fall into the hyperfunctional category of dysphonia.

In earlier literature, SD was considered to have a significant psychogenic basis. For example, Murphy (1964) stated that its onset "may be sudden—following an emotional shock of some kind—or of longer duration. And, although it is usually a hyperkinetic phenomenon, hypokinetic conditions have been observed. We are probably dealing with hysteria in some cases. The disorder may be regarded psychodynamically as a somatization developed unconsciously as a defense against the recognition of unacceptable urges" (p. 71).

Few professionals today consider SD patients to have psychogenic voice disorder. Rather, they are classified more often as having neurogenic etiology with possible psychogenic sequelae (Ross, 2000; Whurr et al., 1998). Most professionals who work with clients having this voice disorder notice that the vocal symptoms are varied, capricious, affected by emotional states, and often absent during laughter, singing, saying "ee" in a high-pitched voice, or engaging in unusual vocal efforts. These factors give the impression that SD is affected significantly by psychosocial and psychodynamic factors, but such evidence does not solve the issue of etiology. As a focal dystonia, SD is generally classified as having a neurogenic etiology. It would appear to be essentially an action-induced dystonia, with the action being speaking; however, the data supporting such a notion of neurogenic etiology are somewhat confusing and controversial.

Brin, Fahn, et al. (1992) reported on 562 patients with laryngeal dystonia and classified adductor and abductor SD with a neurological etiology. The specific focal lesion(s) was not consistently identified, and most cases were further classified as having an idiopathic neurogenic etiology. Brin, Fahn, et al. reviewed the findings of Finitzo and Freeman (1989), who reported on 7 years of research investigating the etiology of SD. Seventy-five patients with spasmodic dysphonia underwent extensive neurological testing, including magnetic resonance image (MRI) scans, auditory brain stem response (ABR) testing, brain electrical activity mapping (BEAM), and single-photon emission computerized tomography (SPECT). Not all of the patients underwent all of these procedures, but the following abnormalities were found:

- Eighty percent of the subjects had multifocal, structural (MRI), metabolic (SPECT), and/or electrophysiologic (BEAM) abnormalities of the central nervous system.

- Thirty-five percent of the patients had abnormal brain stem auditory-evoked responses (ABR).

- Forty-seven percent had abnormal gastric acid secretory responses to sham feeding, indicating vagus nerve dysfunction.

- Forty-six percent had reduced or absent vagally mediated fluctuations in heart rate during deep inspiration.

- Twenty-three percent had brain lesions when imaged with MRI.

- Fifty-six percent had abnormal BEAM scans.

- Seventy-six percent had abnormal brain hypoperfusion on SPECT.

- The most frequent central nervous system lesion sites were in the left frontal/temporal cortex, the subcortical white matter underlying the left frontal/temporal cortex, the medial prefrontal to frontal cortex, and the right posterior temporal/parietal cortex.

Although these data provide a strong indication that all is not well in the central nervous system of many patients with SD, the multifocal nature of findings provides controversy, as stated by A. E. Aronson and Lagerlund (1991), who expressed concern about instrumentation usage and the interpretation of findings reported by Finitzo and Freeman (1989). The dialogue between Finitzo, Freeman, Devous, and Watson (1991) and A. E. Aronson and Lagerlund (1991) provides clear evidence that much more needs to be known about the neuropathology of SD. Additional evidence of possible central nervous system dysfunction in abductor SD, particularly in the brain stem, was reported by Gillespie, Bielamowicz, Yamashita, and Ludlow (1999).

SD appears to be an adult disorder. Blitzer and Brin (1992a) reported the average onset to be 38 years in their series of patients. Their data also indicated that the disorder is more prevalent in females than males, with 59% of cases being female, a gender difference that is similar to that for all dystonias (57% female).

Many patients with SD state that they are pleased to know that the disorder likely has a neurogenic rather than a psychogenic etiology, which raises the question, Why would one be comforted by the fact that something might be wrong in his or her central nervous system? Perhaps such feelings stem from the numerous instances of misdiagnosis in which physicians tell these patients that they can see nothing wrong in their larynx to explain the disorder. I had one female client who suffered from adductor SD for more than 30 years and had numerous diagnoses of a nonorganic nature. She had been through psychotherapy, biofeedback therapy, drug therapy, diet therapy, and hypnosis and had considered acupuncture. She was genuinely relieved to hear that a neurological basis was likely for her disorder. She hated the feeling that she had been given by many professionals that she was not psychologically stable even though she did not feel vulnerable to psychological disequilibrium. No therapy had been helpful until she was introduced to the neurogenic theories and current treatments, which gave her great comfort.

Treatment of Spasmodic Dysphonia

One significant problem with SD is its resistance to treatment. Historically, because of its psychosomatic diagnostic base, patients were subjected to diverse attempts at management, including psychotherapy, voice–speech therapy, acupuncture, hypnosis, biofeedback, relaxation, respiratory therapy, electroshock therapy, meditation, tranquilizers, muscle relaxants, megavitamins, and chiropractic therapies (Dedo & Izdebski, 1983).

In the 32 years I have been treating patients with various dysphonias, I have tried a few strange and esoteric voice therapy techniques without significant success. Many patients have shown slight improvement with traditional voice therapy and have learned to control the vocal symptoms in small units, such as monosyllabic utterances, but rarely in contextual speech. Historically the poor prognosis is one of the most significant symptoms of this disorder and has been pathognomonic and diagnostic to it.

Because of the poor prognosis, an alternative treatment method was developed by Dedo (1976). He reported on 34 patients who demonstrated significant improvement in vocal quality after Xylocaine injection into one recurrent laryngeal nerve to produce temporary paralysis of the nerve and the vocal fold innervated by it. In these 34 patients the recurrent laryngeal nerve later was sectioned to produce permanent paralysis of the vocal fold in an attempt to eliminate the overpressure (hyperadduction) during phonation. With nerve sectioning plus postoperative voice therapy by voice therapists, these patients experienced significant improvement in their voices, with a half gaining near-normal voice. This was the first report of many by Dedo and his associates; many other surgeons and researchers have reported on variations on the technique.

It is difficult to generalize the current status of recurrent laryngeal nerve resectioning for SD. A. E. Aronson and DeSanto (1983) reported that success of any surgery must be viewed according to the long-term results obtained. Of 33 patients who were sectioned, 100% experienced improved voice immediately after surgery, but 3 years later 21 (64%) had failed to maintain improvement and were considered surgical failures. The voices of 10 of these 21 were considered worse than before surgery. Women patients were more likely to experience long-term failure than men, for unknown reasons. Beacuse of data such as these, fewer and fewer of these resections are being done. Although some surgeons still perform the procedure, as reported by Dedo, Izdebski, and Behlau (1993), Fritzell et al. (1993), Izdebski, Ward, and Dedo (1999), and Berke (1999), it has mainly been replaced as a medical procedure by BTX injections.

Use of BOTOX (BTX) Injections for Dystonia

A growing body of literature and clinical experience indicates that injection of BTX into the vocal folds of patients with SD is an effective treatment. BTX is the toxic basis for botulism, a very bad and potentially deadly disease in which muscles are paralyzed by the neurotoxin of botulism. In tiny amounts and under careful medical control, however, BTX does not result in botulism. It has become a therapeutic tool. BTX has been used to reduce extensive muscle contractions in a variety of focal dystonias, such as blepharospasm, oromandibular dystonia, cervical dystonia, and spasmodic torticollis, and it is now being used to treat the specific muscle overcontractions of SD (Brin, Blitzer, Stewart, & Fahn, 1992; Tsui, 1999). BTX is a trade name for botulinum toxin, serotype A (BTX-A). Several subtypes of BTX have been isolated, but only type A toxin is available on the market at this time.

The procedure is rather simple compared with recurrent laryngeal nerve resection. BTX is a neurotoxin that acts at the myoneuronal junction. When tiny amounts of BTX are injected directly into the vocalis muscles (for adductor SD), the neurotoxin acts to stop the neuromuscular transmission or release of acetylcholine, causing varying degrees of muscle weakness of the injected muscles, but usually a flaccid paralysis. It is injected in mouse units (U), and 1 U is sufficient to kill 50% of female mice. The lethal dosage for humans, which is not known and can only be estimated from published reports, is likely around 3,500 times that needed to cause paralysis and death in mice (Brin, Blitzer, et al., 1992). Typically, around 2.5 Us are injected into each vocalis muscle in the first dosage; the amount is physician determined. The effect usually lasts for a few months, but some have reported improvement lasting for years; the typical positive response is between 4 and 6 months. Initially patients experience a dramatically weakened and breathy voice and possibly some slight aspiration and difficulty swallowing; after a few days the voice settles into a more normal quality, devoid of the spasmodic tightness of the disorder. Bielamowicz and Ludlow (2000) reported that unilateral injection also has a positive effect in the noninjected vocal fold, as evidenced by EMG analysis, and speculated that BTX might have a central pathophysiological response as a basis for voice and speech improvement.

The most frequent surgical approach is by needle injection into the cricothyroid membrane (topically anesthetized), monitored by EMG. When the EMG tracing indicates the needle has entered the vocalis muscle, the injection takes place and the surgeon moves to the next vocal fold if the intention is to perform the procedure bilaterally (Blitzer & Brin, 1998).

BTX is used to treat SD in a number of medical centers, and the results appear to be favorable, even with repeated injections. Few sequelae are reported other than the expected slight difficulty in swallowing and vocal breathiness for a short period of time. The patients I have evaluated have demonstrated remarkable and stable vocal control, essentially free of spasmodic voice quality. Patients also report a lessening of a feeling of tightness in the throat, even when the BTX effect is wearing off and vocal symptoms are returning. The more objective findings of Zwirner, Murry, and Woodson (1993) provide documentation of the improvement that results from BTX injections, findings confirmed by Courey et al. (2000).

Patients also are receiving emotional support and encouragement through a national SD support organization (National Spasmodic Dysphonia Association [NSDA], One East Wacker Drive, Suite 2430, Chicago, IL 60601-1905; e-mail address: NSDA@dystonia-foundation.org), and local support groups have been formed in some cities. Speech–language pathologists, otolaryngologists, patients, and related health professionals can receive the NSDA newsletter by writing to the association and thus be kept up-to-date on matters pertaining to SD.

Most of the patients who have been injected with BTX have adductor SD, and the injection is into the vocalis muscles. The less common abductor form, described in the following section, is also being treated with BTX but with a different muscle focus.

Abductor Spasmodic Dysphonia

Whereas adductor SD represents a hyperfunctional form of voice disorder, with vocal stoppage being a primary characteristic, the abductor form represents the opposite problem—spontaneous inappropriate abduction of the vocal folds when phonation is intended. For example, when a patient with this form says the word *puppy*, the unvoiced consonants would likely occasion excessive abduction and little voicing would be heard on the subsequent vowels. The common perception in abductor SD is intermittent but prominent breathiness.

Some evidence exists that classifies abductor SD as quite different from adductor SD, with possibly different etiologies. A literature debate on this question was addressed by Karnell (1992) and Watterson and McFarlane (1992). Whether abductor SD is part of the laryngeal dystonia family as Karnell stated or falls into a different category of dysphonia as posited by Watterson and McFarlane likely will not be clarified in the near future, and abductor SD will probably continue to be classified mainly as a variation of dystonia.

Use of BTX for the treatment of abductor SD is a viable option. The target muscle for injection is usually the posterior cricoarytenoid, the primary abductor, which is thought to be in an overcontractive state in this disorder. Rather than the needle's entering the larynx from the cricothyroid membrane, a side approach posterior to the thyroid lamina is used to provide access to this posterior muscle. This procedure is also EMG guided. Initially one muscle is injected; if a satisfactory result is not obtained, an additional injection is given to the same muscle. If the results remain unsatisfactory, tiny amounts can be injected into the opposite posterior cricoarytenoid muscle (Bastian, 1999; Brin, Blitzer et al., 1992).

There is great hope for patients with either form of SD. Patients who have suffered dysphonia for many years and who have been offered a plethora of treatment modalities, without much success, can now look forward to a life with an improved freedom of vocal expression. For some patients the injection alone is satisfactory, and little help is needed from voice therapy. For other patients voice therapy concentrating on principles of good vocal hygiene increases the latency between injections.

The trail of SD has led from the offices of psychiatrists, where patients received counseling or psychotherapy to help them adjust to having a psychogenic disorder, to the surgeon's table for a nonreversible resection of a major laryngeal nerve, to treatment with neurotoxins. One patient told me about his trip to receive a BTX injection. As he walked the streets leading to the hospital, he saw a man, perhaps homeless, certainly desperate, searching through a garbage can for food. My patient thought, "Here I am approaching a famous hospital to be injected by the neurotoxin (that causes botulism), at great expense, and that man is going to get it for free."

The medical literature contains excellent documentation of the benefits of BTX in the treatment of SD, including reports of voice and speech improvements

(Crevier-Buchman, Laccourreye, Papon, Nurit, & Brasnu, 1997; Izdebski et al., 1999; Lundy, Lu, Casiano, & Xue, 1998; Sherrard, Marquardt, & Cannito, 2000; Stewart et al., 1997). Most of these sources indicate that voice therapy is an important aspect of successful treatment when it occurs before and after the BTX injections. The techniques used vary with the philosophy of the voice clinician, but they generally focus on teaching the patient to produce voice with less hyperfunctional effort and reduced loudness effort, avoid hard attacks, and speak with general body and laryngeal relaxation. These goals can be well achieved under the watchful eye of the speech–language pathologist with voice experience. Often a patient can achieve increased latencies between BTX injections when receiving voice therapy. Merson (1999) also encouraged patients to maintain general principles of vocal hygiene, such as keeping the vocal tract well hydrated and moist; increasing vocal stamina with aerobics and exercise; adopting an easy and melodic vocal style; avoiding shouting, coughing, and smoking; and avoiding a taciturn attitude. Merson also recommended keeping a chart on vocal quality to help document the overall benefit of the treatments, including voice therapy.

There are certainly patients who seem not to benefit from BTX treatment. Bastian (2001) addressed this issue in an NSDA newsletter, stating that when a patient reports "no benefit," there could actually be several ways of interpreting that report. One meaning might be "there was no effect—nothing happened." Another might be "there was an effect, but no benefit." A third possibility might be "there was a big effect, and real benefit, but the side effects were unacceptable or the duration profile was unsatisfactory." A fourth possibility might be "there was the usual effect and benefit profile at the beginning, but the duration was shorter than expected." Bastian gave several explanations for these possibilities, including missed target muscle, immunity to BTX, insensitivity to BTX, and insufficient dosage provided, addressing specific side effect difficulties such as coughing on liquids, shortness of breath, and the possibility that the patient was ill soon after the treatment, which might have shortened the positive effects of treatment. This is an excellent reference for helping patients and professionals understand the multiple issues involved in the use of BTX for treatment of SD.

Although the technical articles referenced are helpful in guiding the professional seeking information on the pros and cons of various treatment modalities, often a more personalized approach is needed, particularly for patients who are struggling daily with the disorder. The NSDA has published in its newsletter and in the book *Speechless: Living with Spasmodic Dysphonia*, by Sowerby, Newcomer, and Schonauer (1999), excellent patient stories of the day-to-day concerns of living with this disorder. An additional reference along these lines is the personal story of Diane Rehm (1999).

Careful management of patients with dystonia requires the cooperation of the medical community and, when communication disorder is involved, speech–language pathologists. I have evaluated and treated hundreds of patients with various forms of dystonia in consultation with medical colleagues and found this professional arena to be most enjoyable. Without medical treatment, I am sure great frustration would have occurred in attempting to ameliorate voice abnormalities. With the advent of BTX and other medical support processes, however, voice therapy augments these treatments to produce excellent results and wonderful patient satisfaction in the majority of cases.

NERVOUS SYSTEM LESIONS AND DYSARTHRIA

To this point, the discussion has focused on lesions that disrupt the innervation of the larynx and pharynx in rather isolated fashion. These disorders are referred to as dysphonias of a neurogenic basis. Neurogenic disruptions affecting motor speech processes more generally are referred to as dysarthrias, as explained by LaPointe (1994a, 1994b), Duffy (1995), and McNeil (1997). LaPointe specified that abnormal neuromuscular control of the sensory and motor processes of respiration, phonation, articulation, resonation, and prosodic aspects of speech should be called dysarthrias. In this section, I discuss many of the dysarthrias that have particular impact on voice.

There have been many classification systems for dysarthrias, beginning with the classic studies by Darley, Aronson, and Brown (1969a, 1969b, 1975a, 1975b). These researchers classified dysarthrias into seven subtypes: spastic, flaccid, mixed spastic–flaccid, ataxic, hypokinetic, hyperkinetic in chorea, and hyperkinetic in dystonia. Because this is a book on voice disorder, not dysarthria, I consider dysarthrias in a more general sense here. My purpose is to describe those dysarthrias that have significant dysphonia as a component. They are described under diagnostic categories such as pseudobulbar, Parkinson's disease, amyotrophic lateral sclerosis, cerebral palsy, and so forth. Some attention is given to the neurological etiology of each dysarthria discussed, but the focus is on symptoms, particularly voice, and treatment considerations.

Dysarthria can result from nearly any insult to the brain when motor control centers are affected. There are numerous central nervous system centers of motor control and extensive peripheral or final common pathways leading to and from the muscles and structures of speech. Often dysarthria results from a specific lesion or pathology in focal areas of the brain, with primary manifestation of the disorder in the structures of speech. Damage at any point on the pathway to and from central to peripheral can manifest a dysarthria. When damage occurs in the central motor control centers, it is considered an upper motor neuron lesion. Damage to the cranial nerves of the peripheral nervous system is considered a lower motor neuron lesion. Sometimes the damage is to both, and a mixed upper and lower motor etiology is manifested.

Upper motor control of the larynx and pharynx is complex, as explained earlier, and lesions anywhere along the entire upper motor pathway can disrupt function. Upper motor neuron lesions usually produce spasticity of function rather than the flaccid form of paralysis caused by lower motor neuron lesions. Upper motor neuron lesions can occur in the pyramidal tracts leading from the cortex, and when they occur bilaterally a form of spastic dysarthria results.

Pseudobulbar palsy is a syndrome caused by lesions that affect the corticobulbar tracts bilaterally. Most often the lesions are caused by vascular disruption (cerebral vascular accidents) and are associated with arteriosclerosis, hypertension, and cerebrovascular disease. Additional etiologies include congenital brain damage in cerebral palsy, neoplasms, and other degenerative diseases such as multiple sclerosis (Crary, 1993; Griffiths & Bough, 1989; Kent, Kent, Duffy, & Weismer, 1998). Such a condition affects motor control to structures other than the larynx, including those involved in respiration, resonation, articulation, and phonation. Thus, these upper motor neuron lesions produce a generalized dysarthria rather than a pure dysphonia. A significant nonspeech characteristic is the uncontrolled and inappropriate laughing and crying that occur frequently in these patients (Crary, 1993; Griffiths & Bough, 1989). Recently Arnold Aronson reported on his own experience with pseudobulbar palsy from a right cerebral vascular accident that resulted in dysarthria and the symptoms of labile crying and laughing that resulted (A. E. Aronson, 1998). This is a fascinating personal account and is highly recommended.

The speech symptoms associated with spastic dysarthria include a slow speaking rate, lowered pitch, reduced pitch inflections (monopitch), excessive nasal resonation on vowel sounds, and a laryngeal tension and aperiodicity during phonation that Darley et al. (1975a, 1975b) described as a harsh, strain–strangle voice quality. The speech–language pathologist thus must be aware of the dysphonic elements of this particular dysarthria, which occurs when there is suprabulbar damage to motor control centers of the central nervous system.

Another dysarthria with dysphonic components involves damaged cerebellar tracts, resulting in ataxic dysarthria. A distinct articulation aspect of ataxic dysarthria is that the random disruption in articulation precision and the staccato stress pattern give listeners the impression of alcoholic intoxication. One client with this condition reported that his main difficulty in daily interaction with people was that he was continually accused of being drunk. Because he was able to drive without difficulty, if he was pulled over by the police, he could count on being tested on suspicion of driving while under the influence. Only a blood test would vindicate him.

Portnoy and Aronson (1982) compared the rate and regularity of diadochokinetic syllable repetitions of /pʌ/, /tʌ/, and /kʌ/ in 30 nondysphonic persons, 30 patients with spastic dysarthria, and 30 patients with ataxic dysarthria and found them to be significantly different. Their data indicated that nondysphonic persons produce 6.4, 6.1, and 5.7 /pʌ/, /tʌ/, and /kʌ/ sounds per second, respectively. Patients with spastic dysarthria produce 4.6, 4.2, and 3.5 sounds per second, somewhat slower than nondysphonic persons. Patients with ataxic dysarthria are the slowest on this task, at 3.8, 3.9, and 3.4 sounds per second.

These findings indicate that the dysarthric groups are slower than nondysphonic persons; further analysis reveals that both dysarthric groups are more variable in their productions. Although the ataxic dysarthric patients manifested the most variability, the researchers were surprised to find significant variability in the spastic dysarthric patients and suggested that variability may not be the discriminating factor between the spastic and ataxic dysarthric patients, as reported by Darley et al. (1969a, 1969b), authors of what is known as the Mayo Clinic system of dysarthria classification. This system has been used for years to discriminate various dysarthrias on the basis of motor speech performance; it has been a stalwart in this respect. However, as testing procedures have become more sophisticated, many of the more subtle aspects of voice and motor performance cannot be discriminated by the Mayo system of classification, as indicated by Kent (1994a) and Kent et al. (1998).

Vocal Tremor

A common characteristic in geriatric populations is vocal tremor. Although an actor or actress might use a slight voice tremor in the role of an older person, vocal tremor is actually an organic condition, often of unknown etiology. It is not merely an aspect of the aging process, because it can be heard in all ages. Organic vocal tremor also is called essential or heredofamilial tremor when tremors of the hands, arms, jaw, tongue, head, or other body parts are involved and other family members are also affected (Hertegard, Granqvist, & Lindestad, 2000). One of the most complete references on essential tremor was provided by Koller and Busenbark (1997), and an excellent reference on uncommon forms of tremor caused by foods and drugs, midbrain tumor, neurotoxins, and psychogenic tremor was provided by Manyam (1997).

Vocal tremor is often heard in a variety of neurological conditions, including Parkinson's disease and essential tremor, adductor and abductor SD of essential tremor, and muscle tension dysphonia (Barkmeier & Case, 2000). When the tremor involves other speech mechanisms, such as the velum, pharyngeal walls, laryngeal mechanisms, diaphragm, and tongue, a condition called palatopharyngolaryngeal myoclonus is present (A. E. Aronson, 1990; Case et al., 1993). Seidman, Arenberg, and Shirwany (1999) reported on palatal myoclonus as a cause of objective tinnitus, or ringing in the ears, caused by rhythmic contractions of the palatal musculature. Ramig and Shipp (1987) compared acoustically the tremor of neurologically involved patients with the vibrato of singers and found more similarities than differences. The patients' typical tremor took the form of both frequency and amplitude (intensity) oscillations occurring at the mean rate of 6.77 Hz ($SD = 2.63$ Hz). Vocal pathological tremor, however, had greater variability and intensity than did musical vibrato. The frequency and amplitude oscillation rate in the tremor group was within the range of 5 to 12 Hz reported by A. E. Aronson (1990). Winholtz and Ramig (1992) suggested integrating frequency and amplitude for more accurate measurement of vocal tremor.

Perceptually, vocal tremor can be difficult to identify, particularly when it is associated with other dysphonias such as adductor and abductor SD. However, Barkmeier, Case, and Ludlow (2001) determined that nonexpert judges such as typical speech language pathologists with limited voice experience could be easily trained to identify predominant speech and voice symptoms of vocal tremor and adductor and abductor SD with 86% of the accuracy of expert judges who had extensive experience in voice.

Essential tremor is difficult to treat, but medical approaches appear to have the best prognosis. Hertegard et al. (2000) treated 15 patients with essential tremor using BTX and found improvement in 50% to 65% of the patients. Improvement in vocal tremor with BTX was also reported by Finnegan, Luschei, Gordon, Barkmeier, and Hoffman (1999) and Warrick, Dromey, Irish, and Durkin (2000) for patients with focal tremor in laryngeal muscles. One of the significant side effects of BTX use includes periods of severe breathiness and sometimes choking on liquids, so often patients would rather deal with the tremor rather than experience the consequences.

Barkmeier (personal communication, February 2001) suggested modifying the speaker's speech pattern to "hide" the tremor, using the variables of pitch, breathiness, and loudness to function as the maskers. Specifically, she recommended shortening vowel duration in speech, encouraging a slightly higher speaking pitch for a female client, and increasing slightly the breathiness in voice quality.

Parkinson's Disease

Lesions can occur in various areas of the basal ganglia to produce dysarthric and dysphonic symptoms. One such disorder is Parkinson's disease (PD). The damaged area in PD is thought to be in the striatonigral (substantia nigra) system of the basal ganglia. One active neurotransmitter in this area is dopamine, and research has demonstrated that dopamine depletion in the striatonigral system is responsible for the neuropathological characteristics of this disorder. The deficiency of dopamine in the striatum of patients with PD intensifies the excitatory effects of the cholinergic system within the striatum. A complete reference on the etiology of PD, including environmental factors, endogenous and exogenous neurotoxins, genetic predisposition, and even a description of the benefit of smoking in the prevention of this disease, is provided by Mizuno et al. (1997).

PD can occur in primary form (idiopathic), secondary to other conditions (drug consequences, postencephalitic states, various toxicities, vascular disruptions, or trauma), or as part of other syndromes (Parkinson's disease plus another syndrome, such as dementia or Alzheimer's disease; Brin, Blitzer, et al., 1992; Mirra, Schneider, & Gearing, 1997). It is often associated with cognitive impairments, including deficits in visuospatial abilities, verbal fluency, set switching, and additional higher level speech and language functions. Difficulty in incidental learning and verbal memory difficulties were reported by Azuma et al. (2000).

Therapeutic administration of drugs to enhance dopaminergic activity or anticholinergic effects has produced remarkable benefits for many persons with PD. The most common drug is levodopa (L-dopa), which replenishes depleted amounts of dopamine in the substantia nigra (Brin, Blitzer, et al., 1992). This treatment is often coupled with the peripheral decarboxylase inhibitor carbidopa (Sinemet). L-dopa substitution has remained the gold standard of treatment modalities for PD, although significant advances have been made, including the introduction of direct-acting dopamine agonists, L-dopa slow-release formulations, and other experimental inhibitors. Also, new concepts of "neuroprotection" have led to the search for drugs that may halt or decrease the progression of nigral cell death in this disease. This science will continue to march forward (Poewe & Granata, 1997). Some of the laryngeal or phonatory concerns of patients with PD do not respond in positive fashion to dopaminergic stimulation (Wang, Kompoliti, Jiang, & Goetz, 2000).

PD is also now treated with stereotaxic surgery, deep-brain stimulation (Vitek, 1997), and transplantation of fetal nigral cells (Olanow, Freeman, & Kordower, 1997). The surgical treatment of PD involves various motor control centers in the basal ganglia. The procedure of choice is a posteroventral pallidotomy (globus palladus) or thalamotomy. Successful results are varied from center to center, surgeon to surgeon, and site of surgical focus. Although initial reports are promising for improved motor control in PD, the long-term outcome data of pallidotomy have not been clearly defined (Vitek, 1997). The impact of motor speech control in pallidotomy has not been as successful as general motor control improvement. Theodoros, Ward, Murdoch, Silburn, and Lethlean (2000) reported on 12 patients who were evaluated pre–post pallidotomy for speech intelligibility. A subgroup of 4 patients also was evaluated on additional speech physiological tests to evaluate respiratory, laryngeal, velopharyngeal, and tongue functions pre–post pallidotomy. Physiological changes in motor speech function postpallidotomy were either negative or nonexistent in the majority of speech subsystems.

Pallidotomy and deep-brain stimulation will likely continue with improved techniques unfolding, but at this point it does not appear that significant positive effects occur to help with the overall dysarthria the patient experiences with this disease. Generally, this same finding was reported by Solomon et al. (2000), who found speech responses to pallidal stimulation, bilaterally and unilaterally, were quite varied and did not match the general movement benefits provided by the procedure. They recommended careful exploration of speech sequelae after pallidal stimulation to develop risk–benefit data for future neurosurgical candidates. This is good advice for pallidotomy as well as pallidal stimulation procedures.

The speech and voice characteristics of patients with PD are well known. A hypokinetic dysarthria results in most instances of this disease (Adams, 1997; Tjaden, 2000). Typically, in 60% to 80% of patients, the voice includes descriptions of low intensity, breathiness, monoloudness, and monopitch that vary considerably during the day and speech that includes short rushes of articulation that affects precision and intelligibility. Deficits in motor speech, motor learning, or programming have been demonstrated in patients with PD (Schultz, Sulc, Leon, & Gilligan, 2000). Hanson, Gerratt, and Ward (1984) showed that the vocal folds of these patients are often bowed to account for the breathiness and other hypofunctional vocal characteristics. This finding was confirmed by Ramig, Bonitati, Lemke, and Horii (1994), who reported that 87% of the patients examined had bowed vocal folds. Lin, Jiang, Hone, and Hanson (1999) reported an increased open-quotient of vocal fold vibration and additional differences in many voice parameters in patients with PD.

The voice characteristics typically found in PD can discriminate patients with ALS from those with other neurological diseases, particularly among male patients (Kent et al., 1994). The respiratory characteristics of patients with PD have been studied by Murdoch, Chenery, Bowler, and Ingram (1989), Solomon and Hixon (1993), and Jiang et al. (1999), who provided evidence for a significant respiratory basis of the dysarthria present in PD.

Until recent decades, little was done to modify these respiratory and laryngeal speech and voice characteristics, but the clinical picture for these patients is improving. Information about the viability of treatment for many of these voice and speech characteristics has been provided by Ramig, Horii, and Bonitati (1991), who studied 40 patients with idiopathic PD to determine the effectiveness of therapy targeted toward improved respiratory support for voice and speech. Improvement was manifested not only in respiration and vocal loudness but also in speech articulation. Improvement occurred under conditions of expected abnormality in vocal parameters and decline because of the progressive and degenerative neurological status of patients with this disease (King, Ramig, Lemke, & Horii, 1994; Ramig, Scherer, Titze, & Ringel, 1988).

Ample evidence indicates that these patients can improve their voice and speech characteristics, or maintain them as deterioration occurs, by being stimulated to increase their speech effort (Ramig, 2000; Ramig, Countryman, O'Brien, Hoehn, & Thompson, 1996). Because speech involves respiration, phonation, and articulation, improvement in all of these areas can occur when proper instructions are given and feedback provided. The program of therapy outlined by Ramig et al. (1991), Ramig et al. (1994), and Ramig (2000) focuses on increasing voice parameters with the expectation that a phonation first approach will have positive impact on other speech parameters in a holistic fashion. The phonation focus is on increasing the loudness of the voice as a function of increased effort. The treatment is administered in 16 individual high-effort sessions over a 1-month period. Biofeedback provides data to indicate improvement. The program, called the Lee Silverman Voice Treatment, has the following goals and characteristics:

- Stimulate patients to increase respiratory effort.

- Stimulate patients to increase phonatory effort.

- Stimulate patients to sustain these effort levels over time.

- These tasks are simple and effective and can be taught to patients with different cognitive levels.

- These tasks can be measured and progress can be objectively documented, and the data involved can provide real-time, online feedback.

- These tasks can be practiced independently by the patients.

- These tasks generalize to improved speech overall when the techniques are mastered to increase phonatory duration and range.

The therapy program is designed to encourage patients with PD to maximize vocal potential. They are encouraged in practice to go "longer and louder" and "higher and lower." Feedback provides documentation that these patients are able to accomplish these maximum tasks. Improvement can be expected even in patients with PD associated with other syndromes and conditions, as evidenced by the data on speech and voice improvement provided by Countryman, Ramig, and Pawlas (1994) and Ramig (2000). The data provided by Ramig and her colleagues are most encouraging and continue to unfold. Patients with PD who are experiencing decline in the effectiveness of speech communication should be encouraged to enroll in therapy. Although this therapy will not stop the ravaging effects of their neuropathology, it can improve their communication abilities as they live with this disease.

Amyotrophic Lateral Sclerosis

The complex and delicate nature of laryngeal function makes the larynx highly vulnerable to abnormalities resulting from numerous diseases. A common example is ALS, popularly known as Lou Gehrig's disease. This progressive, degenerative neuromuscular disease involves both upper and lower motor neurons of the cerebral cortex, the brain stem, and the lateral spinal tracts or the pyramidal tracts of the spinal cord. It is the most common among a group of motor neuron diseases and results in both spastic and atrophic muscular symptoms. The cause of ALS is unknown, although histopathologic examination reveals widespread atrophy and loss of motor cells at all levels in the central nervous system. Viral and immunologic theories of etiology are numerous, with about 5% positing a familial basis. Males are more likely to develop it than females, at a 2:1 ratio. Median age of onset is about 55 years (Duffy, 1995). It is often reported that patients with ALS do not experience altered cognitive functions such as dementia, but many patients do manifest difficulty in this arena and should be tested in neuropsychological fashion as reviewed by Mathy, Yorkston, and Gutmann (2000).

The classical presentation of ALS is progressive muscular atrophy of the arms, legs, and trunk muscles, with weakness, cramping, fasciculations, and tremors, leading to eventual dysfunction in swallowing, digestion, respiration, and all other motoric biological systems. The prognosis in ALS patients is poor; in most cases it is a terminal condition. Only 10% of patients survive 10 years, and death usually results from aspiration pneumonia or respiratory paralysis (Duffy, 1995; Garfinkle & Kimmelman, 1982; Mathy et al., 2000; Younger, Lange, Lovelace, & Blitzer, 1992). ALS patients are typically divided into those with bulbar ALS and nonbulbar ALS (Duffy, 1995).

The generalized dysarthria of ALS involves all aspects of speech and has been well documented by Ramig, Scherer, Klasner, Titze, and Horii (1990) and Yorkston, Strand, Miller, Hillel, and Smith (1993). Respiration progressively deteriorates until it is unable to sustain life. Phonation disorders parallel the respiratory deterioration, producing an aperiodic voice, sometimes tense and sometimes breathy, but certainly less efficient in the delicate maneuvers of voicing in speech segments of voice–voiceless contrasts in human speech (Kent et al., 1994), particularly among male ALS patients. The vocal quality often sounds as though excessive mucus is present on the vocal folds, resulting in a wet hoarseness. This is caused by poor oral management of saliva and discharge from mucous membranes of the vocal tract. Delorey, Leeper, and Hudson (1999) studied velopharyngeal functions in subgroups of ALS patients and found issues of hypernasality present, particularly in patients with bulbar ALS. Klasner, Yorkston, and Strand (1999) reported that nasality was not a significant issue affecting speech intelligibility in many speakers with ALS compared to the issue of voicing concerns. However, when patients experience severe hypernasality because of weakness of the velum, the use of a palatal lift has been recommended in these instances (Esposito, Mitsumoto, & Shanks, 2000; Roth, Poburka, & Workinger, 2000).

The vocal characteristics, like overall speech patterns, vary considerably from patient to patient, as reported by Strand, Buder, Yorkston, and Ramig (1994). However, the following are typical findings. The pitch usually is low and monotonic. Speech phrasing is fragmented because of poor respiratory control. The intensity of the voice is soft and lacks variability, particularly in the late stages of the disease. One of the most striking features of the dysarthria involved in ALS is poor articulation, resulting from slow and inaccurate lingual and labial movements. Pressure consonants are articulated improperly, also because of velopharyngeal insufficiency that results in nasal air emission.

In the final stages of this disease, speech is essentially anarthric. Intelligence and complete awareness remain in ALS patients up to death, so their ability to maintain communication with family and friends is important because they may pass months in this condition. Often the intelligibility of the patient becomes such an issue that only a spouse or someone very familiar with the speaking style can understand the patient as deterioration occurs (DePaul & Kent, 2000). The speech–language pathologist must be aware of the special needs of ALS patients and be prepared to augment their communication efforts during the late stages when speech is unintelligible and anarthric.

Several communication aids are available to the speech–language pathologist for this purpose. Silverman (1989) thoroughly reviewed communication aids for persons unable to speak intelligibly regardless of the etiology involved, including dysarthrias, apraxia, aphasia, glossectomy, laryngectomy, and mental retardation. Aids that are gestural (no instrumentation needed) and gestural assisted (containing a readout device or auditory or written display activated directly or indirectly by muscle gestures or movements) are described in detail. Beukelman, Yorkston, and Reichle (2000) provided a comprehensive reference and description of augmentative and alternative communication (AAC) aids for patients with various forms of neurological impairment, and Mathy et al. (2000) described the progressive deterioration that accompanies an ALS diagnosis and suggested appropriate AAC support for the stages of change. Yorkston et al. (1993) reported that more than half of their patients in a large study exhibited speech or voice abnormalities sufficient to warrant augmentation support for communication. Gorenflo and Gorenflo (1991) and Raney and Silverman (1992) stated that patients have better attitudes about augmentation of voice and speech when the system used is sophisticated and provides a full range of communication potential. This is particularly important in that the language and cognitive abilities of ALS patients remain normal even in the final stages of life. This philosophy was confirmed by Mathy et al.

Mathy et al. (2000) described stages of dysarthria in ALS and recommended specific AAC support in the latter stages. For example, their Stage 4 indicates the patient might have some natural speech function remaining but will in all likelihood require AAC support, such as alphabet supplementation, an alerting signal for gaining attention, augmented telephone communication, and portable writing systems. Stage 5 indicates that no useful speech is possible, and speakers at this stage may include establishing a reliable yes-or-no signal, eye-gaze systems, communication systems dependent on ventilators, and integrated, multipurpose AAC systems. Such systems are described clearly in this reference. It should be kept in mind that in the Stage 5 category, hand control for writing and manipulating AAC objects is highly restricted or nonexistent.

Medicare has established new policies for coverage and payment of augmentative and alternative communication (AAC) devices and has changed the terminology for these services. Instead of AAC devices, Medicare now refers to *speech-generating* devices. The change in terminology is a response to concerns that the use of *augmen-*

tative or *alternative* would lead administrative law judges in Medicare Part B appeals to cover items that Medicare did not intend, such as Braille or TTY devices for the hearing impaired. The intent is that Medicare cover only those devices that generate speech.

As one can imagine, there are huge quality-of-life issues that a patient and family members must face when given a diagnosis as bleak as ALS. It has been my experience with these patients that adjustments do occur and appropriate modifications to lifestyle issues emerge that, in many cases, enhance quality of life. This topic was addressed by Young and McNicoll (1998) in their appropriately titled article "Against All Odds: Positive Life Experiences of People with Advanced Amyotrophic Lateral Sclerosis." Certainly, help with the communication concerns of these patients and family members constituted a significant factor in maintaining a positive focus. This same philosophy was expressed by Olshan (2000) in his personal account of ALS diagnosis and voice–speech deterioration, which was greatly improved by AAC support.

Multiple Sclerosis

One common neurological disorder is multiple sclerosis (MS; called disseminated sclerosis by the British and *sclerose en plague* by the French), a disease characterized by scarring or sclerosis of the white matter in various parts of the central nervous system. When MS develops, episodes of involvement occur and recur, interspersed with long periods of latency in some cases. Lesions can involve the cerebral cortex, the brain stem, the cerebellum, or the spinal tracts, with symptoms mirroring the site of involvement. The lesions of MS range from less than 1 mm to several centimeters, and they cause a loss of myelin (demyelination) on the involved neurons while the axons, or dendrites, remain intact (Gosselink, Kovacs, & Decramer, 1999; Guberman, 1994; G. R. Moore, 1998; Murdoch, 1990). There are several theories of etiology, most centering on unspecified viral infections. Complete studies of the epidemiological considerations of etiological factors were provided by Riise and Wolfson (1997), Compston (1997), and Ebers and Sadovnick (1998). Some of the factors mentioned are nutritional matters, exposure to organic solvents, infections, and genetics.

Several clinical manifestations have been related to MS, many of which are pathognomonic to its diagnosis: ataxic gait; spastic paralysis of the legs; hyperreflexia; unilateral loss of vision; ataxic nystagmus; nystagmus of various types (central, vertical, positional, horizontal); vertigo; a tingling, heaviness, or numbness of the extremities; diplopia; bladder disturbances (incontinence); tinnitus; hearing loss; and trigeminal nerve neuralgia. Many patients exhibit symptoms related to mood changes and negative affects in memory and higher cognitive functions (Patty & Ebers, 1998). Various forms of dysarthria are also seen (Kent et al., 1998; Murdoch, 1990).

One of the most thorough studies of the dysarthria often associated with MS was reported by Darley, Brown, and Goldstein (1972). They said that of 168 patients with MS, 99 (59%) had speech that would be considered normal. Only 21 had a speech disorder judged to be more than minimal in severity. The following specific speech deviations were found among the patients (from most frequent to least common): impaired loudness control, harshness, defective articulation, impaired emphasis, impaired pitch control, decreased vital capacity, hypernasality, inappropriate pitch level, breathiness, increased breathing rate, sudden articulation breakdown, nasal escape of air, and inadequate ventilation. Hartelius, Buder, and Strand (1997) provided data showing significant phonatory instability in patients diagnosed with MS. Gosselink et al. (1999) described the respiratory contributions to life-sustaining processes, coughing for pulmonary protection, and motor speech functions and stated that respiratory difficulties can be seen at all stages of the disease, although they are more significant in the terminal stages.

No cure is known for MS, but symptomatic treatment has improved quality of life by providing patients with physical therapy, audiological amplification, visual prostheses, nutrition advice, psychiatric support, and speech pathology services for the dysarthria. Hartelius, Wising, and Nord (1997) provided an excellent study of the effectiveness of therapy to improve speech function among patients with MS. In pre-post testing of individuals who received therapy services over 10 months, 5 of the 7 patients followed produced better speech on the variables of articulatory precision, vocal accuracy, and overall naturalness. This is significant because MS is generally a disease of deterioration. Rontal, Rontal, Wald, and Rontal (1999) reported an interesting case study of a patient with MS who experienced dysphonia from vocal fold immobility. This patient was treated with BTX in an attempt to rebalance vocal fold vibration. Unexpectedly, instead of simply having the immobile vocal fold return to midline, the patient regained normal laryngeal mobility and voice. Although many patients with MS do not have significant communication disorder, speech–language pathologists must be prepared to help those who do.

Myasthenia Gravis

Myasthenia gravis (MG) is an autoimmune neuromuscular disease characterized by weakened (striated) muscles, easily fatigued muscles, and prolonged latency of the return of muscle strength (Younger et al., 1992). The locus of neurological impact of the disease is at the myoneuronal junction. In its classic presentation MG is caused by autoantibodies that work against the acetylcholine receptors, leading to a decrease in the number of receptors at the motor end plate. Several conditions or states, such as infection, excitement, general fatigue, menstruation, and increased carbohydrate intake, tend to aggravate the muscular characteristics.

Muscular manifestations of MG include ptosis (droopy eyelids); diplopia (double vision); weakness beginning in the legs and spreading to other muscles over time;

generalized fatigue; weakness in the facial muscles, producing a smooth, immobile visage (facial expression); dysphagia (difficulty swallowing); unnatural smile with lips elevating but not retracting; and generalized dysarthria (Younger et al., 1992). MG is caused by a biochemical abnormality at the junction of the motor end plates of the somatic nervous system and the muscle cells of the striated fibers. Although no muscle atrophy is involved, clinical and experimental findings indicate that reduced availability of acetylcholine in the myoneuronal junction is the basis for the disease.

The diagnosis of MG is based primarily on patient response to anticholinesterase agents, such as edrophonium (Tensilon), which can be administered under control conditions to determine muscular response. For example, when there are objective signs of muscular weakness in the eyes (ptosis), low voice volume, hypernasality from soft palate weakness, or poor articulation, the patient is first given an intravenous control injection of saline or calcium chloride. No improvement should occur. Following this, 2 mg of Tensilon is administered; if no undue hypotension or hypersensitivity is observed, an additional 8 mg of Tensilon is administered. If clinical weakness in observed muscle groups abates within the next 1 or 2 minutes, a positive diagnosis of MG is highly likely (Guberman, 1994). Shulman (2000) reported an interesting case in which MG was ruled out as the etiology of dysarthria, demonstrating the difficulty of differentially diagnosing patients with neurological disease.

A. E. Aronson (1990) described the dysarthria of MG as involving a breathy, hoarse voice weak in loudness and manifesting increased hypernasality that leads to nasal air emission on pressure consonants as speaking increases. There also are non-speech symptoms of dysphagia, nasal regurgitation of food or liquids during swallowing, and, in severe states, inhalatory stridor and dyspnea. The voice quality often is of the wet hoarseness variety because of poor oral management of liquids and oral–nasal secretions. Mao et al. (2001) reported on 40 patients diagnosed with MG in which the presenting symptom was dysphonia as the initial and primary complaint. The authors concluded that MG can often focus in the larynx in initial stages and should be included in the differential diagnosis of dysphonias. The dysphonic presentation in this study was manifested in several different forms, including hoarseness, vocal fatigue, difficulty with pitch control, decreased volume or projection in the voice, breathiness, aphonia, and miscellaneous additional complaints.

Besides these symptoms, which can be observed clinically or by EMG, there is abnormal articulation function secondary to muscle weakness of the lips, tongue, and mandibular muscles in a flaccid dysarthria (Duffy, 1995). Distortions of consonants resulting from these weakened articulation muscles are compounded by poor velopharyngeal closure for oral-breath pressure. These articulation distortions increase as speaking becomes continuous, until in severe cases it becomes unintelligible.

The MG symptoms of muscle weakness can often be improved after administration of physician-controlled medications. As the physician manages the disease process with medication, to ameliorate the condition as much as possible, the speech–language pathologist must be prepared to evaluate the motor speech systems affected by the disease and provide care or augmentation as warranted.

Cerebral Palsy

Although much has been written about cerebral palsy (CP), a brief analysis of the dysarthria involved is appropriate. CP is an umbrella term for several congenital and early developing neurological disorders of the motor system. It is now considered to be more of a developmental dysarthria or group of dysarthrias than a separate neurological disorder (Hardy, 1994; Mecham, 1996).

The developmental dysarthria of CP manifests itself in spasticity, athetosis, ataxia, rigidity, tremor, and dystonia—separately or combined—in all degrees of severity. Hearing loss, visual abnormalities, mental retardation, emotional abnormalities, and developmental language delay can contribute to the motor dysfunction. When language is normal or near normal, the most striking speech characteristic in CP often is some form of dysfunction in respiration, phonation, articulation, resonation, and/or speech prosody, with intelligibility dependent on the severity of these motor speech dysfunctions. In severe cases, the brain damage that generates these symptoms can completely shut down verbal communication, producing a condition called anarthria.

When vocal symptoms of the dysarthria affect intelligibility significantly, particularly when vocal difficulties are of the hyperfunctional nature, BTX-A has been used. This treatment is common in SD but has only recently been attempted in CP. Lapco, Forbes, Murry, and Rosen (1999) reported a case study of a 34-year-old woman with spastic cerebral palsy and severe communication articulation and dysphonia. She was treated with BTX and obtained significant improvement in voice control. Her intelligibility improved to 85% at the single-word level and 94% for sentences with familiar listeners. Although her improvements were temporary, as is typical with BTX treatment, the results of this case study provided evidence that this may be a viable treatment option for patients with spastic CP. AAC aids should also be considered in patients with cerebral palsy where intelligibility issues are significant (Beukelman et al., 2000).

THERAPY FOR NEUROGENIC VOICE DISORDERS

When a patient with some form of neurogenically based dysphonia, in isolation or in some combination with other motor speech processes, is referred to the speech–language pathologist, the evaluation process must involve determining the effect that specific valves have on the speech and voice process. LaPointe (1994a, 1994b) elaborated on his Point-Place system of motor speech evaluation and management, indicating that it is a useful strategy for determining what components in the motor speech system need to he managed. He likened the movement of air in and out of the lungs as one point or place (Point 1), the headwaters of the speech Nile, which must be evaluated and perhaps modified. As the air moves from the lungs into the trachea, the next point or place of concern, a valve along the Nile, is the laryngeal valving mechanism (Point 2). This is perhaps the most important point to the speech–language pathologist. Point 3 is the valve along the Nile for velopharyngeal closure. This valve is another significant area of concern in voice evaluation and treatment. Other valves or points in La Pointe's Nile system are concerned with articulation and resonance and are less significant to the topic of this book. Points 1 through 3 are discussed in detail in the following paragraphs.

1. *Respiration.* Technical aspects of respiration are covered in Chapters 2 and 3. The focus here is on more general yet clinically relevant concerns about breathing for voice. The speech–language pathologist must ask the following questions with regard to Point 1, the lungs and processes involved in voice breathing:

- Does this patient have sufficient vital capacity to sustain voice? If not, can this be modified by improved breathing techniques and feedback?

- Does this patient have a breathing pattern that maximizes respiratory support for voice? If not, can I modify it?

- Does this patient have respiratory support for voice that does not involve abdominal and diaphragmatic support? If not, can I teach it?

- Is there significant upper thoracic or clavicular involvement in breathing that might be interfering with maximal respiratory support for voice? If so, can I eliminate it?

- Does voice (speech) begin with the lungs nearly full of air to support phonation, or is there a tendency to speak with the air tank nearly empty? If the latter, can I provide instructions and feedback to point this out and modify it?

- Does this patient attempt to speak too long on one breath? If so, can I point this out and modify it?

These are a few of the questions involved in targeting respiratory behaviors that might improve voice. In some cases of neurological disorder, such modification is difficult and progress might be limited. Respiratory support for significantly impaired individuals might be necessary by posturing or girdling, as explained by Johns (1985), Duffy (1995), McNeil (1997), and Andrews (1999).

2. *Phonation.* Because the major focus of this book is on the larynx and how it works in phonation, much is said about modifications of voice pertaining to the larynx. However, with regard to the neurologically impaired person with dysphonia,

specific questions must be addressed. Some of these questions also apply to nonneurologically involved patients.

- In the case of hypofunctional phonatory function, is this patient's larynx sufficiently managed (thyroplasty, Gelfoam, etc.) to allow efficient impedance of the airstream to produce voice? If not, can I do something in therapy to change how it is working? Can I touch, move, press, or in some way physically manipulate the larynx to produce a better tone?

- In the case of hyperfunctional phonatory function, can the tension in the voice be further modified after medical management (BTX, etc.)? Does changing the pitch help?

- Is excessive musculoskeletal tension present around the larynx? Can relaxation therapy help eliminate that tension? Is the patient aware of the tension? Does the tension really affect the voice? When more relaxation is present and the tension is reduced, does voice quality improve? Does physical manipulation of the larynx to eliminate tension change the voice? How much time should I spend in teaching relaxation as part of voice therapy? Is biofeedback of muscle activity needed?

3. *Velopharyngeal closure*. The valve for velopharyngeal closure is the primary structure of voice quality resonance. Additionally, good voice therapy often involves instruction about open-mouth, open-throat resonance as explained in this book and by Boone and McFarlane (2000) and Stemple (2000). (More about teaching voice production with a more open vocal tract appears in later chapters.) Also, a primary focus of Chapter 8 is voice disorder related to abnormalities in the velopharyngeal mechanism. With regard to the neurologically impaired patient, however, the possibility exists that insult will result in a paralysis or paresis of the velum, producing improper oral–nasal resonance from insufficient velopharyngeal closure. The following general questions help the speech–language pathologist focus on this valving concern:

- Do I hear consistent nasal resonance on vowels? Does it occur when I measure it with the Nasometer or similar equipment? Can the patient modify the nasal sound when provided with feedback of occurrence (e.g., by the Nasometer)? How much does the vowel affect the amount of nasal resonance?

- In addition to nasal resonance on the vowels of speech, do I hear perceptual evidence of nasal air emission on pressure consonants? If so, does it happen on all pressure consonants? On only the stops? Fricatives? Affricatives? Blends? Voiceless more than voiced consonants?

- If there is sufficient evidence of velopharyngeal difficulty, would it be important to objectively evaluate the velopharyngeal mechanism? (See Chapter 8.)

- Is there evidence of inadequate nasal resonance on the nasal sounds /m/, /n/, and /ŋ/? If so, can I determine the source of the denasality? Is it nasal obstruction from infection, allergy, or structural abnormality such as swollen turbinates? Should an otolaryngologist evaluate this patient as part of voice management?

- Is there a mixed resonance concern, such as excessive nasal resonance on the nonnasal sounds (vowels and consonants) and insufficient nasal resonance on the nasals /m/, /n/, and /ŋ/? Can I account for such mixture? (See Chapter 8.)

Often when voice is affected negatively by improper resonance because of velopharyngeal insufficiency in neurologically involved individuals, the velum is paralyzed or in a state of poor movement (paresis). The pharyngeal flap, explained in Chapter 8, rarely helps such a patient because of inadequate movement around the flap. Therefore, a palatal prosthesis (lift), also detailed in Chapter 8, is a more appropriate form of management.

SUMMARY

This chapter has reviewed normal laryngeal innervation (central and peripheral) and many disorders that can disrupt neurological functioning in the motor speech system, with special emphasis on laryngeal aspects. Various forms of laryngeal paralysis, dysarthria, anarthria, and specific disease processes or disorder types have been analyzed. Also discussed was current literature on the etiology, epidemiology, symptomatology, and medical and nonmedical treatments of these disorders.

Psychogenic Voice Disorders

Although the larynx is a well-organized and stable biological structure with complex neurological control (as described in Chapter 5), its vulnerability to changes in the individual's emotional or psychological state makes it an excellent barometer of mental and psychological stability. Persons anxious and under stress often can hide the condition in every way but vocally. The pitch may go higher and the voice may acquire a slight vocal quiver or unsteadiness, or even stop suddenly in a moment of spasm, or in some other subtle way betray attempts to appear calm and in control.

Most persons have experienced the frustration of losing vocal control in an emotional situation, no matter how hard they tried to avoid it. For example, I was asked by family members to speak at my father's funeral. He was old when he died and his death was not sad; he had lived a long and productive life and had died peacefully. My brother and sisters asked me to represent the family because they knew I was used to speaking in front of large crowds of people. I resisted, but they prevailed. Moments before I was to speak, I self-analyzed my emotional state and felt that everything was fine. I felt calm. I was going to be able to express the many wonderful thoughts I had planned about my father. Then I stood before this large assembly and made the mistake of looking into my sister's eyes. The look on her face was a mixture of sadness and happiness, but mostly of sorrow from saying goodbye to our beloved father. When I saw that look, in an instant I was vocally paralyzed. No sound came from my mouth. I could not utter even a sigh. I thought, "No one in this room knows the voice and the larynx better than I do. I know every muscle, every nerve, and every theory of how the voice works. I also know what is happening to me." The look on my sister's face had negated all of that knowledge and experience. I could do nothing about it. I was emotionally and psychogenically stopped in my communication effort by my sister's eyes. Descartes would have been proud of this example of dualism in mind and body, and even though I believed his philosophy as expressed in the statement, "I think, therefore I am," I was faced with the reality that sometimes mind controls the body, and only thinking is possible when body functions are locked in (Descartes, 1637/1968).

Many persons have had similar experiences when voice could not be produced, when speech was stopped, or when voice was affected negatively so that the emotional state could not be hidden or masked. Whether the emotional state is one of fear, anger, or happiness, the human voice generally communicates the condition. Indeed, it is almost impossible for individuals to mask their emotions from the voice. The voice is the barometer of the psyche. The quality of voice is intrinsically tied to the concept of self and self-worth, as stated by Andrews (1999).

Under emotion or stress, the biological functions of the larynx usually are not affected, because swallowing water or some other liquid or food does not jeopardize the integrity of the protective valving mechanisms. In an emotional state, the lungs are protected by the larynx but the psyche is not.

All of this vocal symptomatology involving stress, fear, anger, or happiness is experienced by everyone and is normal. However, in many individuals these vocal effects are the standard, not the emotional exception. The symptoms vary from a slight but rather consistent quiver or tremor in the voice at one extreme to complete aphonia at the other. The common factor in each disorder is the absence of any physical basis that can explain the voice symptoms. A laryngoscopic examination reveals essentially normal structures, but the voice function is abnormal. Such a person has a psychogenic, or nonorganic, voice disorder. This chapter details this process of functional or psychogenic loss of vocal control so that the speech–language pathologist will have sufficient background to evaluate, treat, or refer the person with this disorder.

Psychogenic voice disorder occurs when vocal control over pitch, loudness, quality, or resonance is disrupted sufficiently to impede communication effectiveness rather continuously because of psychological disequilibrium. Such disequilibrium can result from unrealistic fear, anxiety, depression, anger, unresolved conflicts, personality abnormalities, psychosexual or gender dysphoria and confusion, conversion reactions, interpersonal relationship disruptions, poor self-confidence, and puberty adjustment difficulties. To qualify as a psychogenic voice disorder, (a) one of the foregoing factors or similar conditions must be present; (b) the voice must be affected fairly continuously, rather than in minor episodes of extreme emotion; and (c) no physical or structural bases in the speech system (particularly the larynx) can account for the disorder.

One significant word of caution is appropriate at this point. Psychogenic voice disorder often is referred to as nonorganic. The diagnosis of nonorganic voice disorder can be inaccurate, and many individuals so diagnosed in actuality have significant organic disease. Yang and Mu (1989) reported on 333 patients diagnosed as having functional or nonorganic dysphonia. Only 16 of these patients (4.8%) were found to have functional or nonorganic disorder after careful scrutiny (laryngoscopic, electromyographic, and spectrum analysis). The majority of these patients (317, or 95.2%) had organic disease with various degrees of laryngeal nerve paresis, usually idiopathically caused. Speech–language pathologists must be careful not to consider a patient or client to have a nonorganic or functional voice disorder until organicity has been carefully eliminated by competent medical evaluation, regardless of the similarity of vocal symptoms to psychogenic disorder.

A. E. Aronson (1990) reported a patient diagnosed as having "functional aphonia" when the symptoms actually stemmed from myasthenia gravis, a myoneuronal junctional disease that produces a generalized dysarthria (see Chapter 5). Only after case history examination and endurance speech testing was the vocal deterioration noted, prompting the neurological testing that determined the actual etiology.

Another example of an organic condition misdiagnosed as functional or psychogenic was that of a 73-year-old woman seen in our clinic at Arizona State University. She had been referred by an ears–nose–throat physician who believed her significant dysphonia was psychogenic. She presented with a weak and breathy voice, not atypical of many forms of psychogenic dysphonia with which I was familiar. The onset of her dysphonia was sudden and had occurred about 3 months before her appointment with me. In my case history, because of the physician's referral diagnosis, I spent considerable time exploring possible psychological bases for her dysphonia. After several minutes of inquiry, I said something to this effect: "We have been exploring several areas regarding your psychological background and mental health issues that have been related to voice disorder in many people. I have found nothing so far to explain why you are having this difficulty. Perhaps if we spent more time, something of significance would emerge. I would rather try to help you change your voice if possible. I would like to try some techniques that might help produce a better voice." I then attempted facilitating approaches to modify her dysphonia, such as relaxation, tone focus, modifying pitch, and digital manipulation of her larynx. Nothing helped and her dysphonia remained.

I came to the conclusion that perhaps there was an organic basis to her dysphonia notwithstanding the negative finding from her physician and decided to visually examine her larynx. She was difficult to examine, but with a flexible scope I was immediately able to see the physical basis for her dysphonia. She had a paralyzed left vocal fold in a fairly abducted position. I showed her the videotape of her larynx and indicated that for some reason her physician had not detected this paralysis. When I viewed the tape with her physician, he recognized that his next task was to identify the etiology, if possible, of her paralytic vocal fold. Radiological examination of her chest revealed an 8-mm tumor in her left lung that was thought to be malignant and that had disrupted the innervation of her left recurrent laryngeal nerve, producing her paralysis and dysphonia. The patient was from Iowa and spent her winters in Arizona and decided to return to Iowa for medical management. I do not know the long-term results of her case, but it certainly illustrates the importance of recognizing a possible organic basis to a suspected psychogenic dysphonia (Case, 1999).

Another consideration is that many individuals consider themselves to be reticent speakers. They are shy, rather quiet, and have a general feeling that what they have to say does not need to be said and that more is to be lost than gained by talking. They are likely to have a rather flat voice, with little pitch variation (monotone), little loudness variation (monoloud), and reduced inflection patterns to emphasize their speech suprasegmentally. Generally, they would not consider themselves as having good communication skills. They might speak at a slower rate and be less fluent. Rekart and Begnal (1989) studied the acoustic characteristics of such speakers who classified themselves as reticent speakers for placement in a speech class and found many of the characteristics common to nonorganic voice disorder. The acoustic characteristics of Rekart and Begnal's reticent speakers included differences from normal in terms of fluency and perceived pitch. The reticent speakers had greater pause durations, fluency difficulties, and, in the case of females, a narrowed frequency range (monotone). In addition, male reticent speakers tended to have a higher pitch (F_0) than nonreticent male speakers. More research is needed in this area because many persons find themselves in employment that requires good communication skills and have difficulty matching such expectations (Rosen & Sataloff, 1997).

SYMPTOMS OF PSYCHOGENIC VOICE DISORDERS

Although the literature comparing specific voice characteristics to specific psycho-logical states is extensive, as reviewed by A. E. Aronson (1990) and Rosen and Sataloff (1997), few speech–language pathologists have the experience and skill necessary to differentially diagnose a particular psychological state by evaluating only the voice. Moses (1954) stated, "Whoever diagnoses neurosis is consciously or unconsciously affected by the patient's voice" (p. 1). Moses contended that specific neurotic states can be diagnosed accurately by evaluating only vocal features (respiration, range, register, resonance, rhythm, melody, intensity, speed, accents, emphasis, pathos, mannerism, melism, exactness, pauses between words). His analysis continues to be quoted by writers on psychogenic voice disorders, although few authorities claim to have the skill necessary to use his diagnostic system.

Williams and Stevens (1972) compared actors' simulations of various emotional states with recorded examples of voice and speech patterns of speakers under actual circumstances of emotion to determine acoustical correlations in relation to the emotional state. For example, the destruction of the German dirigible *Hindenburg* in 1937 was recorded by an announcer, excerpts of whose vocal patterns were compared before and during the crash by spectrograms (narrow band). Significant differences were noted in contours of the F_0 for up-and-down inflection. The average F_0 was considerably higher during the crash, with a greater range of F_0 change. Some evidence of tremor and irregularities reflecting a loss of precise control of the speech musculature and breathing control were noted spectrographically.

An actor's simulation of this event revealed similar patterns, even though the actor had never heard the broadcast. The Williams and Stevens (1972) study covered the emotions of anger, fear, sorrow, and a neutral condition in a similar manner and provided spectrographic data on the acoustic patterns in these emotional states. Their data revealed how vulnerable the speech and vocal systems are to changes from psychological balance.

PHYSIOLOGICAL CHANGES UNDER STRESS

What happens physiologically under conditions of anger, fear, sorrow, grief, hysteria, elation, or any of the typical states of emotional change? First, it must be determined whether these emotions have different biochemical or psychophysiological bases. According to most psychophysiologists, the nervous system responds differently to rage, to fear, and to positive emotions such as joy or sexual arousal. However, the differences are not sufficient to account for the variety of emotions experienced by humans during social, sexual, competitive, and other daily interactions. Essentially, to understand changes that typically occur in the body under various conditions of emotion, speech–language pathologists must comprehend the workings of the autonomic nervous system, particularly the limbic aspect, and the manner in which the nervous system interacts with the endocrine system (Webster, 1999).

Autonomic Nervous System

The autonomic nervous system is a functional component of the entire nervous system and has sympathetic and parasympathetic aspects. These divisions of the autonomic nervous system, along with the limbic system, are under the direct and primary control of the hypothalamus. Although the hypothalamus is a relatively small structure in the nervous system, it is the major integrating center for visceral and hormonal functions of human physiology, including emotions, and thus plays a significant role in every aspect of human self-concept and interpersonal interactions. It is a vital structure for understanding the processes of voice disorder outlined in this chapter.

With the help of the endocrine system, the autonomic nervous system with all of its connections controls body homeostasis. Homeostasis refers to a state of balance maintained by biological processes ongoing in daily bodily physiology. The internal environment of the body must be regulated with regard to temperature, hunger, thirst, blood pressure, oxygen content in the cells, acid–base balance, blood sugar levels, and all other metabolic functions. When some aspect of the internal environment is out of balance, a homeostatic drive occurs to achieve balance (i.e., to seek water, change temperature, etc.).

All of the cells of the body in their own specialized manner are regulated by the nervous and endocrine systems to maintain homeostasis by regulating the basic metabolic rate (BMR) of cellular function. The sympathetic and parasympathetic divisions of the autonomic nervous system are responsible for either increasing (sympathetic) or decreasing (parasympathetic) the BMR by stimulating the endocrine system to maintain homeostasis. For example, the thyroid gland, under stimulation of the autonomic nervous system, is the master controller of the BMR by means of thyroxine secretions. The thyroid is stimulated to increase thyroxine secretion under the direction of the anterior lobe of the pituitary gland, which secretes thyrotropin (or thyroid-stimulating hormone, TSH). TSH directly stimulates the thyroid. This is one example of the complex interaction between the nervous system and the endocrine glands in maintaining homeostasis (Kolb & Whishaw, 1990; Webster, 1999).

Limbic Lobe or System

The section of the brain thought to be responsible for regulating emotion is the limbic lobe. This is a set of forebrain structures that form a border around midline structures in the brain, thus the term *limbic* (from the Latin *limbus*, meaning border). The system includes the amygdala; a portion of the deep temporal lobe; the cingulate gyrus just above the corpus callosum on the medial aspect of the brain; the parahippocampal gyrus of the medial temporal lobe; the hippocampus, bulging into the lateral ventricle in the temporal lobe; the septum or septal area just under the genu of the corpus callosum; and other small portions of the forebrain (Kolb & Whishaw, 1990; Webster, 1999).

Another little-understood structure of the human nervous system is the insula. The human insula is covered by the opercula of the inferior frontal gyrus, the superior temporal gyrus, and the inferior parietal lobe. It has been characterized as a paralimbic structure because it has numerous connections and association tracts with both the neocortex and older limbic structures, even leading to a consideration that the insula is really the limbic cortex in humans. The insula has been identified as having neurophysiological involvement in emotion; visceral responses such as vomiting, belching, chewing, and swallowing; taste and smell sensations; and auditory, visual, and vestibular functions. It has also been identified as having significant speech and language functions. The more one studies the brain, the clearer it becomes how intertwined brain functions really are (Bennett & Netsell, 1999).

Through direct stimulation to animal and human brains, as well as through postmortem studies, sections of the limbic system have been found to be directly related to many emotional aspects of pleasure and displeasure. For example, electrical stimulation to the septum, hippocampus, and cingulate gyrus of rats produces penile erection, self-grooming, and related pleasurable responses. Damage or stimulation to certain nuclei in these areas produces increased aggressiveness in animals and humans, whereas damage or stimulation to other nuclei of the same structure causes tameness and passive behavior or placidity (L. R. Aronson & Cooper, 1979; Webster, 1999). Thus, it can be seen that humans' emotional status is dependent on the regulation of many nervous system and endocrine interactions.

What happens to the human body when some environmental (internal or external) change occurs to upset homeostasis, and how does that change relate to speech and voice processes? Only a partial answer can be provided here as a foundation to generally understanding psychogenic voice disorders, but some sources mentioned in this chapter provide additional information on the psychophysiological processes of emotion.

From Basic Level to Excitation

Essentially, when a person is resting and not digesting food, the metabolic rate is at its basic level. Heart rate is normal, blood pressure is normal, cellular metabolism is normal, respiration cycles of inhalation and exhalation are steady and regular, and the person generally is experiencing a sensation of calmness. However, should an environmental change generate an emotional response, several changes occur to offset homeostasis and physiological balance.

In the case of a stress signal causing fear, rage, or anger, for example, the sympathetic nervous system acts to prepare the person in the classic "flight-or-fight" reaction. The nervous system stimulates the adrenal gland to secrete epinephrine and norepinephrine. Epinephrine raises blood pressure by cardioacceleration, and norepinephrine does so by vascular constriction of the blood vessels leading to the skin and viscera. Epinephrine output by the adrenal medulla also elicits adrenocorticotrophic hormone (ACTH) output from the anterior pituitary gland, which increases carbohydrate metabolism and nervous excitability. Respiration cycles increase to provide more oxygen for cellular metabolism, blood sugar levels rise, a feeling of "butterflies in the stomach" is created because of blood drainage from it, arteries of the digestive system contract and somatic muscle arteries expand to divert blood where it is needed, bronchial tubes to the lungs dilate to accommodate increased respiration, pupils of the eyes dilate, sweating increases to cool the body, stomach and intestine muscles stop digestion, and mucous membranes that line the body cavities such as the mouth and throat dry significantly. There is also evidence that vocal tremor increases under conditions of high stress (Mendoza & Carballo, 1999). The degree of these effects depends on the significance of the emotional stimulus (Kolb & Whishaw, 1990; Webster, 1999).

Many of these reactions are part of the well-known phenomenon of "stage fright," but to a lesser degree than is seen in the flight-or-fight sympathetic nervous system—endocrine reaction. A later section of this chapter discusses the common phenomenon of stage fright.

The examples that follow illustrate how an emotional experience can affect the voice beyond the duration of the triggering experience.

CASE EXAMPLES OF PSYCHOGENIC VOICE DISORDER

R. T. was an 18-year-old woman who was referred because of a severe voice disorder. She had been robbed while working late one night as an attendant at a gasoline station. The robber stood behind her, held a knife to her throat, and told her to empty the cash register and place the money in a sack. After she complied, he took the money, but before leaving he ran the knife across R. T.'s throat. Although her throat had been cut, she was able to summon help. She was taken to the hospital and examined for possible laryngeal damage. Only a superficial cut of external tissue was found; there was no laryngeal damage. A laryngoscopic examination revealed normal form and function of her vocal folds. However, R. T. could produce only a weak and breathy voice even 3 weeks after the incident. She was essentially aphonic. This is an example of true psychogenic aphonia. (The resolution of her situation is discussed in the aphonia case example later in this chapter.)

Another example is a child who had his tonsils and adenoids surgically removed. On the child's awakening from the anesthesia, the physician told him not to talk for a few days or else he could "hurt his throat real bad." This boy was very conscientious and would not make a sound. He gestured and pointed to his throat as though to say, "I can't talk." After a few days his physician told him he could start talking, but the boy could not make a voice. Encouragement from his physician and parents did not seem to help. Luckily, after a few days the boy spontaneously began to use his voice, which is functioning normally today. Boone (1966) reported similar examples involving a child after surgery and an adult after prolonged illness, both of whom required therapy to restore voice.

Another example involves an older woman with aphonia of 3 years' duration. Hospital records revealed that 3 years before the examination she had undergone thyroid surgery for tumor removal. After the surgery she lost her voice completely. While reading the hospital record as part of the voice evaluation, I noticed that the patient continually coughed strongly and cleared her throat with a phonated grunt. The hospital records indicated that her laryngology examination showed normally functioning vocal folds in every respect.

When asked to speak, the woman moved her lips as though attempting to speak, but no sound emerged. During the evaluation I pressed on her neck in the general area of the larynx, asked her to cough, and said, "Oh, yes, I can see what the trouble is; you cannot bring your vocal folds together to produce voice. Let me help you and I think your voice will be fine." In the next few minutes, the woman produced many examples of normal voice in words and short phrases, but no functional communication was established even after an hour of intense effort.

The next day in therapy she was not able to produce any voice at all. I also noticed she was holding her breath for several seconds, then quickly breathing to catch up, then holding her breath again. Her daughter said this was new behavior that, as far as she knew, her mother had not done before. I soon learned that the woman was on welfare because of her voice disorder and had been for 3 years. The psychological mechanisms underlying her aphonia then were clear, as were the reasons why the woman was resisting reestablishment of her voice: She seemed to be afraid, consciously or unconsciously, of losing the welfare payments if she regained her voice.

A final example illustrates the delicate relationship between hidden fears and voice control. A 45-year-old woman was referred to me by an otolaryngologist for a dysphonia that had lasted several months. The patient indicated in the case history that medical consultation had not been able to determine why she had been coughing for 4 months and had been dysphonic for a similar length of time. The pattern of voice was typical of psychogenic dysphonia, and I suspected this as the etiology of her difficulties. Her cough was not typical of an organically based coughing reflex from upper respiratory infection or allergy. Her vocal pattern was unusual and based in the larynx, but not typical of phonation patterns seen in laryngeal organicity.

I was so confident about a psychogenic basis of the patient's dysphonia that I did not inspect her larynx in the evaluation. Most of the time was spent taking case history information. Her overwhelming concern seemed to be the fear that no physician had been able to tell her why she was coughing and dysphonic. She reviewed her medical history, which was extensive. As she spoke of her medical history, I did not hear anything that seemed related to her current condition.

As I listened to her story, I kept thinking that therapy would be successful in restoring her voice. I had seen many patients with psychogenic voice disorder, and I believed the prognosis was excellent for a quick restoration of her voice. She was married, and her husband was with her, providing excellent support. I explored many aspects of her life in an attempt to uncover the psychogenic basis of her dysphonia. Nothing emerged. She was happy with her husband, children, lifestyle, and daily routine, and she expressed no disappointments in life. Finally, I felt enough time had been spent in psychological pursuits, and I said, "I feel that your voice disorder is not based on any physical or structural problem, and I believe therapy will restore your voice. I would like to try a few things now and see if a better voice is possible."

I used a few facilitating techniques, which will be explained later. In a few minutes I was able to elicit a much improved voice in a rather high-pitched humming fashion. I thought it would be necessary to merely maintain that quality and slowly lower her pitch to a more appropriate level, but that did not work.

I ended the evaluation session with the instruction for her to go home, practice producing voice with the high-pitched hum, and attempt to lower the pitch. I thought this might occur in the comfort of her own home. As she left, I felt confident that in the next session 2 days later, with more time to spend, her voice would be stabilized at a more appropriate pitch level if she was unable to accomplish it on her own at home. The next therapy session went about as poorly. She achieved some good voice but was unable to sustain it at lower pitch levels. Then I also noticed her dysphonia occurring at the high-pitched hum level. I began to suspect that her voice was giving her some secondary gain that she was unwilling to give up. My confidence in a quick cure began to wane.

After three sessions of therapy with little improvement, my confidence that her dysphonia was completely psychogenic was beginning to change. Because she could not seem to produce a clear voice in her normal speaking range, I decided to look at her larynx.

She was very difficult to examine, but eventually I was able to examine her larynx endoscopically under normal lighting conditions. She was too dysphonic to obtain a good stroboscopic signal; however, I showed her the video recording of her larynx, which appeared normal in every aspect that could be seen under nonstroboscopic conditions. As she looked at her larynx on the video recording, I noticed tears in her eyes. She said, "I am so relieved to see that my larynx is normal. I was sure I had laryngeal cancer." The most shocking aspect of this statement was that she was speaking with a normal voice. Her dysphonia was gone.

I reviewed with her some of the information she had provided in her case history, which in the present context of sudden voice improvement was very revealing. She had been diagnosed in the past with uterine cancer and underwent a hysterectomy. She had also been diagnosed with breast cancer and underwent a bilateral mastectomy. She then stated that a family friend had just undergone a laryngectomy for laryngeal cancer prior to the beginning of her dysphonia and coughing. At the time her dysphonia began, she had a serious episode of the flu, after which her cough did not go away. That was also when her dysphonia began. It became clear that she had lost her uterus and her breasts to cancer, and she felt her larynx was about to be lost to this same dreaded disease. She had been told by physicians that her larynx was normal, but to her these were just words. She had been told the same about her breasts and uterus. It took visual proof that her larynx was normal for her to finally accept what her physicians had been telling her. When she saw the proof herself, her emotions were unleashed and her fears dissipated. Her voice restoration was complete. I saw this woman 1 year later at a gas station. She was interacting with her family and did not recognize me. I was pleased to hear her speaking to her husband and children in a beautiful and clear voice (Case, 1999).

These case examples illustrate the relationship between the mind and the voice. (Details of therapeutic management of such cases are provided later in this chapter.)

Specific psychogenic voice disorders should be examined in terms of symptoms, etiology, evaluation, and treatment considerations. Many psychological or psychiatric disorders can and do affect communication processes, many of which have a specific effect on the voice. The American Psychiatric Association (APA, 2000) classifies mental disorders according to the primary symptom associated with a given condition. Some of the categories include mental retardation, learning disabilities, motor skill disorders, communication disorders, pervasive developmental disorders, attention-deficit and disruptive behavior disorders, feeding and eating disorders, tic disorders, elimination disorders, delirium, dementia, alcohol-related disorders, various drug-induced and substance-related disorders, schizophrenia and other psychotic disorders, mood disorders, depressive disorders, anxiety disorders, somatoform disorders, factitious disorders, sexual disorders, gender identity disorders, sleep disorders, and various personality disorders. The fourth edition and text revision of the *Diagnostic and Statistical Manual of Mental Disorders* (DSM–IV–TR; APA, 2000) has modified the listing somewhat from previous editions, but the only modifications pertaining to this chapter are in the general area of gender dysphoria, which will be discussed later. One additional intriguing modification of the 2000 edition is the inclusion of communication disorder as a category. However, no mention is made of the many voice disorders of psychogenic origin discussed in this chapter. Some of the disorders also involve communication dysfunctions that are not treated as a separate aspect of the disorder because improved status in the condition is paralleled by improved communication skill. This chapter deals only with psychogenic disorders that have communication (particularly voice) disorders that are treated as separate aspects of the conditions.

It is often difficult to separate organically based changes in personality and behavior from those that are nonorganic. Most of the psychogenic voice disorders covered in this chapter do not have an organic or physiological etiology. In some instances, however, the etiology of the personality and behavioral components is unclear. Professionals working with such patients use the DSM–IV–TR (APA, 2000) to clarify symptoms and diagnostic processes, and I recommend that every speech–language pathologist have a current copy of this manual on the shelf.

CONVERSION APHONIA

A conversion aphonia can involve one of the somatoform disorders listed in the DSM–IV–TR (APA, 2000). Essentially, somatoform disorders are those in which symptoms suggesting physical etiology occur and for which no identifiable organicity can be demonstrated, no physiological basis is inferred, and symptoms are linked through positive evidence or strong presumption to psychological disturbance or conflict.

The essential features of somatoform disorders are that the patient often seeks medical care from many physicians, sometimes simultaneously, and presents a complicated medical history in which numerous diagnoses of possible conditions have been made. Somatoform disorders can involve any of the organ systems but typically are pseudoneurological (blindness, deafness, paralysis), gastrointestinal (abdominal pain), female reproductive (painful menstruation), psychosexual (sexual indifference), or cardiopulmonary (dizziness). In any event, the physical symptom serves to reduce or eliminate anxiety from some sort of unresolved conflict. In the patient with conversion aphonia, the striking symptom is the absence of phonation during attempts to communicate. The patient often uses only a whispered voice in a functional turnoff of phonation, producing only articulated air. Some patients with the same psychogenic etiology are classified as conversion dysphonic because a slight amount of voicing can be heard in speech attempts, but the striking feature is a breathy voice, weak in intensity. The conversion at times is so effective in reducing the anxiety that caused it that the patient displays an attitude of unusual calmness considering the severity of the symptomatology, a phenomenon called *la belle indifference* (A. E. Aronson, 1990).

The question is often asked, Why in the patient with conversion aphonia or dysphonia does the physical symptom occur in the voice rather than some other organ system, such as the eye or ear? There is no clear answer, but at least two characteristics in the case history of the typical patient provide some clarification:

1. There usually is evidence of a breakdown in communication between the patient and some other person of importance, such as a spouse, parent, child, or person of authority. The loss of voice seems to serve the function of eliminating the burden of attempting to continue, maintain, or reestablish the communication that has become so psychologically painful to the patient.

2. There often is evidence that at the time of onset of the aphonia, or just prior to it, the patient experienced actual loss of voice from a cold, upper respiratory infection, episode of laryngitis, or severe allergy condition.

The relationship between this actual dysphonia and the conversion aphonia can be explained in part by the following dialogue between a speech–language pathologist (SLP) and a patient with conversion aphonia (PT).

SLP: When did you first lose your voice?

PT: [Whispering] During May of this year, I caught a bad cold and became very hoarse. This cold lasted for several days and then I started to feel better, my nose stopped running, and I no longer had aches and pains, but my voice never improved. It kept getting worse and worse until I couldn't make any sound at all . . . like this today. I saw my doctor and he gave me some pills, decongestants I think, but that didn't help at all. They just made me sleepy and I felt worse, so I stopped taking them. I don't know, maybe I shouldn't have stopped. But my voice has been like this all the time since.

As the interview continued, the patient reported that at the time this cold was developing she was experiencing extreme interpersonal difficulty with her mother. It seems her mother had been unusually protective and demanding of high moral values and behavior, embarrassing her in front of boyfriends by asking them about their physical intentions, and in general accusing her of being "loose" with sex.

The patient had learned, at about the same time her cold had developed, that throughout her dating years her mother had been a prostitute. She said, "I could not understand how my mother could demand such moral perfection from me and be living a life of a prostitute at the same time. I can never forgive her for that." She confronted her mother with her inconsistencies, arguments developed, and communication broke down. It was easy to deduce that the development of her cold and actual hoarseness became a means of avoiding these verbal conflicts, resulting in her conversion aphonia once the cold was over.

Conversions can take the form of conversion aphonia (no voice but articulated airstream), conversion muteness (no attempt to produce voice or articulate, or perhaps the lips are moved as though attempting to speak without exhaling), or conversion dysphonia (some voice but abnormal quality, pitch, or loudness function). Even situation muteness occurs, in which a person speaks in one situation, such as at home, and is not able to speak in any other social situation because of some psychological difficulty. A recent example was seen in a school district in Arizona. A child spoke clearly and normally at home, but in school and other social situations would not even whisper, only gesture. She seems happy with her social interactions but remains mute. The speech–language pathologist working with this child is attempting to encourage speaking indirectly by having the child speak through a puppet. At the time of this writing, that has not worked, but the speech–language pathologist is encouraged by the child's apparent desire to speak (Mattson, personal communication, January 2001).

Conversions have been reported in the literature as being caused by strong suggestions not to talk after surgery (Boone, 1966), adjusting to divorced parents, adjusting to the death of a loved one, difficulty accepting being involved in an extramarital affair, difficulty adjusting to the role of being a tough policeman, and difficulty accepting that an only daughter is annoying (A. E. Aronson, 1990). This is only a sampling of the many etiologies that can produce conversion aphonia, muteness, or dysphonia.

One case of a 40-year-old woman who developed a significantly high-pitched voice (320 Hz) was labeled hysterical conversion dysphonia. Voice therapy (symptomatic) using a modification of the pushing approach (Boone & McFarlane, 2000) was successful in lowering the woman's voice to a normal habitual pitch level of 213 Hz. Although the DSM–IV–TR (APA, 2000) regards hysterical neurosis as another term for conversion disorder, A. E. Aronson (1990) considered the two as separate entities and provided criteria for the differences between them.

It is clear, therefore, that conversion aphonias or dysphonias can have varied vocal symptomatology in pitch, resonance, and hyperfunctional laryngeal valving. The most common form, however, is hypofunctional laryngeal valving. Loudness can be affected by psychological states so that the person speaks in a very soft voice. Some adults present abnormal pitch inflections. All of these voice dimensions can interact in subtle ways to produce a complex of symptoms of underlying psychological disorder.

One unique characteristic of many forms of psychogenic voice disorder in the conversion area is the variability of voice symptomatology in the same patient. Within the same voice sample, the trained speech–language pathologist often can detect vocal hyperfunction, vocal hypofunction manifested as breathiness, and even instances of normal vocal fold vibration. These symptoms occur randomly during a communication utterance and can be so unusual that no organic condition could affect the larynx and vocal system in such an extreme and variable manner.

Another unique characteristic in conversion aphonia or conversion muteness is the presence of phonation during coughing, laughing, or throat clearing and its absence during speech. Typically, the person with this sort of voice disorder does not seem to realize that the sound produced by the vocal folds during coughing, laughing, or throat clearing uses the same mechanism as in speech phonation. The following dialogue demonstrates the typical manifestation of this phenomenon in conversion aphonia:

SLP: What happened to your bank job while you were confined to the state hospital?

PT: [Whispering] Well, they kept me on the payroll.

SLP: For 3 months, even though you started working there only 1 week before you went to the hospital?

PT: [Whispering] Yes, they have been very good to me.

SLP: I'm impressed with that bank. I think I will switch banks!

PT: [Laughs loudly with phonation, then again whispers] I don't know why, but they seem to want me back.

SLP: When I open my new savings account with that bank, I will tell them why I am switching.

PT: [Laughs again with phonation and gives no indication she has just produced voice, then again whispers] Thanks, that might help them keep me forever.

EVALUATION PROCEDURES

Before proceeding with evaluation and management of a patient with some form of psychogenic voice disorder, the speech–language pathologist should be sure the client is evaluated medically by an otolaryngologist or other physician. Organic conditions of a neurogenic nature (see Chapter 5) produce voice symptoms similar to psychogenic voice disorders, so medical referral is necessary to diagnose the etiology properly.

When a medical examination has eliminated organicity as the basis for the voice disorder, the speech–language pathologist should begin the evaluation by taking a thorough case history (see Chapter 3). Beyond the questions outlined in Chapter 3 for a general case history, further questions should explore background and general aspects of lifestyle to identify possible interpersonal or environmental sources of stress and conflict. In a general and nonthreatening manner, the speech–language pathologist should discuss with the client such areas as family and marital relationships, employment stress factors, attitudes about self-worth and self-acceptance, financial concerns, and general lifestyle considerations. Many of these areas are private, emotionally laden, difficult to express, embarrassing to the client, and in general highly sensitive. It is not necessary to probe deeply into the individual's private life ("Tell me how happy you are in your sex life," etc.), and that would be inappropriate for voice symptom management. Rather than probing, a general atmosphere of communication, encouragement, and acceptance is appropriate.

The speech–language pathologist should begin something like this:

> It has been found that persons with voice patterns similar to yours are experiencing conflicts and stresses that might be affecting the voice. Is anything happening in your life that might be important for us to understand? What about your family life? Your marriage? Job? Financial concerns? These or any other areas? Tell me what you think.

An encouraging attitude can stimulate communication about these areas. The client at first may deny any such conflicts, but time and rapport in an encouraging atmosphere usually provide the forum for the person to start talking about these sensitive concerns.

Why should the speech–language pathologist ask about such areas? Is he or she playing psychiatrist or psychologist by asking such questions? Should the clinician merely deal with vocal symptoms and leave the psychology to the psychologist or psychiatrist? These are significant and legitimate questions. The answer lies in the fact that the speech–language pathologist often is the first professional to see a person with a psychogenic voice disorder. If that is the case, it is important to determine the psychological status of the client in a general sense to determine when referral for psychological or psychiatric services is necessary. Rollin (1987) and D. C. Rosen and Sataloff (1997) have written extensively on the psychological aspects of communication disorder, including dysphonia, and have provided excellent guidance to the speech–language pathologist in dealing with this aspect of professional life.

Speech–language pathologists often treat clients with psychogenic voice disorder who are referred by a laryngologist who has examined them, determined that the voice disorder is not organic, assumed it is functional or psychogenic, and referred them for voice therapy. It then is necessary for the speech–language pathologist to determine how critical the psychological or psychiatric symptoms are: Can symptomatic voice therapy remove the dysphonia before psychological or psychiatric referral? Or must the patient be seen immediately by another professional and referred back later for symptomatic voice therapy? Such a determination can be made only after the speech–language pathologist has heard a client discuss his or her background. The more background a speech–language pathologist has in psychology, the more comfortable he or she will be in determining the psychological status of clients. Nevertheless, that determination must be made. In my experience therapy to eliminate abnormal symptomatology in psychogenic voice cases usually is effective only with patterns that are extremely distinguishable from the patient's emotional or psychological status. The patient who has dysphonia only when crying or having an emotional confrontation with some other person is unlikely to be helped by symptomatic voice therapy. Such a client would benefit more by immediate referral for psychological and psychiatric services.

By the end of the evaluation period, it should be clear whether the significant aspects of the client's voice disorder are nonorganic or psychogenic. Medical evaluation should have produced a diagnosis of functional or psychogenic dysphonia, and the speech–language pathologist should expand on that diagnosis with an analysis of the vocal symptoms. Therapy then can begin to remediate the dysphonia. The therapy procedures recommended in this chapter involve removal of vocal symptoms found to be abnormal in the evaluation, without much attention to underlying psychological or psychiatric dysfunction. If the therapy is successful, the person will continue to have stress, interpersonal relationship difficulties, coping difficulties, or emotional disorder, but with a better voice. Such a therapeutic process has been called symptomatic voice therapy (Boone & McFarlane, 2000) because only symptoms are removed, not causes.

THERAPY PROCEDURES

The prognosis for removing abnormal symptoms in conversion aphonia or dysphonia depends on several factors. One of the most important is the time between the onset of vocal symptoms and the initiation of therapy to remove them. The sooner the speech–language pathologist is consulted after the origin of the voice disorder, the better the prognosis for improvement. However, several months or even years may elapse before the client seeks help. Under such conditions it is more difficult to eliminate the abnormal symptoms. The passage of time seems to stabilize the need for the symptoms. Another prognostic factor is the severity of the symptoms. The more extreme they are, whether hypofunctional or hyperfunctional, the better the prognosis for improvement, particularly when managed soon after onset. Aphonia, whispering, and extreme tension all are easier to modify than slight vocal quivering or tremor that is psychogenic and not neurologically based.

Symptomatic voice therapy with an adult or child with newly developed and extreme patterns of voice production, such as in aphonia, can be managed in a direct and straightforward manner. One of the most effective facilitators is to use a simple coughing pattern of voice initiation. Adults with psychogenic aphonia, as mentioned earlier, often do not realize that the sound heard in a cough involves the same valving and vibration principles as true phonation. The sound of the cough is the sound of vibrating vocal folds. When asked to cough, the aphonic client produces "voice" without realizing it. By extending the cough phonation into normal vowel production, normal phonation is facilitated.

Once the person can cough and prolong it into a vowel, the speech–language pathologist can suggest that the client drop the cough while continuing to produce the vowel. The individual may have trouble doing that without dropping the cough phonation. If that is the case, the speech–language pathologist should suggest that the client think of beginning to cough without actually doing so. The person should feel the "set" of a cough without actually coughing, then prolong the set into a normal vowel. A suggestion to grunt as though lifting something heavy can produce the same valving action of the vocal folds as is heard in coughing or normal phonation. This form of voicing then can be prolonged into a vowel in the same manner as the coughing method. The client also can be asked to demonstrate a forceful hum.

Coughing, grunting, and humming are all techniques of distraction. The client suddenly is producing voice without being aware of it. Whichever technique is used, it is important that the speech–language pathologist move the client quickly through steps leading to normal voice usage in communication:

1. Coughing or similar technique
2. Prolongation into a normal vowel with the cough
3. Production of all vowels
4. Monosyllabic words
5. Any word
6. Simple phrases
7. Oral reading
8. Simple conversation
9. Conversation about anything and with anyone in the clinic setting
10. Generalization to everyday communication

Because several suggestions or techniques are workable, I have a word of caution regarding how to proceed. Before trying any particular technique, such as coughing or grunting, the speech–language pathologist should make a general statement such as, "You have not lost your voice. You have merely lost the ability to make it work. We are going to try a variety of things to help you regain this ability. Let's see how they work. Let's begin by having you. . . ." With such an approach, the speech–language pathologist is not limited to just one of the techniques, as he or she would be with narrowly focused statement such as "You will speak as I have you cough." A general statement permits one technique to be attempted and if it fails another tried without discouraging the client.

I recently worked with a woman who had a psychogenic dysphonia that was based on her being terminated from employment because she was ill too often. Because she was in litigation with the company, I was not sure how successful the therapy would be.

After an extensive case history, which identified the basic psychogenic nature of her dysphonia, I decided to begin the therapy to remove her dysphonia. I started with the statement, "I am going to try some techniques that have proven helpful in eliminating voice disorder like you have, and there is a good chance that something will work." I then asked her to hum, thinking this might produce a voice that was normal. When that failed, I shifted to another technique that involved lightly touching her larynx, suggesting that if I pushed on her thyroid cartilage gently, her vocal folds would be brought together better. That did not work. Then she said, "I have noticed that when I sing I have a normal voice." I immediately said, "Good, I would like you to sing a note that you have noticed comes out well." She sang an "ah" sound at the note of E above middle C (330 Hz). Her voice was clear and beautiful. I matched her note in my falsetto voice and said, "Good, that means your larynx is working well. Keep singing that note and move it into a hum. Now notice that the tension in your voice is gone. Notice the sound is resonating nicely in your head and is not being forced in your larynx. Now, I want you to follow me down." I then hummed a tone one note lower and asked her to match it. She did so nicely. Then another note down, and another. At each step, I reinforced her effort because her voice was normal. Of course, I realized she was in a singing mode rather than speaking, but my task was first to keep her singing and move her into a pitch that was closer to a normal speaking pitch for a woman.

When we approached the note of G below middle C (around 196 Hz), I asked her to continue humming but to add a vowel to it (/mi/, /ma/, etc.). I modeled the task, still in a singing mode. Then I asked her to hum "mymymy" and slowly changed my model from a singing mode to a speaking mode, as one would say the word "my." She followed my modeling very well. I then added words to "my," such as "my man, my mother, my father," and continued in this fashion to move from the facilitating technique of singing, which she cued me to use, to speaking. In approximately half an hour, she was reading in a normal voice. One hour later, she was engaged in conversation with a normal voice. The whole therapy experience was video recorded, and it provides a marvelous tape for training. The lesson I learned was to listen to the client and respond to any cues offered about when voice is normal and use such information as perhaps a novel facilitating technique.

Once the client can communicate with voice in the therapy session, it is important to move as quickly as possible into conversation by following the steps listed. When the aphonia has been of rather short duration, the client often can move quickly into a conversation mode without the aphonia. The speech–language pathologist should accept such rapid change and say something such as, "There, you have your voice back! You have done the right thing(s) to get it going again, and you do not need to worry that you will ever lose it again."

The speech–language pathologist should continue the conversation mode until convinced of vocal stability, then make an appointment for a checkup in a few days. It is a good idea to have the client speak with normal voice with someone in the clinic setting in addition to the clinician who facilitated the voice change. Telephone contact between appointments is helpful to ensure client voice stability away from the clinic. When rapid and successful change occurs, the speech–language pathologist should remember that only the symptom of psychological disturbance has been removed, not the disturbance itself. It is a good idea to refer the client to a psychologist or psychiatrist to help with unresolved conflicts and adjustments, if such a relationship has not been established. In any case, the speech–language pathologist can have confidence that the aphonia is neither likely to return nor be replaced with some other symptom. Symptoms have been known to recur, but the common clinical finding is that they do not.

The following example illustrates the therapy approach recommended for conversion aphonia. It is the case, introduced earlier, of R. T., the 18-year-old female victim of a gas station robbery.

CASE EXAMPLE OF PSYCHOGENIC APHONIA TREATMENT

R. T. was referred because of a recently developed severe aphonia. After the robbery, as mentioned earlier, the robber cut R. T.'s throat superficially. Laryngoscopic inspection revealed an intact laryngeal neuromusculature. However, from then until her evaluation 3 weeks later, R. T. had been "unable" to produce voice; she could only whisper.

At her evaluation, I decided that no long case history about her emotional status was necessary because it seemed obvious that she suffered a conversion aphonia from a specific incident. General questioning of the mother indicated that R. T. had been a well-adjusted person before the robbery, with no evidence of voice disorder. I decided to initiate symptomatic voice therapy immediately.

I instructed R. T. to cough. She gave a loud and abrupt cough. I told her to cough again and prolong it into a vowel /a/, which I demonstrated. She accomplished this without difficulty. Several other vowels were attempted in this same manner, and the cough was eliminated without difficulty. Next, I asked her to repeat several words from a list, then to count from 1 to 20. Following the counting, I asked her to name the days of the week, months of the year, and items that could be purchased in a department store; to describe how to scramble eggs; and finally to tell what her plans were for the next few days. She explained in a clear and strong voice ("This is my normal voice") that she was planning a wedding and that she was glad to have her voice back before her wedding day.

After a few minutes of conversation about the wedding plans, I was convinced that R. T.'s voice was entirely normal and no further therapy would be needed. An appointment was made for her to return in 3 days for a checkup to ensure stability. I also mentioned that she might experience some horror memory from the robbery and that it might be helpful to see a psychologist or psychiatrist, even though her voice had returned, to help her cope and adjust. I was aware that should she be in a similar situation late at night, or see a person who reminded her of the robber, she might experience once again the same fear. I told her that should this happen, she might experience fear but would not lose her voice. That would not happen again. She was not sure how she felt about the suggestion to see a psychologist or psychiatrist but said she would consider it. When the time came for her next appointment, R. T.'s mother called to say that because of the wedding pressures, she did not want to come for the checkup and that her voice was entirely normal and expressed thanks for the help. The case of R. T. clearly represents successful voice therapy for conversion aphonia.

Therapy for Conversion Dysphonia

Many forms of conversion dysphonia, and even some aphonia cases, are not managed as easily as R. T.'s was. For example, when considerable time has passed between the development of the voice disorder and the initiation of therapy, the prognosis for quick improvement is diminished. When the client has had the voice symptoms for several months or even years, it is as though they become an integral part of everyday coping strategies. The voice pattern seems to become part of the client's communication personality and, as a result, is more resistant to easy modification. This should not discourage the speech–language pathologist, because such resistance to easy change is more typical of the everyday clinical experiences in communication disorders. Quick and easy solutions are the exception rather than the clinical rule in any therapy of communication disorders, so why should voice therapy be different?

With patients who have experienced significant, long-term psychogenic change, a simple cough, hum, or grunt technique will likely not produce voice, although these techniques should be attempted. Change will likely come only when the client learns how to produce voice; how to regulate such factors as tension, pitch, loudness, and quality; and how to cope with stress. The client must become informed and aware that although personality, emotion, and voice are highly intertwined, considerable conscious control can be exerted over the vocal system, even in emotional states. This control will not develop easily, but with careful instruction and therapeutic direction, vocal stability can be achieved by those who really seek such improvement.

Several techniques have been reported in the literature as clinically effective in achieving control over long-term psychogenic voice disorders. Most of these are directed at reducing the hyperfunctional aspects of voice production. When tension exists and the voice manifests it, it is not enough to suggest that if the person could relax when talking, the voice would improve. Rather, the individual must be taken through systematic stages of control over the muscles involved in the hyperfunctional basis of phonation. The following sections describe techniques that have been used to accomplish this control.

Progressive Relaxation

E. Jacobson (1978) proposed a method of training clients to learn to contrast states of tension in the body with its elimination through progressive relaxation. Although

Jacobson introduced this general technique many years ago, variations on the theme he established remain in contemporary approaches. The specific method of obtaining muscle relaxation in the person with psychogenic voice disorder is not as critical as focusing on the laryngeal mechanism once general body relaxation has been achieved. In Chapter 4, in a case of contact ulcers, part of the therapy involved directions for achieving relaxation by means of progressive control. This is a specific example of how progressive relaxation therapy can be integrated with voice disorder of any form when excessive muscular tension is present.

Digital Manipulation of Phonation

Although it is difficult for the typical person with a hyperfunctional psychogenic voice disorder to understand, normal phonation should be an easy process. The speech–language pathologist should demonstrate that the larynx does not work efficiently under tension but does its best when little or no effort is involved. Easy, relaxed phonation should result in the client's feeling vibration not so much in the larynx but in the resonance chambers above it. Most of the vocal energy during phonation should be felt in the oral and nasal cavities, referred to by music teachers as the mask of the face.

This balance of resonance in the mask of the face can be demonstrated by having the client feel the vibrations in the speech–language pathologist's face during normal phonation. The person should place one finger lightly on the side of the clinician's nose, another finger on the face around the lips, and another lightly on the side of the larynx around the thyroid laminae. As the speech–language pathologist phonates an /m/ sound, the client should be able to detect a balance of vibration in all three areas, with most of the sound concentration felt in the mask of the face around the lips. The client then can phonate an /m/ sound and feel the results in the same manner. The client also should experience a tingling sensation generally throughout that area and around the lips. If this is felt, chances are excellent that the larynx is being vibrated efficiently without excessive tension. The speech–language pathologist should point out how phonation in this manner seems devoid of effortful vibration in the larynx. Boone and McFarlane (2000) strongly recommend this method of monitoring normal phonation in clients with hyperfunctional voice disorders.

If management of laryngeal effort cannot be modified with the techniques mentioned here, the speech–pathologist can employ A. E. Aronson's (1990) and Roy's (2000) more aggressive physical management of eliminating musculoskeletal tension, outlined in Chapter 4 and further explained in the next section.

Muscle Tension Dysphonia

Excessive musculoskeletal tension in the extrinsic and intrinsic laryngeal structures is present even when the primary vocal symptom involves hypofunctional voice (breathiness or aphonia). Tension can be detected in the masseter, sternocleidomastoid, and mylohyoid muscles. Most other strap muscles manifest similar tension, but the masseter, sternocleidomastoid, and mylohyoid muscles are easier to palpate and thus identify the tension. The hyoid bone and thyroid cartilage often rise excessively during phonation attempts. The speech–language pathologist should not be confused by these seemingly incompatible symptoms. These disorders have been called vocal hyperfunction and muscle tension dysphonia (Barkmeier & Case, 2000; Dworkin, Meleca, & Abkarian, 2000; Stemple, 2000).

Muscle tension dysphonia is often difficult to distinguish from the vocal tension heard in adductor spasmodic dysphonia and other hyperfunctional voice disorders. It is considered a disorder devoid of neuropathology, suspected or observed, and is a manifestation of excessive laryngeal musculoskeletal tension and hyperfunctional true and false vocal fold involvement in voice. The pitch of the voice is typically extremely high as a function of the overall tension present in the vibratory system. Often there is pain associated with the excessive tension in the muscles of phonation. The etiology is considered generally unresolved psychological conflict, and treatment must combine behavioral management of the psychological conflict and techniques to correct the physiological functions of voice that are abnormal (Dworkin et al., 2000).

Laryngoscopic examination of the laryngeal structures may reveal slight swelling or reddening (edema or erythema) of the vocal folds, giving the impression that there is an organic or structural basis for the voice disorder. However, it should become apparent that the severity and extreme variability of vocal symptoms are inconsistent with the slight organic factors. The edema or erythema most likely results from the general tension associated with psychogenic voice disorder and can be considered a slight vocal abuse factor. In any case this abuse factor is not sufficient to explain the presence of the voice disorder.

Roy (2000), augmenting the original work of A. E. Aronson (1990), described techniques for assessing and treating patients with muscle tension dysphonia. This was done through an extensive case presentation of a patient with chronic mild-to-moderate dysphonia with episodes of acute difficulty bordering on aphonia. The patient was a 55-year-old woman who reported a persistent ache and tightness in her neck, larynx, and shoulder regions. She had been treated for a variety of disorders, including asthma, depression, tension headaches, gastroesophageal reflux disorder, and temporal mandibular joint dysfunction. Her employment was described as significantly stressful. Rigid videolaryngostroboscopy revealed no evidence of structural or neurological pathology. The closed phase of vocal fold vibration dominated the vibratory cycle. Musculoskeletal tension was assessed manually and found in several areas around her larynx. Pain was noted when these areas were manually palpated, and it was noted that her larynx was excessively elevated by supralaryngeal musculature in hypercontracted states. The larynx was lowered and muscle tension reduced through use of the techniques of circumlaryngeal massage as described by A. E. Aronson (1990) and explained in this book. The patient's voice immediately improved, and with only one significant relapse, which required a repetition of the circumlaryngeal massage techniques, she remained symptom free at 3- and 6-month follow-up visits. Roy reported this same success in 25 patients with various forms of functional voice disorder with these techniques.

Vocal Abuse as a Psychogenic Voice Disorder

Several writers have classified dysphonia resulting from vocal abuse (vocal nodules, contact ulcers, acute laryngitis from abuse, etc.) as a form of psychogenic voice disorder. A. E. Aronson (1990) indicated that because clients who develop vocal nodules and contact ulcers tend to fit the same type of personality profile (highly vocal and intense in verbal interactions, hard driving, perfectionistic, loud speakers, etc.), they should be classified as having psychogenic voice disorders. I believe most cases of vocal abuse occur in clients or patients with aggressive or intense personalities, but to classify vocal abuse clients as having a psychogenic disorder confuses the issue of the nature of psychogenic voice disorder.

Case Studies of Psychogenic Voice Disorder

Several excellent case studies of the evaluation and treatment of patients with psychogenic voice disorder, often called functional voice disorder, are found in the literature. Stemple (2000) edited a book that contains numerous examples of case management of psychogenic voice disorder from many authorities. The case examples by Andrews, Glaze, Casper, Hufnagle, Lee, and McFarlane and Von Berg, Stemple, Case, and Stone all contribute significantly to the literature on management of these psychogenic dysphonias and aphonias. Each case example provides subtle variations on the themes presented in this chapter and will aid the speech–language pathologist in management techniques. Andrews (1999) presented another interesting case, involving a gay male whose self-evaluation of voice was that it "sounds like a young kid's voice," although he wanted to "sound like Walter Cronkite." Stemple et al. (2000) discussed the various disorders generally classified under the umbrella of psychogenic dysphonia/aphonia and presented case studies that involved treatments that, although effective, were unnecessary and perhaps unethical because false statements were issued regarding the cause of the disorder. For example, it would be misleading and unethical to examine a patient and state something to the effect that "a 'little piece of cartilage' is out of place in your larynx, and if you will 'raise your arms while I push on the cartilage,' it will be fixed and your voice will be fine." It is clear that such deceit is unnecessary because straightforward and correct statements about how the larynx is being used improperly would facilitate the therapy techniques necessary to improve the voice.

PUBERPHONIA

One of the most easily corrected psychogenic voice disorders is puberphonia, also called mutational falsetto. During puberty, the typical male experiences significant body transformations as a result of hormonal changes that produce growth spurts and the development of secondary sex characteristics. Failure to adjust the voice to reflect these changes is the basis for puberphonia. Chapter 1, in the section on age and sex differences in fundamental frequency, refers to the specifics of laryngeal change during pubescence. The growth changes in the larynx during this time essentially parallel general body development. Kahane (1982) discussed these changes in terms of (a) vocal fold length, (b) vocal fold mass or thickness, and (c) cartilage and tissue weight. The interaction between the changes reflected in pubescence, which is the biological change, and adolescence, which is the psychological change, constitutes the basis for the development of psychogenic voice disorder at that age.

The process of biological growth is a gradual one, beginning around age 11 for girls and age 12 for boys. In girls, breast and pubic hair development and height increase all begin about age 12. Their growth spurt peaks at about age 12½, and by age 16, the average girl has reached adult height. Menarche (menstruation) in girls generally begins around the peak growth spurt of age 12½ (in the United States) but often does not start until age 16. In boys the testes begin to grow at about age 11½ and are adult size by age 16. Penis growth begins about age 12 and usually stops at about age 15. The growth spurt for height and general body size in boys begins about age 12 and peaks as a spurt at about age 14. By age 17, the typical male has achieved adult height. There may be significant variations in individual differences, because these figures reflect only averages (Offer, 1980; Wierzbicki, 1999).

Most adult hormonal levels are achieved by age 16 in both sexes. The interaction between the hypothalamus of the central nervous system and the pituitary, thyroid, ovaries, and testes of the endocrine system in producing the hormonal bases of puberty, associated growth, and secondary sex characteristic development is complex and cannot be treated in significant detail here. However, full details can be found in Offer (1980), Wierzbicki (1999), and Webster (1999). Generally, the factors are as shown in Table 6.1 and are based on the early and classic work of Kalat (1981) and confirmed by Webster (1999).

With an understanding of the complex growth (body and larynx) and hormonal changes associated with puberty, one can better understand the effect of abnormalities

TABLE 6.1

Factors in Sexual Maturation

Organ[a]	Hormone Secreted	Hormone Function (Partial)
Hypothalamus (part of CNS)	TRF (thyrotropin-releasing factor)	Causes pituitary to release TSH (thyrotropic hormone or thyroid-stimulating hormone)
	LRF (luteinizing hormone-releasing factor)	Causes pituitary to release LH (luteinizing hormone)
Pituitary gland (endocrine)	TSH	Stimulates thyroid gland
	LH	In female: causes ovary to produce progesterone In male: causes testes to produce testosterone
	FSH (follicle-stimulating hormone)	In female: causes ovary to produce estrogen In male: causes testes to produce sperm
	Oxytocin	Affects mammary glands and uterus
	ACTH (adrenocorticotrophic hormone)	Stimulates adrenal gland to secrete steroid hormones
	STH (somatrophic or "growth" hormone)	Promotes muscle and bone growth and metabolic processes (utilization of glucose for fuel)
Thyroid gland	Thyroxine and triiodothyronine	Increases metabolic rate; promotes growth, bone development, sex gland maturation, maturation of nervous system
Ovary glands	Estrogens, including estradiol	Affects female secondary sexual characteristics, including breast development, female sex drive, ovulation
	Progesterone	Maintains pregnancy
	Androgens (small amounts)	Not clearly understood in females
Testes	Androgens, including testosterone	Affects male secondary sexual characteristics, including penis size, pubic hair, body hair, sex drive, sperm production
	Estrogens (small amounts)	Not clearly understood in males

Note. Adapted From *Biological Psychology*, by J. W. Kalat, 1981, Belmont, CA: Wadsworth. Copyright 1981 by Wadsworth Publishing Co. Adapted with permission.

[a]Only the organs and glands pertaining to the topic of this chapter are included here.

in biology or psychological pressures of adolescence. With regard to puberphonia, the psychological pressures of adolescence seem to have more of an effect on the genesis of the disorder than do the biological changes of puberty.

During puberty, the typical male experiences major body changes due to growth and hormone factors. The larynx similarly changes rapidly. Voice quality and pitch change significantly, often in a matter of a few months. The pitch of a young man's voice manifests the most significant and noticeable vocal change. As a result of rather sudden increases in vocal fold length and mass, the typical young male's pitch will drop about one octave, or eight whole tones. The voice also becomes more resonant and acquires a richer and fuller quality. Essentially, in a few short months the boy's voice becomes a man's. This is also true of female voices but to a less drastic degree (Ferrand, 2000).

In some instances the transition from boy to man is not easy. Not only is it difficult to handle increased responsibility in life, but the rapid body changes can also be confusing and difficult to understand. When a boy has difficulty in making these adjustments, puberphonia or mutational falsetto can develop. Kaplan (1982) described mutational falsetto as the psychological failure of the adolescent's voice to descend or maintain its descent to a normal adult pitch at puberty. Instead, the adolescent (usually male) raises his voice above its prepubertal pitch and consistently speaks in a falsetto voice. Untreated, the symptom may be lifelong. Kaplan contrasted mutational falsetto voice with what he called persistent pubertal voice, which involves symptoms beyond voice that suggest the possibility of an endocrinologic disorder manifesting itself as delayed puberty. Welch, Sergeant, and MacCurtain (1988) and Andrews (1999) provided information on the speech and voice characteristics of the male falsetto speaker. In my experience, this voice disorder of puberty and adolescence can have the following characteristics:

- A pitch level that is typical of the prepuberty voice and is maintained after the boy has essentially completed the biological changes of puberty

- A pitch level that is excessively higher (usually falsetto) than that of the typical prepuberty voice after the biological changes of puberty have occurred

- A pitch level that is typical of the prepuberty voice when the biological changes of puberty have not occurred at an age at which they normally would be completed

- A voice that is unusually high for a mature male but is compatible with the size of the laryngeal structures but incompatible with body size

The first three of these disorders are functionally based, the last is structurally or organically based, and all have psychogenic components. In all cases the pitch and overall quality are the dramatic characteristics of dysphonia. One recently seen client was a 15-year-old male with significantly high-pitched and somewhat aperiodic voice quality. On evaluation it was immediately apparent that his voice was typical of puberphonia. However, on laryngeal inspection a unilateral vocal fold paralysis was noted. His mother said, "Oh, I remember he was born with that." It was not clear from my case history whether this maternal statement was true, but in all likelihood it was. I supposed he had spoken with a paralyzed vocal fold most if not all of his life and developed a high-pitched voice because an elevated pitch helped with overall voice quality. I also speculated that when he went through puberty, his dysphonia was magnified by growth changes and he continued to maintain an elevated pitch. When I lowered his pitch to a more appropriate level, his voice was breathy and dysphonic as a result the paralysis. I recommended an examination by an ears–nose–throat physician who might perform thyroplasty type I to improve medialization of his paralyzed vocal fold. This was done. Following a period of healing, therapy was resumed and the boy was able to stabilize his voice at an appropriate level.

Voice Factors in Puberphonia

The most common form of puberphonia occurs when a male goes through the biological changes of puberty and experiences body and laryngeal growth changes but does not allow the pitch of the voice to descend to its adult level. This functional voice disorder results when a boy is not able to make the vocal transition to manhood. The perceptual effect is a boy's voice in a man's body. The development of this disorder is not understood clearly other than from the perspective of clinical experience. Several cases I have seen provide the profile described here.

The male who develops puberphonia usually is shy and somewhat insecure in personal relationships. Case history data from parents and clients verify this point. I think that most males experience some embarrassment about the rapidly changing voice during puberty, although this seems to be a momentary concern for most. During this period, pitch breaks and other voice adjustment problems occur, but they seem to have a significant effect only on the male who has a poor self-image or who is shy and insecure.

For example, should a pitch break occur in a boy around a friend or group of peers, teasing may result. Nobody enjoys being teased, but the boy who has a poor self-concept and is not secure in peer relationships can be devastated psychologically by it. The boy is likely to become concerned about a recurrence. It is almost as though he becomes so worried about a pitch break that it is on his mind each time he begins to talk, especially if he is in a socially difficult situation, such as being with a girl or with peers. He may think such thoughts as, "I wonder if my voice will squeak or break if I talk to her. I hope it doesn't happen here."

This concern about pitch stability before speaking sets the stage for the development of puberphonia. To obtain pitch function and ensure that breaks will be unlikely to occur, the boy may attempt to keep his pitch at the level he has always used (i.e., his prepuberty level). It is not long before his old pitch becomes stabilized and the puberphonic dysphonia has been established. The following sections describe typical voice characteristics of the male who has developed puberphonia.

Pitch Factors

Few data are available regarding the pitch of individuals with puberphonia. Although Welch et al. (1988) presented data on vocal and laryngeal characteristics of male falsetto singers (countertenor or male alto), the only group pitch data specific to puberphonia before and after therapy have been presented by Case (1987). Pitch levels of 7 clients with puberphonia were recorded before and after therapy on high-quality instrumentation (Nakamichi 550 DualTracer Stereo Recorder). All clients were male (mean age = 16.8, range = 14 to 18 years) and indicated (self-report or parental report) that essential completion of physical puberty and secondary sex changes had occurred. All therapy was accomplished in one or two sessions, with an average time of 4 hours. Although checkups were scheduled and maintained, no relapse was found.

The audio recordings of pre–post therapy speech samples were computer analyzed, digitized at a sampling rate of 10 kHz/sec. Figure 6.1 provides the results for the 7 clients. Fundamental frequency is represented along the ordinate (y-axis) and the subjects are represented along the abscissa (x-axis). Individual subject means (before and after therapy) are provided, as well as group means.

The group mean before therapy was 250.4 Hz. These data indicate that the pre-therapy mean was well above the mean-acceptable F_0 for 16-year-old males (150 Hz, acceptable range 125 to 180 Hz; Kent, 1994b) and even above the acceptable level for 16-year-old females (215 Hz, range 180 to 255 Hz; Kent, 1994b). In other words, these male clients had a mean pitch level at the upper end of what Kent described as acceptable for females. The highest mean for subject J.O. was 377 Hz, which is not acceptable for a person of any age or sex. The group mean after therapy was 126.9 Hz. As a group these clients were well within normal limits of pitch and even at the lower end of the range of normal expectations as reported by Kent. The lowest subject mean was 105 Hz, which is lower than the expected mean of 18-year-old males.

The typical pitch level of a young male with puberphonia is more closely matched to that of a female who has completed puberty, about 200 Hz. This is the lowest habitual pitch level that the typical client with puberphonia uses, although instances of extremely high pitch (falsetto) are common. By contrast a postpuberty 17-year-old male has a normal pitch around 135 Hz, with an acceptable range from 98 to 150 Hz (Kent, 1994b). The pitch frequently breaks upward or downward. The young man may even experience moments of "low voice" that occur when he is relaxed and not threatened by the speaking situation or during a spontaneous laugh.

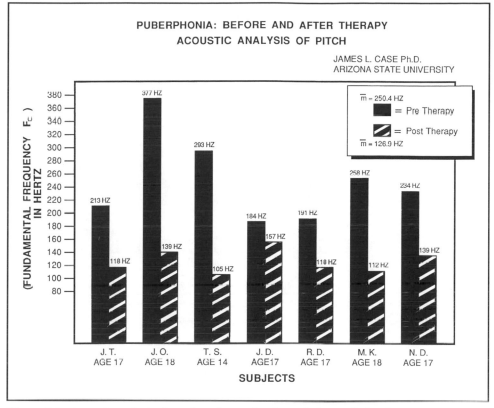

Figure 6.1. Acoustic analysis of vocal pitch in puberphonia before and after therapy.

Except for the breaks, the habitual pitch level of the boy with puberphonia is monotonic and devoid of natural inflections. Diplophonia (double pitch) is common. However, the unnaturally high voice is the striking characteristic of this disorder. Sex confusion over the phone is common; when the male with puberphonia answers the phone and the caller asks, "Hello, is your husband home?" fuel is added to the psychogenic factor.

Quality Factors

The voice of the puberphonic speaker usually is of normal quality in terms of laryngeal vibration and resonance. Hoarseness is rare. Slight tension is heard at times, but it is a minor concern and probably results from the speaker's use of a pitch level that is not appropriate for his larynx, so that increased effort is necessary to maintain voice continuity.

Loudness Factors

The speaker with puberphonia has essentially normal loudness ability in conversation but sometimes complains of not being able to yell. This is related to using a pitch level that is not compatible for the larynx under normal conditions and thus limits its projection potential. It also is related in many cases to a shy personality that is nearly incompatible with yelling in social situations.

Resonance Factors

Puberphonia does not produce any significant alteration in vocal resonance. Hyponasality or hypernasality in the vocal signal probably results from an independent factor (see Chapter 8). Therefore, resonance is expected to be normal.

THERAPY FOR PUBERPHONIA

Therapy for puberphonia in most instances begins in the evaluation session after it is clear that puberphonia is the diagnosis.

Case History

Obtaining appropriate case history information for a client with puberphonia is fairly straightforward. The speech–language pathologist asks questions about when the pitch disorder first occurred, when the onset of puberty was, what was happening socially during the puberty change, whether there were instances of speaking avoidance because of embarrassment about pitch breaks, and whether any conscious attempt was made to keep pitch at a high level.

Generally, it is necessary to gain perspective only about the relationship between puberty and the current state of the voice. A. E. Aronson (1990) wisely suggested exploring additional factors such as delayed maturation of the laryngeal structures because of endocrine imbalance; severe hearing loss, which makes pitch monitoring difficult; neurological disease during adolescence change; and general debilitating illness during puberty. From this information, the speech–language pathologist can determine whether medical referral is necessary. If any question exists after such a case history as to the possibility of a physical basis for the pitch disorder, it is important to obtain current medical information by appropriate referral.

The client's voice characteristics of pitch, quality, and loudness are rated. This is important in obtaining a measurement of the habitual pitch level, using procedures outlined earlier. The speech–language pathologist should obtain an audio or video recording of a 5-minute conversation sample during which the client reads a short paragraph. Any instances of low-pitched voice should be noted.

In most instances, after a case history and voice evaluation have been completed, it should be apparent that puberphonia is the basis for the disorder. It is particularly helpful to have medical information on the client, either before or shortly after the evaluation, indicating that the laryngeal structures are normal for voice production.

Voice Stimulation Techniques

Once puberphonia is established as the basis for the pitch disorder, the speech–language pathologist should explain to the client the likely relationship between the onset of puberty and the voice problem. The professional then uses one or both of the techniques that follow to try to find the client's true pitch.

• *Cough.* A human cough creates a sound that is a result of air vibrating the closed vocal folds. It is a rough form of phonation using the same mechanisms as in normal voice production. Because coughing, compared with normal phonation, is a biological act, it is not subject to the emotions associated with phonation in human communication. Therefore, when the client coughs, the sound usually reflects the condition of the vocal folds in a natural state. The pitch of the cough roughly approximates the normal pitch. A cough can facilitate the use of a more appropriate pitch.

• *Digital manipulation.* Gentle pushing on the thyroid cartilage of the larynx during phonation suddenly relaxes the vocal folds, and the pitch drops approximately one whole tone. The technique is to have the client relax and say "ah" as the speech–language pathologist pushes gently on the thyroid cartilage. The pitch goes down, and when the dropped tone is heard, the client is instructed to hold on to it as the pressure on the thyroid cartilage is released. The process is repeated as the client lowers his pitch in whole-tone steps.

An additional technique for obtaining an appropriate pitch in clients with puberphonia by using vocal fry is provided by Pinho, Navas, Case, and LaPointe (1993). When the client has a pitch that is appropriate for his age, the speech–language pathologist stabilizes it and shapes it into conversation using techniques explained next.

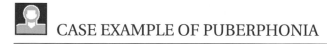 CASE EXAMPLE OF PUBERPHONIA

This case illustrates how evaluation and treatment procedures for puberphonia can be handled. R. D., a 15-year-old male, was referred by an otolaryngologist because of persistent diplophonia (double-pitched voice) and an inappropriately high-pitched tone. He also had been treated by another physician who had diagnosed R. D. as having contact ulcers on his vocal folds.

R. D.'s case history revealed nothing of significance about his pitch disorder other than that his "voice did not change when it was supposed to." It seemed apparent that, because recent examinations by otolaryngologists indicated normal laryngeal structures and the case history was devoid of significance other than the delayed voice change at puberty, R. D. had puberphonia. The recording of the language I used in explanation to R. D., which follows, is an example of voice management of this disorder.

> Let me explain what has happened to your voice. During the years of puberty change, as your body was growing and changing, you probably experienced some frustration handling the pitch of your voice. This frustration led you to keep the pitch of your voice with which you were most familiar rather than let it change. We are going to try some techniques to help you find your best pitch. It may be easy; it may be hard. Let's find out.
>
> First, I want you to cough like this. [I demonstrated a cough.] Did you notice that the sound of your cough was low, much lower than your speaking voice? That is because your vocal folds were vibrating at a pitch that was natural for them.
>
> Now try it again. [R. D. coughed at around 147 Hz.] Good, try it again . . . and again. Now cough and prolong the cough into an "ah" sound like this. [I demonstrated. R. D. coughed, followed by an "ah" at the same pitch level.] Good. Notice your pitch stayed low with both the cough and the "ah." Do it again . . . and again.
>
> Now I want you to "think" of a cough without actually coughing and say "ah" at that pitch. [R. D. did.] Good. Do it again. Now say "ah" like you have been, then go into an "o" sound like this. [I demonstrated. R. D. did it.] Good. Now you can say any sound at that pitch level. Say the following sounds after me. [R. D. repeated 10 different vowel sounds after I modeled.]

In a few minutes, using a biological state of the larynx to facilitate normal phonation at an appropriate pitch level, R. D. learned to control his pitch and left the therapy session with a new voice. As he became comfortable with his new pitch, he relaxed and his voice lowered to an appropriate habitual pitch of 110 Hz. During the first session, he was able to read orally, converse with me about school, then chat for 20 minutes with his sister, who had accompanied him. I monitored this conversation to determine that he maintained his new pitch level.

As he left the clinic, I instructed R. D. to use his new pitch in any situation in which he felt comfortable. I called him a few hours later and he reported difficulty using his new pitch in all speaking situations, including those with close friends. He mentioned that several persons had commented on his new voice, but he dismissed these comments by saying he had a cold. Four days later R. D. returned to the clinic and I recorded him in conversation. All aspects of his voice were judged normal, including pitch, quality, and loudness. He was using his voice in all speaking situations and felt comfortable with it.

Special Considerations in Puberphonia

Although puberphonia is a functional voice disorder and easy to remediate when handled properly, there are a few cautions to be aware of. As the speech–language pathologist begins to change the client's voice, care should be taken not to indicate to the client that if one specific technique is used, the proper pitch level will occur (e.g., telling the client to cough and the proper pitch will emerge). Rather, the professional should indicate that several methods will be attempted to help the client find his new pitch and that one of them should work. Then, if failure occurs on the first technique, the client will not become easily discouraged.

When the client hears his new low-pitched voice, he may comment that he does not like it. This is understandable because he has never heard himself speaking at a low level. Because he is not used to it and so does not like it, he may be somewhat reluctant to try it with others, assuming that they will not like it either. The speech–language pathologist should tell him that he soon will be accustomed to it and that others will like it immediately. He should test his new voice with strangers, such as store clerks, and he will notice no negative reaction to his pitch. Such experiences will help him develop confidence that his new pitch is normal.

Care also should be taken not to lower the client's voice too much; rather, an appropriate pitch level about three or four tones from the basal should be sought. This new level will allow downward inflections in the client's voice without approaching the basal, which would likely produce excessive laryngeal tension if used often. Even when the pitch still seems somewhat high after it is lowered, it should be kept in mind that, as the client matures into adulthood, his voice will become deeper in pitch and richer in resonance.

If the client expresses concern about using his new pitch around persons other than the speech–language pathologist, it may be necessary to carefully control the process of generalization from the clinic or school therapy to other situations. This can be done through ranking all speaking situations according to task difficulty. This is called hierarchy analysis of typical speaking situations (Boone & McFarlane, 2000) and is done by assigning the student to speak with his new voice first in situations low on the task hierarchy before moving on to the more stressful levels.

It is important that the change of pitch from puberphonic to normal occur quickly relative to the typical school communication disorder therapy durations of weeks and months. Within 2 or 3 days, the change should be complete. Even in settings such as the school, where the student might usually be seen by the speech–language pathologist only a few minutes a week, it is important to change the student's schedule to accommodate intense therapy. The speech–language pathologist must be assertive in expecting the student to use the new pitch in situations that may be rather uncomfortable at first. The youth should be told that any discomfort he experiences will be momentary and that people soon will not even notice the change.

Working with clients who have puberphonia can be most satisfying to the speech–language pathologist, who is accustomed to only slight change when working with most clients with communication disorder. To hear a boy, in a few hours or days, significantly change a voice pattern that has caused so much concern and embarrassment can compensate for more-frustrating therapy efforts.

Literature Review in Puberphonia

In addition to the factors already discussed, A. E. Aronson (1990) identified several etiologies of puberphonia:

- Delayed maturation in endocrine disorders that retard laryngeal development, perpetuating a high-pitched voice that then becomes difficult to abandon because of longer-than-normal persistence into adolescence, even after the larynx has attained normal size.

- Severe hearing loss, preventing the individual from perceiving the voice during adolescent voice change.

- Weakness or incoordination of the vocal folds or of respiration during puberty because of neurologic disease.

- General debilitating illness during puberty, which not only may delay overall growth during puberty but also, because of the physical restrictions of being bedfast, reduce the range of respiratory excursions and consequently tidal air volumes, preventing the development of adequate infraglottal air pressure.

Aronson also indicated that several patients have been seen as adults (in their 50s and 60s), often for the first time, in an attempt to change their voice. The prognosis for changing even these adults' voices is excellent using the methods outlined.

Kaplan (1982) presented a unique case of mutational falsetto that appears to be different from the typical profile. In this case, a 15-year-old boy who had been speaking in a falsetto for 2 years was treated for the dysphonia by psychotherapy. The client was able to demonstrate to the psychotherapist that he was capable of speaking in a lower voice but failed to understand why his parents were so concerned that he did not speak using it. He persisted in speaking in a falsetto. After two sessions of psychotherapy directed toward helping the client understand his motivations for using the falsetto, the boy began speaking in his low voice. Therapy was terminated after five sessions with the boy's using the low voice consistently; a 6-month follow-up revealed the pitch was maintained at the low level.

Six months after the follow-up, the boy began to develop symptoms of behavior deterioration in school and social coping, with auditory hallucinations that people were calling him a homosexual and telling him to physically assault classmates. He was diagnosed as developing a psychotic disorder and was admitted to an inpatient psychiatric unit with a diagnosis of schizophreniform disorder. On the night of admission, he physically assaulted staff members because he felt that his display of physical prowess would communicate to the voices (hallucinations) that he was a man. He was treated with high-dose phenothiazine medication and was released after 2 months. Although this case appears unique and is the first reported in the literature in which mutational falsetto preceded schizophrenia, it serves as an alert to professionals who treat this disorder to monitor the psychological or psychiatric status of these clients during and following voice therapy.

Hartman and Aronson (1983) reported an interesting case of psychogenic aphonia that masked itself as mutational falsetto. A 14-year-old boy experienced aphonia because of laryngeal inflammation that persisted as a psychogenic aphonia after the inflammation subsided. The psychogenic aphonia became superimposed on the unstable pitch of adolescent voice change. The details of treatment in the case are consistent with the procedures outlined earlier.

Peppard (2000) presented two cases of puberphonic treatment. One was a 15-year-old boy with a pitch level around 260 Hz. The boy was significantly hearing impaired, and his voice was changed to an appropriate pitch level in approximately three sessions. The second case was of functional falsetto (ranging from 205 to 860 Hz) in a woman whose voice was changed using a hard glottal attack, which produced the deepest and loudest tone that she had ever heard emanate from her mouth. The sound that emerged, which was appropriate for her, shocked and puzzled her, and she could hardly believe Peppard when he explained that the sound she heard was appropriate (around 196 Hz).

A final example, a 15-year-old boy with hearing impairment thought to be etiologically related to the development of his puberphonia, was provided by Peppard (2000). He had a bilateral, symmetrical, moderate-to-profound sensorineural hearing loss averaging 95 dB HL (hearing level). His loss was acquired after he had developed speech and language. He wore binaural, ear-level hearing aids. A voice evaluation determined that he spoke with a voice around 260 Hz with reduced intensity and used a fairly monotone voice. In three therapy sessions his voice was stabilized at around 140 Hz, with increased loudness projection.

Organic Puberphonia

In some cases of voice disorder, for organic reasons the larynx fails to develop to its adult size and the voice remains at prepuberty pitch, quality, and resonance. Endocrine imbalance must be suspected in such cases, and the only reasonable treatment is medical. When pubescence, general development of secondary sex characteristics, and changes in voice and larynx size are delayed, such endocrine imbalance must be considered as an etiology and must be evaluated by an endocrinologist or other physician.

The ancient custom of castration of male adolescents and adults for a variety of reasons provides evidence of the effect of endocrine imbalance on the voice. For example, castration was done to produce eunuchs as slaves in brothels, harems, and the courts of royalty; for religious excommunication; for revenge on prisoners of war; and to produce a certain singing quality in early religious music. St. Paul wrote, "Let your women keep silence in the church" (1 Corinthians 14:34); therefore, women could not be used in church choirs. Much has been written about the famous castrate voice; one excellent reference is Brodnitz (1988).

It is difficult to know how common puberphonia is as a voice disorder. I would assume most young men go through the process of puberty and have only minor and somewhat nuisance experiences with pitch breaks and stability. However, because puberphonia is devastating to the young man vocally trapped by it, and its management is so straightforward and successful, it is unfortunate when speech–language pathologists do not treat it appropriately. I had a recent case involving a young man with puberphonia who had been treated for nearly 8 months without any success. Within 2 hours, his vocal pitch was lowered to an appropriate level and stabilized in conversation using the techniques discussed in this chapter. I have not experienced one example of this disorder that was not successfully treated within a few sessions following these therapy strategies.

PARADOXICAL VOCAL FOLD DYSFUNCTION

Christopher et al. (1983) introduced the medical world to a functional voice disorder that mimics attacks of bronchial asthma ("pseudoasthma"). They reported on 5 patients who presented with symptoms of dramatic episodes of wheezing and who had been diagnosed as having uncontrolled asthma. Paroxysms (sudden recurrence or intensification) of wheezing and dyspnea persisted despite aggressive medical management, including bronchodilators and long-term steroid therapy. The terms used to describe this disorder include *paradoxical vocal fold function, laryngeal dyskinesia, pseudoasthma, functional upper airway obstruction,* and *stridor,* and many authorities, particularly pulmonologists, now refer to it as *vocal cord dysfunction* (VCD). I prefer the terms *paradoxical vocal fold dysfunction* (PVFD) or *paradoxical vocal fold movement* (PVFM) because they describe more exactly the nature of the disorder (Stemple, 2000). The essential aspect of this disorder is that the vocal folds are closed or adducted to some degree during respiration, particularly when inhalation is attempted. In some cases the constriction occurs in the supraglottic regions of the larynx or in the ventricular folds (Powell et al., 2000). This is the paradox of vocal fold (cord)

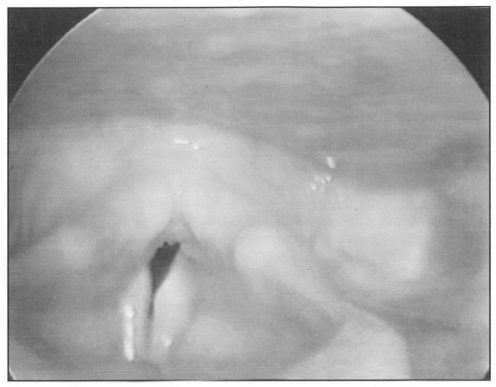

Figure 6.2. Paradoxical vocal fold movement. (Larynx shown during inhalation.)

movement. Therefore, dyspnea is the most critical aspect of this disorder. Often the voice is essentially normal, but it is not uncommon to find various degrees of dysphonia. PVFD is often episodic, sometimes in a predictable manner, other times capricious and unpredictable. It is typically seen in women (Andrews, 1999), but it is also seen in juveniles (Trudeau, 1998). Patients usually report predictable factors that trigger the episodes. Rammage, Morrison, and Nichol (2001) reported a relationship in some patients between PVFD and the irritable larynx syndrome, which manifests itself in many ways, including as PVFD. PVFD is typically described as a psychogenic disorder, but Blager (2000) reported on possible subcategories of patients that might present with CNS laryngeal dysfunction. Figure 6.2 demonstrates the dysfunction of a patient's vocal fold during inhalation.

PVFD is often associated with asthma because patients suffering from various degrees of asthma alter their respiration pattern (Lee, 2000a). Blager (2000), in an excellent review of the literature pertaining to this disorder, reported that as many as 10% of patients with recalcitrant asthma have PVFD. Because breathing difficulty is so much a part of their daily existence, it is understandable why patients with a history of asthma are more vulnerable to the development of PVFD. Loudon, Lee, and Holcomb (1988) studied 10 healthy individuals and compared them with 14 patients with various degrees of asthma. Their protocol involved conversation, monologue, and counting at two loudness levels while measuring respiration patterns with a Respitrace. They found that asthma patients used a greater percentage of their reduced vital capacity, had a slower inspiratory flow rate and a faster expiratory flow rate, and spent a greater amount of the total respiratory cycle time on inspiration. When necessary, asthma patients favored respiratory needs over communication needs and would cease speaking to maintain necessary ventilation. Couple this daily or episodic struggle and breathing concerns with any stress factors present in a person's life, and it is easy to see how PVFD could develop.

PVFD is often also associated with athletic activity and persons required to perform physically under stressful conditions, such as military personnel (Blager, 2000; Powell et al., 2000). I recently worked with an 18-year-old female from Michigan who attended Arizona State on an athletic scholarship. She was an excellent long-distance runner and had won several awards and achievements in Michigan at the high school level. However, she struggled to compete at the higher levels of the PAC 10 Conference. She began to experience dyspnea in her races, forcing her to drop out of many of them. She was referred to me by an athletic pulmonologist who was suspicious of PVFD, which was confirmed by my evaluation. Her background, evaluation procedure, and treatment considerations were similar to those for the patients reported by Swift (2000), Andrianopoulos (2000), and Powell et al. (2000) regarding excellent athletes who had difficulty and anxiety competing at higher levels of performance at major universities or who were experiencing other aspects of psychosocial difficulty.

Case (2000) presented a case of PVFD that had been referred with a diagnosis of "functional upper airway obstruction." The patient was a 33-year-old woman who had been hospitalized several times for chronic airway obstruction. No proper diagnosis was made until she was seen at the Mayo Clinic in Scottsdale, Arizona. She was referred to Arizona State University for therapy.

The patient presented with severe stridor during breathing and dysphonia. Spectrographic, laryngographic, and stroboscopic documentation confirmed the diagnosis, and therapy was immediately instituted. By demonstrating to the patient endoscopically on videotape how the vocal folds were being misused functionally, then teaching relaxation during breathing and voice production, I was able to help the patient eliminate the dysphonia and the stridor in one therapy session. Follow-up by phone for several months provided documentation that this functional disorder was no longer a problem for this patient.

Some patients with paradoxical vocal fold movement present with breathing difficulty but no dysphonia; in other instances, both breathing stridor and dysphonia are present. The treatment is straightforward. The speech–language pathologist can document the disorder by using endoscopy recorded on videotape. The recording can be shown to the patient and instructions provided as to how the larynx works in respiration and phonation. If necessary, flexible endoscopy can be used for real-time feedback. With the scope in place, the patient can be taught to relax and allow the vocal folds to abduct for breathing, close for phonation, then open again for breathing. The real-time feedback is powerful in this teaching process. Once control has been established, negative practice can be introduced in which the patient is encouraged to deliberately adduct the vocal folds during inhalation and then relax the larynx so that abduction occurs, facilitating normal inhalation.

The treatment protocol for this disorder, as explained by the cited authorities, follows similar patterns. A nice summary protocol was presented by Von Berg, Watterson, and Fudge (1999) and involves four general categories of treatment:

1. Patient education: anatomy and physiology of the laryngeal mechanism
2. Relaxation of the jaw, shoulder, and neck muscles
3. Placing focus of breathing at the oral/nasal cavities away from the glottis
4. Identifying and reducing the number of precipitators to the PVFM episodes

PVFD is often difficult to diagnose, particularly when the professional involved is not familiar with this disorder. The case study by Andrianopoulos (2000) illustrates this difficulty, with the patient's being referred to several medical specialists (otolaryngology, gastroenterology, allergy, pulmonology–respiratory) and finally to a speech–language pathologist, who provided treatment. It is necessary to explore many facets of life when treating a person with PVFD because it is such a complicated disorder. Treatment requires attention to patient education about phonatory anatomy and physiology, normal and abnormal respiratory processes, psychological and psychosocial considerations, muscle tension locations on the body affecting voice and breathing, factors that trigger the episodes, and support along the therapy highway of desensitization and control. PVFD is a challenging disorder but one that responds nicely to properly directed therapy.

GENDER DYSPHORIA AND REASSIGNMENT

In the third edition of this book, this section on gender presentation and reassignment referred to the issue as transsexualism. Much has changed since 1996 in this arena. It is now clear that *transsexualism* refers to only one small aspect of a person who is unhappy with his or her gender. The phrase *gender dysphoria* connotes someone who is uncomfortable with his or her socially and culturally assigned gender role. The phrase *sexual dysphoria* connotes unhappiness or discomfort with one's biological makeup or sex. There are several continua along which people fall with regard to how they are perceived by society. No one is entirely dichotomized into gender. The term *unisexual* describes cultural, sociological, and personal phenomena that are not clearly dimorphic with regard to sexual identification. Whether it is in dress, vocations, avocations, hairstyles, jewelry, or a variety of other elements, the unisex concept applies more and more to today's society.

One continuum along which a person falls is biological, ranging from strongly male to strongly female. Various traits place most individuals somewhere along the continuum. With regard to gender presentation, rather than sexual biology of being male or female, there is the continuum ranging from strong masculinity to strong femininity. Most individuals can identify traits that confuse the gender continuum. Additionally, in a strict biological sense, along the continuum of sexual orientation, many individuals fall somewhere between strongly heterosexual and strongly homosexual (Andrews, 1999). Many have some degree of bisexuality. The developing embryo has clearly defined unisexual potential until the endocrine system makes its mark and the infant becomes sexually defined. This is the role of the Y chromosome and its genes in the XY pair of sex chromosomes, which distinguishes males from females, who have two XX chromosomes. Hermaphrodites, who are intermediate between normal male and female in anatomy, or have genes of one sex and anatomy of another, are common abnormalities (Durden-Smith & Desimone, 1984). The term *hermaphrodite* refers to biological disparity of gender and perhaps is an antiquated term. It does not address the issue of mind, self, personality, and gender satisfaction. Hausman (1995) conceptualized that when an incompatibility exists between mind and body, either the body must be made to fit the mind and self, or the mind and self must be made to fit the body. The degree to which this disparity cannot be adjusted provides the basis for gender dysphoria.

With all of this sexual confusion, it is a wonder that more people do not experience difficulty with gender identity. Certainly, most of the traits other than physical distinction, which identify gender, emerge through the development years. No behavior or trait is clearly gender specific during the first year of life.

Brodnitz (1988) indicated that voice professionals are seeing increased numbers of individuals with forms of gender dysphoria. One such category of voice concern more commonly seen by speech–language pathologists is the client with gender and sometimes sexual dysphoria who seeks some degree of transformation and reassignment. In most speech and hearing clinics where services to help in this process are available, clients are typically attempting to move from the gender of male to female. Clients are seen in various stages of transgender reassignment. Some clients are thinking about the process and realize that their present voice and speech patterns would make it difficult to present as female, and others have begun the psychological and physical processes of change, such as counseling, hormonal support, electrolysis, breast augmentation, and cross-dressing. Others have done everything except genital surgery. Some have completed all of the stages of transformation, including the transgender genital surgery.

There are guidelines that have been provided for professionals who are involved with clients who are experiencing gender dysphoria. The Harry Benjamin International Gender Dysphoria Association (HBIGDA) has provided the most comprehensive guidelines on this topic. I would recommend that anyone involved with this population become familiar with these guidelines. (For further information contact HBIGDA, 1300 South Second Street, Suite 180, Minneapolis, MN 55454; e-mail: hbigda@famprac.umn.edu)

Most authors writing on the topic of gender dysphoria state that such individuals are identified by society as members of one sex but who wish to change to the opposite sex. *Gender identity* refers to an individual's self-perception as male or female, and *gender dysphoria* denotes strong and persistent feelings of discomfort with one's assigned sex, the desire to possess the body of the other sex, and the desire to be regarded by society as a member of the opposite sex. This must be considered separately from the notion of sexual orientation, which refers to erotic attraction to males, females, or both (APA, 2000). Persons with gender dysphoria seek gender changes at many levels, including cross-dressing and general adoption of behaviors considered typical of the gender being sought. These early gender modifications may be followed by surgery or hormone therapy to make the body appear and function like that of the opposite sex. The DSM–IV–TR classifies the typical person with gender dysphoria as having a gender identity disorder from childhood, particularly males, who usually first experience these feelings beginning in childhood or early adolescence. This is confirmed in my experience with many male-to-female clients with gender dysphoria. Most state that their feeling of being female in a male body existed from early youth.

A male who wishes gender reassignment to female can do so in appearance through cross-dressing, hormonal treatment (estrogen), and electrolysis to remove body hair. Estrogen therapy will help the male to develop breasts and have a more female presentation, but the male larynx will not be altered by this hormone therapy. Surgical alteration of the penis to form a vagina has been done successfully in many cases, and patients report normal sexual satisfaction after this surgery. Only 1 in 30,000 adult males and 1 in 300,000 adult females seek sex reassignment surgery (APA, 2000). When this process is contemplated, extensive psychiatric treatment is usually recommended so that such persons can confront directly any negative side of their wish to physically change sex.

For the male-to-female client, the voice and communication style are often the most troublesome aspects of the change. Increased testosterone lowers the voice in the female-to-male person, but increased estrogen does not change the larynx and cause it to produce a higher pitched voice in the male-to-female person. The hormone does increase breast size but does not reverse laryngeal size. Gender identify can be identified by perceptual measures of fundamental frequency and other acoustic variables, but clear gender identification in male-to-female transgender individuals can be difficult to achieve. Gelfer and Schofield (2000) studied 15 male-to-female transgender individuals on several acoustic and perceptual features and compared them with typical males and females. Results indicated that subjects perceived as female had a higher mean fundamental frequency and higher upper limit of pitch than subjects perceived as male. Ten of the 15 male-to-female transgender individuals were identified perceptually as male, and only 3 were clearly identified as female. The discussion section of this article is excellent and communicates clearly how complicated gender identification is from a voice perspective. These findings illustrate the difficulty of gender presentation without careful modification of vocal pitch factors to increase the fundamental frequency, upper and lower limits of frequency range, intonational variability, and possibly resonance characteristics.

Surgical alteration of the larynx has proved successful in providing a higher pitch for the male-to-female client. Blaugrund et al. (1992) reported a thryoplasty type IV procedure, which is known as the cricothyroid approximation technique. Following this procedure the vocal folds are increased in longitudinal tension, which will raise the pitch. This technique, an extension of the early work of Isshiki, Taira, and Tanabe (1983), can be successful when carefully done. Gross (1999) reported a technique of depithelizing the vocal folds in the anterior commissure and suturing the vocal folds together at that juncture, thus shortening the vibrating mass of the vocal folds and producing a higher pitched voice. Ten patients were reported and found to increase fundamental frequency of the voice by a mean of 9.2 semitones, with a reduction of lower frequencies of the voice range. This was a desired effect, because in uncontrolled situations, no deep voice was possible.

Wolfe, Ratusnik, Smith, and Northrop (1990) evaluated 20 male-to-female persons with transsexualism (transgender) to determine frequency and intonation patterns that would be judged as female or male. Of the 20 participants, 9 were judged as female and 11 as male. Those judged as female had significantly higher pitch levels (mean F_0 = 172 Hz, range = 155.5 to 195 Hz) than those judged as male (mean F_0 = 118 Hz, range = 97.2 to 145 Hz). The researchers also found that subjects rated as male had more significant and extensive downward inflections of the voice, whereas those subjects rated as female had a higher percentage of upward inflections than male-rated subjects.

It is important to remember, as illustrated by Wolfe et al., that raising the pitch alone is not sufficient to communicate female sexual gender (Gelfer & Schofield, 2000). Laing (1992) presented useful information about how females communicate and provided many helpful suggestions to the speech–language pathologist who might be working with a transgender client. Some factors that distinguish the sexes in communication style include raised pitch in the female; increased use of modal constructions (can, will, may, shall, must) in the female; and intonation patterns of pitch, stress, and duration of phoneme production that appear to be more feminine. Females often use a softer voice and more precise articulation contacts. Female body language factors also need to be considered. Because I am male and cannot provide a very good model of many of these characteristics, I ask my female graduate students to guide clients with male-to-female transgender goals in these female forms of presentation.

A complete listing of the literature dealing with gender and transgender issues up to early 1990s was provided by Denny (1994). This reference documents hundreds of scholarly articles and books as well as popular magazine articles pertaining to the many issues of gender dysphoria. Andrews (1999), Hooper (2000), and Gelfer (1999) presented excellent overviews of many of these principles that go far beyond changing the speaking pitch. Gelfer's conclusion to her article is salient: "Behavioral change is not an easy process, but it does offer possibilities for the male-to-female transgendered client. We have found by carefully selecting and habituating a target pitch, by moving from chanting to speech intonation at the word level, by targeting natural-sounding intonation at the phrase level, by practicing different styles of emotional expression and intensity levels at the sentence level, and by monitoring nonverbal and paralinguistic behaviors in connected speech, good results can be obtained" (p. 208).

My clinical experiences with male-to-female transgender clients have been most challenging but fascinating. One significant challenge has been to determine how much about the noncommunication aspects of this life-altering change should be understood and addressed versus leaving these areas to the psychologist or psychiatrist. When a father comes to the clinic with his children but is in the process of gender change, I have resisted the questions regarding how these transformations in family structure have affected the client. Often, however, they come up naturally, and one must be prepared to understand and support the client. It would be unwise to assume an attitude of merely changing communication factors without recognizing how communication is affected by social, familial, psychosocial, and psychosexual aspects of life. I have never asked a client to discuss her sexual life since the male-to-female transformation occurred. One client, however, presented a major challenge in this regard because she informed me that she had been married 3 years and her husband did not know she was transgendered. After therapy provided her with the necessary communication changes to present more successfully as female, I videotaped an interview with her as she discussed her move to the United States from Mexico, her employment as a hairdresser, and general life questions having nothing to do with gender issues. I played this tape in a class of undergraduate majors, asking whether her Spanish accent affected English intelligibility. Not one student questioned her female gender, although there was lively discussion about her accent. She was always referred to as "she" or "her" in their comments, and I considered this a successful conclusion to a challenging case.

Working with transgender clients is an interesting aspect of voice management. It is also very challenging because the issues are so complex and involve every dimension of the client's life. It is important that the speech–language pathologist understand these complexities, be comfortable with the processes of transformation, communicate a clear attitude of nonjudgment, and focus on the areas of voice and communication style that facilitate rather than hinder the process. Not all speech–language pathologists will be able to do this and must refer to others who can. When I present this information in my graduate classes in voice disorder at Arizona State University, I always ask the students to indicate whether or not they would be comfortable working with clients who have gender dysphoria. Typically, about one fourth of the students indicate they would not. I do not try to persuade, because that would be judgmental on my part. They would not, however, be assigned to help me manage such a client in clinical practicum.

STAGE FRIGHT

Many persons experience in daily life or in formal performance the physiological changes associated with stage fright. The physiology behind these body reactions to "performance," whether in speaking or singing, was previously discussed. It is very disconcerting to even the experienced professional when anxiety prior to speaking or performance causes physiological changes that affect vocal and speech control. Shakespeare was correct when he said, "All the world's a stage, and all the men and women merely players. They have their exits and their entrances" (*As You Like It*). It is perhaps the natural state to experience anxiety (stage fright) when one is about to enter one of these stages and speak in an unusual situation with strangers or before large groups. Most persons merely struggle through it, often with voice quivering, with tension apparent in a slightly higher tone, and perhaps with thoughts somewhat cluttered.

Persons who are to perform or speak before audiences often experience a lack of control over body functions and experience increased sweating, rapid heartbeat, flushing of the skin, dryness of the mouth and throat, and a general feeling of anxiety and nervousness. It does little good to say, "Be still my heart!" When about to speak or sing, persons might focus particularly on how dry the mouth and throat are, because such dryness affects the phonation and articulation processes significantly. These feelings of insecurity have been designated as aspects of performance anxiety (D. C. Rosen & Sataloff, 1997, 1998). These reactions can be experienced by the seasoned professional or the next-door neighbor who is about to make a comment at a community town hall meeting. Most speakers who have had stage fright, upon the conclusion of the speaking event and after the parasympathetic nervous system has countered the effects of the sympathetic nervous system and brought the body back to homeostasis, tend to say, "Let me do it again; I could do so much better now." An individual who has trouble speaking because of these reactions is having a psychogenic speech–voice difficulty. However, such a psychogenic reaction, notwithstanding its reality and effect on the communication process, is not considered a communication disorder in the clinical sense.

Beta-blockers are often used by performers and athletes to modify objectionable preperformance feelings of anxiety or stress, particularly those related to muscle tremor or heart palpitations. Some performers, particularly those with extreme anxiety, might benefit from medically supervised low-dosage use of beta-blockers. However, Gates and Montalbo (1987), Sataloff (1998b), and Sataloff et al. (1998) have questioned the positive benefits of beta-blockers on performance and discourage their use, particularly for singers. A physician can help a performer decide whether such drug treatment would be helpful. Use of mucolytic agents might be helpful under physician direction to counter mouth dryness resulting from environment or stage fright. Excellent references by Sataloff (1998b, 1998c) and Vogel et al. (2000) and articles in *The Journal of Voice* often present information regarding medicines used by the professional voice performer.

THE SPEECH–LANGUAGE PATHOLOGIST AND THE PSYCHOLOGY OF VOICE

As discussed in this chapter, the voice is intricately intertwined with the psyche. When aphonia or dysphonia occurs because of psychological or psychiatric disintegration, the speech–language pathologist can be effective in improving voice as part of the overall therapy team. Many speech–language pathologists have extensive training in psychology, are comfortable with the psychogenic bases of communication disorders, and have no difficulty knowing when to treat and when to refer. Others may not have the slightest idea when symptomatic voice therapy is appropriate and when it is not.

The speech–language pathologist should refer for psychological or psychiatric consultation whenever in doubt about the appropriateness of treatment for psychogenic voice disorder. When dealing with such clients, it is important to consider that, whether intended or not, symptomatic voice therapy is treating both the voice and the psyche. One of the most significant analyses of voice and psychological considerations was written by Brodnitz (1988):

> The success of vocal rehabilitation depends to a large degree on the search for emotional dynamics that have produced the disorder of the voice. Just to act as a kind of "vocal gymnastics teacher" who puts the patient through vocal routines, manipulates pitch, and corrects faulty breathing, is to treat the symptoms of a disorder instead of its etiology. Of course, such attempts to normalize vocal

production have their place in voice therapy, but they have to be supplemented by a deeper understanding of psychological dynamics. A quiet hour of probing into the background of vocal difficulties, covering such essential facts as family situations, professional problems, and emotional conflicts will go far in obtaining a proper perspective for the understanding of dysfunction of the voice and for the handling of vocal rehabilitation. (p. 24)

Brodnitz ended by describing Rembrandt's *Christ Preaching,* in which Jesus is preaching to 25 or more people and not one of the listeners is looking directly at him. Rather, each is in a state of attention, contemplation, and reflection in an attempt to understand what is being said. They are receiving the message entirely through their ears.

All speech–language pathologists can learn from this example, particularly when working with clients with psychogenic voice disorders. They must tune in to the messages the patients are communicating and attempt to understand their significance. Only then can the speech–language pathologist be effective in knowing when to treat, when to refer, and what effect specific management procedures are likely to have on clients with psychogenic voice disorders.

SUMMARY

This chapter has covered the many interrelationships between voice and psyche. Several forms of psychogenic voice disorder have been described, including conversion aphonia and dysphonia, vocal abuse, puberphonia (mutational falsetto), gender dysphoria and transgender issues, and stage fright. Voice characteristics and treatment considerations have been analyzed. The interactions between the nervous system and the endocrine system in the pathogenesis of psychogenic voice disorder have been presented in general terms. With this background, the speech–language pathologist should understand the nature of psychogenic voice disorder and treatment considerations.

Alaryngeal Communication

E ach year since around 1887, when the first laryngectomy was reportedly performed (Duguay, 1989, 1998), thousands of persons throughout the world have lost to surgery their vital organ of voice—the larynx—because of cancer or trauma. In the case of cancer, the patient's larynx must be sacrificed surgically to stop the spread of malignant cells in the hope of saving the person's life. In the case of trauma, the larynx is removed surgically because it has suffered damage that has incapacitated laryngeal valving mechanisms necessary to protect the respiratory tract from aspiration of food, liquids, and saliva, or its patency for respiration has been compromised (Veivers & Laccourreye, 2000). Regardless of why the larynx must be removed, life for the person involved is altered significantly: psychologically, sociologically, economically, often in employment, and particularly in communication (Shanks, 1999). One whose larynx is removed surgically becomes a laryngectomized person. The term *laryngectomee* is used to identify such individuals, but the trend is to use the designation laryngectomized person. Laryngectomy is the surgical procedure involved.

Laryngectomized persons have many adjustments to make in life after surgery, often in all of the areas just identified. The speech–language pathologist working with such an individual must understand the overall significance of laryngeal amputation on the client and family members, particularly as to the impact on communication. Only then can the speech–language pathologist function competently in the rehabilitation process of restoring communication. This chapter provides perspective to the speech–language pathologist on the overall impact of laryngectomy, with particular emphasis on alaryngeal communication training.

LARYNGEAL CANCER

Cancer of the larynx can begin in any location of intrinsic or extrinsic laryngeal tissue. Laryngeal tumors are classified as being supraglottal (above the vocal folds but in the larynx), glottal (on the vocal folds), and subglottal (below the vocal folds but still in the laryngeal region). The supraglottal zone involves the epiglottal region, including the valleculae, the aryepiglottic folds, the arytenoid cartilages, the ventricular folds, and the ventricular cavity. Glottal tumors arise on the vocal folds and on the anterior commissure or posterior aspect. Transglottal tumors appear both above and below the ventricle. Subglottal tumors are rare and arise more commonly from the lower margins of the vocal folds.

The location of the tumor is called the primary site. Any cancer that spreads from a primary to a secondary site is an indication of metastasis, which means the disease has transferred from one organ or part to another not directly connected with it. In the case of laryngeal cancer, metastasis occurs through the cervical lymphatic node system. The most common type of laryngeal cancer is squamous cell carcinoma.

Several methods are used to classify laryngeal carcinomas. Most are based on the physical examination of the physician and tests such as endoscopy, fine-needle aspiration biopsy, CT scanning, MRI, chest films, and blood chemistry tests (Benninger & Grywalski, 1998). Table 7.1 presents the classification system of the American Joint Committee for Cancer Staging and End-Results Reporting (1988) and is commonly referred to as the TNM classification system: location of tumor (T; supraglottis, glottis, subglottis), nodal (N) involvement, and evidence of metastasis (M). With this classification system, physicians can determine the effectiveness of various treatments in terms of survival and recurrence.

In many ways, any discussion of laryngeal cancer must involve head and neck cancers generally. The focus of this chapter, however, is on laryngeal cancer and its management. Cancer is second only to heart disease as the major cause of death in the United States, and head and neck cancers account for approximately 10% of all cancers and 5% of cancer deaths. An estimated 12,000 new cases of laryngeal cancer occur each year in the United States, and there are approximately 4,000 deaths (Franco & Har-El, 1999). Although the gender ratio of general head and neck cancers is only 1.5:1 males over females (Hoffman, Karnell, Funk, Robinson, & Menck, 1998), the gender relationship in laryngeal cancer demonstrates increased vulnerability to males. This ratio has changed over the decades from 10:1 (males to females) in the 1970s to a present estimated ratio of approximately 7:1. There has been a dramatic increase in the prevalence of laryngeal cancer in females attributed to increased smoking among females in the past decades. The majority of laryngeal cancers are glottal (55% to 75%). The next highest location of tumor development is in the supraglottal region (24% to 42%), and subglottal tumors are rare (1% to 6%) (Benninger & Grywalski, 1998; Meyerhoff & Rice, 1992).

Laryngeal cancer is considered a disease of adulthood, with the majority of cases occurring in the fifth through seventh decades of life. However, although rare, laryngeal cancer can occur in childhood. Because it is rare, often the diagnosis is late in coming because physicians are not expecting malignancy (McDermott et al., 2000). Ferlito, Rinaldo, and Marioni (1999) reported on 47 cases of laryngeal malignant

TABLE 7.1
TNM Classification for Laryngeal Cancer

Staging

Primary Tumor (T)

T_x	Tumor that cannot be assessed by rules
T_0	No evidence of primary tumor

Supraglottis

TIS	Carcinoma in situ
T_1	Tumor confined to region of origin with normal mobility
T_2	Tumor involving adjacent supraglottic site(s) or glottis without fixation
T_3	Tumor limited to larynx with fixation and/or extension to involve postcricoid area, medial wall of pyriform sinus, or preepiglottic space
T_4	Massive tumor extending beyond the larynx to involve oropharynx, soft tissues of neck, or destruction of thyroid cartilage

Glottis

TIS	Carcinoma in situ
T_1	Tumor confined to vocal cord(s) with normal mobility (including involvement of anterior or posterior commissures)
T_2	Supraglottic and/or subglottic extension of tumor with normal or impaired cord mobility
T_3	Tumor confined to the larynx with cord fixation
T_4	Massive tumor with thyroid cartilage and/or extension beyond the confines of the larynx

Subglottis

TIS	Carcinoma in situ
T_1	Tumor confined to the subglottic region
T_2	Tumor extension to vocal cords with normal or impaired cord mobility
T_3	Tumor confined to the larynx with cord fixation
T_4	Massive tumor with cartilage destruction or extension beyond the confines of the larynx, or both

Nodal Involvement (N)

N_x	Nodes cannot be assessed
N_0	No clinically positive nodes

(continues)

259

TABLE 7.1 *Continued*

Staging

Nodal Involvement (N) (*Continued*)

N_1	Single clinically positive homolateral node less than 3 cm in diameter
N_2	Single clinically positive homolateral node, 3 to 6 cm in diameter, or multiple clinically positive homolateral nodes, none over 6 cm in diameter
N_{2a}	Single clinically positive homolateral node, 3 to 6 cm in diameter
N_{2b}	Multiple clinically positive homolateral nodes, none over 6 cm in diameter
N_3	Massive homolateral node(s), bilateral nodes, or contralateral node(s)
N_{3a}	Clinically positive homolateral nodes, none over 6 cm in diameter
N_{3b}	Bilateral clinically positive nodes (in this situation, each side of the neck should be staged separately: that is, N_{3b}: right, N_{2a}: left, N_1)
N_{3c}	Contralateral clinically positive node(s) only

Distant Metastasis (M)

M_x	Not assessed
M_0	No (known) distant metastasis
M_1	Distant metastasis present

Stage Grouping

Stage I	$T_1N_0M_0$
Stage II	$T_2N_0M_0$
Stage III	$T_3N_0M_0$
	T_1 or T_2 or T_3, N_1, M_0
Stage IV	T_4, N_0 or N_1, M_0
	Any T, N_2 or N_3, M_0
	Any T, any N, M_1

Residual Tumor (R)

R_0	No residual tumor
R_1	Microscopic residual tumor
R_2	Microscopic residual tumor

Note. From *Manual for Stages of Cancer* (2nd ed., pp. 38–39), by American Joint Committee for Cancer Staging and End-Results Reporting, 1988, Philadelphia: Lippincott. Copyright 1988 by Lippincott. Reprinted with permission.

neoplasms in children and adolescents, with the most frequent neoplasm being the embryonal variant of rhabdomyosarcoma. Most were successfully treated with radiation and chemotherapy, but partial or total laryngectomy was done on rare occasions. Squamous cell carcinoma accounted for 27.6% of the malignant tumors of the larynx in this population.

Etiology of Laryngeal Cancer

Several factors have been identified as being etiologically related to the pathogenesis of laryngeal cancer. Smoking and excessive alcohol consumption are significantly correlated with its development, particularly in supraglottal and glottal cancers. Heavy alcohol intake has been shown to significantly increase the risk of laryngeal cancer as long as smoking is also present. When no tobacco usage is present, alcohol intake does not appear to increase the risk of laryngeal cancer (Benninger & Grywalski, 1998; Doyle, 1994; Lawson, Biller, & Suen, 1989). Carcinoma of the larynx has been induced teratogenically in laboratory animals exposed to cigarette smoke (Meyerhoff & Rice, 1992). Gastroesophageal reflux disorder (GERD) has been found to be a comorbid condition for some cancers, particularly cancer of the larynx (Koufman & Burke, 1996; Sataloff, Castell, et al., 1999). The American Cancer Society estimates that each year approximately 3,000 nonsmoking adults die of lung cancer, and 150,000 to 300,000 infants and children have lower respiratory tract infections such as pneumonia and bronchitis from secondhand smoke exposure. Secondhand smoke also increases the number of asthma attacks and the severity of asthma in about 20% of the 2 to 5 million asthmatic children (American Cancer Society, 2001). Secondhand smoke exposure is likely a growing factor in the development of laryngeal cancer among those who have been diagnosed with it but who have never smoked themselves.

Types of Laryngeal Cancer

Head and neck cancers account for 10% of all cancers. Laryngeal cancer accounts for approximately 1% to 2% of all cancers and 20% of all head and neck cancers. The most common form of laryngeal cancer is squamous cell carcinoma, making up 90% of the cancers that affect the larynx (Benninger & Grywalski, 1998). As indicated in Chapter 1, the true vocal folds have a covering of stratified squamous epithelium. In carcinoma in situ, the epithelium of the vocal folds is replaced by a full thickness of cells with malignant cell features that can be detected by microscopic analysis. In the carcinoma in situ classification, there is no invasion of these malignant cells beyond the squamous epithelium.

When these cells develop beyond the epithelium, the carcinoma invades the underlying muscle and other tissues of the larynx. Simple squamous cell carcinoma (in situ or invasive) represents the uncontrolled growth of squamous cells. Laryngeal carcinoma often is preceded by laryngeal keratosis (also called hyperkeratosis, squamous cell hyperplasia, or epithelial hyperplasia; Benninger & Grywalski, 1998; Meyerhoff & Rice, 1992).

Symptoms of Laryngeal Cancer

As indicated, laryngeal cancer can arise in the supraglottal, glottal, or subglottal regions, and its symptoms depend on its location. Fortunately, cancers in the glottal region present an almost immediate symptom of hoarseness, one of the danger signals identified by the American Cancer Society. Brodnitz (1988) stated, "As long as we have no drug that cures cancer, everything depends on early detection. There is no excuse for the many cases of laryngeal cancer that still come to the doctor in a late stage. *Nobody should be hoarse for more than two weeks* without having his or her vocal folds examined by a competent specialist" (p. 124).

Dyspnea (difficulty in breathing) and stridor (voice heard on inhalation) are late-appearing symptoms caused by bulky tumors or vocal fold fixation. When the patient responds to early hoarseness symptoms and seeks medical attention that leads to prompt diagnosis and treatment, the prognosis for survival is excellent. In supraglottal cancers early symptoms are dysphagia (difficulty in swallowing), weight loss, halitosis, neck swelling, bloody discharge, and pain. Many times the pain associated with laryngeal tumors is referred to the ipsilateral ear via the sensory portions of the vagus nerve (cranial nerve X). In subglottal tumors the most common symptoms are pain and dyspnea.

TREATMENT OF LARYNGEAL CANCER

The treatment of laryngeal cancer involves radiation, surgery, chemotherapy, or combinations of those procedures. The treatment of choice depends on the bias of the physician, based on experience and research data directed by clinical staging data. The most conservative treatment for specific laryngeal cancers is radiation only. In such cases the basic voice is preserved and respiratory airway remains oral and nasal; tracheostoma is avoided. There is also a trend toward treatment of laryngeal cancers using chemoradiation with the intent of larynx preservation. Voice is also preserved in such treatment, but voice is generally affected in a negative manner by the radiation whether in combination or as a separated treatment modality (Honocodeevar-Boltezar & Zargi, 2000). Orlikoff, Kraus, Budnick, Pfister, and Zelefsky (1999) reported on 12 patients treated with chemoradiation for advanced stage laryngeal carcinoma and moderate to severe dysphonia. These patients were studied from a voice perspective. Although acoustic indicators showed significant improvement after 1 month of chemoradiation treatment, none of the patients achieved normalcy in voice as compared with control subjects. Also, some patients are unable for health reasons to undergo surgery, and combinations of radiation and chemotherapy provide the best solutions (Orlikoff et al., 1999; Stemple et al., 2000).

When surgery is required, the surgeon has several options, depending on the stage of the cancer. These options range from surgeries that remove the cancer but retain the laryngeal valving structures of the larynx for biological and phonatory functions on the conservative end to total removal of the larynx on the aggressive end. Kirchner (1998) provided an atlas of color photographs of surgical specimens of tumors in various stages of cancer with indications on how cancers spread and barriers to cancer extension during the early stages. Laryngeal cancer surgeries range from cordectomy to partial laryngectomy, to hemilaryngectomy, to total laryngectomy, with a variety of techniques and surgical approaches employed. It is important for speech–language pathologists to understand basic principles of laryngeal cancer management in order to aid the patient in rehabilitation following surgery.

Weinstein, Laccourreye, Brasnu, and Laccourreye (2000) presented surgical techniques for organ preservation in laryngeal cancer. Many of the techniques covered include endoscopic surgeries that preserve the functions of speech and swallowing without a permanent tracheostomy. The surgical technique of partial tissue removal requires consideration that the tumor can be removed but the patient will be left with sufficient laryngeal valving to swallow well during eating and drinking without aspiration. When this is achieved, some voice potential is usually possible. If conservative surgery provides a condition in which aspiration occurs and cannot be managed postsurgically, more aggressive surgery is likely regardless of the voice concerns. Doyle (1994) and Benninger and Grywalski (1998) outlined the medical and surgical options using language and photographs that the speech–language pathologist can easily understand.

The specifics involved in total laryngectomy are well described in the literature (Blom, Singer, & Hamaker, 1998; Doyle, 1994; Meyerhoff & Rice, 1992; Myers & Suen, 1989; Thumfart et al., 1999) and need not be repeated in detail here. The speech–language pathologist should, however, understand the basic anatomical and physiological changes involved in this procedure. This understanding may be facilitated by studying the differences between the man drawn in Figure 7.1 (before laryngectomy) and in Figure 7.2 (after total laryngectomy).

The general procedure for total laryngectomy has changed little since early times. Basically, in a total laryngectomy the larynx is removed along with all cartilages, intrinsic muscles, membranes, and the hyoid bone. The upper tracheal rings usually are sacrificed and the exposed trachea is brought forward and provided with external attachment in the neck region just above the sternal notch. This external opening is

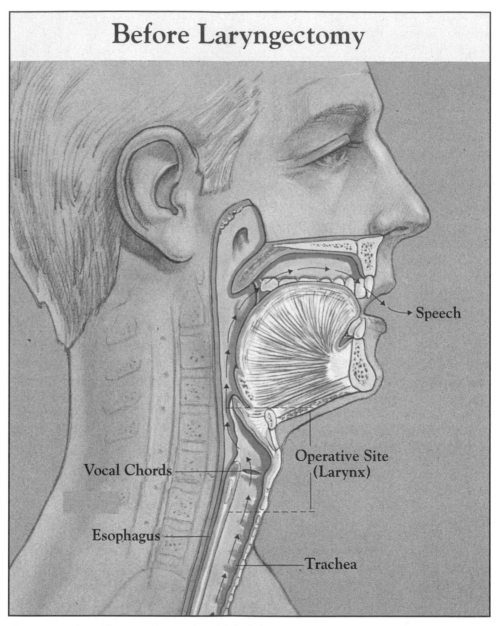

Figure 7.1. Sagittal view of normal individual before laryngectomy. (Illustration courtesy of International Healthcare Technologies.)

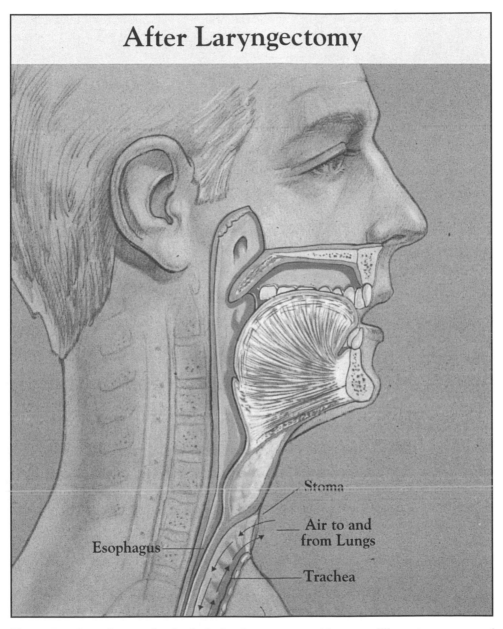

Figure 7.2. Sagittal view of individual after laryngectomy with stoma. (Illustration courtesy of International Healthcare Technologies.)

called the tracheostoma, or stoma, and is the orifice for all respiration following the surgery. The stoma creates a permanent change for all patients in that they become neck breathers for the remainder of their lives. Total laryngectomy often involves unilateral or bilateral radical neck dissection of strap muscles when there is evidence of metastatic disease (Ferlito & Rinaldo, 1998), or sometimes radiation therapy also is used. These options are physician determined. In the past, radical neck dissection was commonly done with total laryngectomy, but as more conservative surgical approaches to disease management have emerged, a more conservative attitude has also emerged with regard to neck dissection. The speech–language pathologist working with laryngectomized individuals should be familiar with all of the possibilities of surgery, radiation, and combination treatments because options of speech and voice rehabilitation are often influenced by these options.

The primary role of the speech–language pathologist in working with laryngectomized persons is to facilitate alaryngeal communication or, in the case of partial laryngectomy, to facilitate the best voice possible with residual tissues. In the case of total laryngectomy, typically there are three general categories of direction for the speech–language pathologist to take in pursuing the goal of facilitating alaryngeal speech for the patient:

- Traditional esophageal phonation
- Artificial or electrolaryngeal devices
- Tracheoesophageal puncture (TEP) and prosthetic processes

The trend in this new century is certainly toward the surgical placement of a prosthesis that will facilitate alaryngeal phonation for speech. However, choices remain as to how rehabilitation should unfold. The choice of procedure after surgery for communication restoration should be determined by the patient after extensive consultation and direction from the medical team involved and the speech–language pathologist. The role for the speech–language pathologist is one of providing excellent information on the choices available and then helping the patient decide how to proceed.

Iversen-Thoburn and Hayden (2000) surveyed 110 laryngectomized individuals to determine primary alaryngeal voice and speech status. Their results indicated that all three of the methods of alaryngeal speech listed earlier were being used. Just over 40% of the respondents used traditional esophageal voice; 34.6% used some sort of artificial larynx; 12.7% used some prosthetic-assisted alaryngeal voice, such as TEP; 9.1% used a combination of esophageal speech and an artificial larynx; and a few, 2.5%, used writing or gestures for communication. Data from Hong Kong (Ng, Kwok, & Chow, 1997) showed that Cantonese-speaking laryngectomized persons also use a variety of the above methods, including several who use pneumatic devices (e.g., the Tokyo artificial larynx) in which air from the stoma is directed into a reed-sound generator, which is then directed into the mouth for speech purposes. Blom et al. (1998) reported successful acquisition of tracheoesophageal voice in 75% to 92% of more than 1,500 patients.

Extrinsic and intrinsic alaryngeal sources of voice are available to help facilitate alaryngeal phonation. Extrinsic sources of phonation include all devices used external to the body to generate a pseudolaryngeal sound. These include a variety of battery-driven electrolarynges, examples of which are discussed later in this chapter. Intrinsic sources of alaryngeal phonation include generation of voice by tissue vibration in the buccal cavity, in the pharyngeal cavity, and at the junction of the pharynx and the esophagus or by means of some surgically constructed shunt that connects the trachea to the esophagus. These processes also are discussed in detail later.

EXTRINSIC SOURCES OF ALARYNGEAL PHONATION

The commonly used extrinsic sources of alaryngeal phonation are discussed in the following sections. Several varieties previously available, including the AT&T neck-type artificial larynx, are no longer being manufactured and are not discussed.

Intraoral Artificial Electrolarynx

Figure 7.3 shows the Cooper–Rand Electronic Speech Aid, which is an electrolarynx. It is an intraoral device that consists of a battery-powered pulse generator and battery case that is approximately 3 × 4 inches (7.62 × 10.16 cm) and fits into a shirt pocket. The pulse generator and battery case are connected by a heavy-gauge wire to a handheld tone generator that produces the alaryngeal voice. Connected to this tone generator is a plastic tube that fits into the oral cavity. The tone produced is channeled into the oral cavity for articulation and resonance purposes. Two dials on the top of the pulse generator control loudness and pitch. The speech–language pathologist must keep in mind that the two-pronged connector on the cord must be plugged into the handheld transducer in only one direction; plugging in reverse results in a significant impedance mismatch and a noticeable reduction in loudness.

Many patients using the Cooper–Rand have difficulty at first coordinating the voicing with articulation. The placement of the tubing becomes a mild obstruction to the rapid movements of articulation until practice provides proper positioning. Once the individual becomes used to articulating with tubing in the oral cavity, good intelligibility is obtained. The lingual–velar consonants /k/ and /g/ are not produced well because the tubing placement is not far enough back in the oral cavity to facilitate the stop portion of these consonants. Context usually is sufficient to produce intelligible

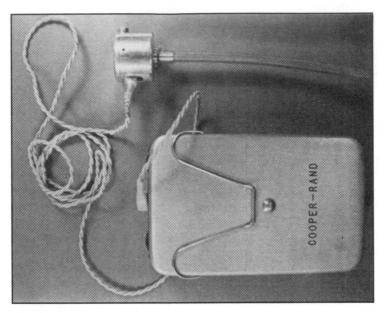

Figure 7.3. Cooper–Rand Electronic Speech Aid, an electrolarynx.

speech even in the absence of these consonants. The Cooper–Rand intraoral artificial larynx can also be adapted for use by wheelchair-bound patients or patients with the need for hands-free activation for voice (Andrews, 1999).

A primary advantage of the Cooper–Rand is that it is an intraoral device. Because a laryngectomy in most cases does not involve the oral cavity, the client can use the device immediately after the operation. Other extrinsic devices held against the neck are not as comfortable to use at that time because of soreness and tissue healing. The Cooper–Rand is an excellent alternative to writing during the first few days of postsurgical rehabilitation and is used by clients as a primary means of alaryngeal phonation. A pneumatic device similar in usage to the Cooper–Rand is the Toyko artificial larynx. This device involves a mouthpiece (similar to a trumpet mouthpiece) that contains a diaphragm sound generator. The mouthpiece is attached to a plastic tubing that ends with an insertion mouthpiece that is placed in the oral cavity so that sound generated can be articulated (Casper & Colton, 1998; Salmon, 1999).

Neck-Placement Artificial Devices

A neck-placement artificial device is a battery-driven sound generator such as the one illustrated in Figure 7.4. Each uses a rechargeable battery system, and some have an adaptable intraoral extension. The sound is produced when a piston strikes a fixed diaphragm at a high velocity. The quality of the tone can be adjusted slightly. Pitch and loudness control also are adjustable but not in a variable manner during speech. These are expensive electronic devices, but the overall quality makes them worth the price. Addresses for these companies or distribution sources are available at the end of this chapter.

INTRINSIC FORMS OF ALARYNGEAL PHONATION

Pharyngeal Speech

Pharyngeal speech involves pseudophonation in which the locus of vibration is posterior in the oropharyngeal cavity but superior in placement to esophageal voice. It is produced by forcing air through a constriction between the back of the tongue and the posterior pharyngeal wall. It is easy to accomplish, and clients often generate this sound early in the therapy process when trying to achieve esophageal speech. It also is rather unintelligible; the likely reason for this is that the tongue is involved in both phonation and articulation in pharyngeal phonation (Diedrich, 1999).

One patient seen at Arizona State University was a 49-year-old man who was laryngectomized as a result of cancer of the upper esophagus. His surgery was rather atypical in that both his upper esophagus and larynx were removed. This required construction of a pseudoesophagus by displacing stomach tissue upward to connect it to his pharynx, a surgical procedure called gastric pull-up (Hartley, Bottrill, & Howard, 1999).

Before learning esophageal (pseudo) phonation, this man developed excellent pharyngeal speech. Although the vibration source was not studied by means of radiography, it was thought to be the back of the tongue against the posterior pharyngeal wall. His fundamental frequency was 85 Hz, and his speaking rate was 90 words per minute. His intelligibility was rated at 85% on the *Rainbow Passage*. In therapy this man later learned superior pseudoesophageal phonation.

The man's pharyngeal speech served him well and was understood by most everyone except when he talked on the phone. As an executive for a large national company, he frequently had to make long-distance calls. Because of this unintelligibility, many times the answering party would hang up on him, thinking it was a prank call. This frustration prompted him to attempt to learn another form of phonation.

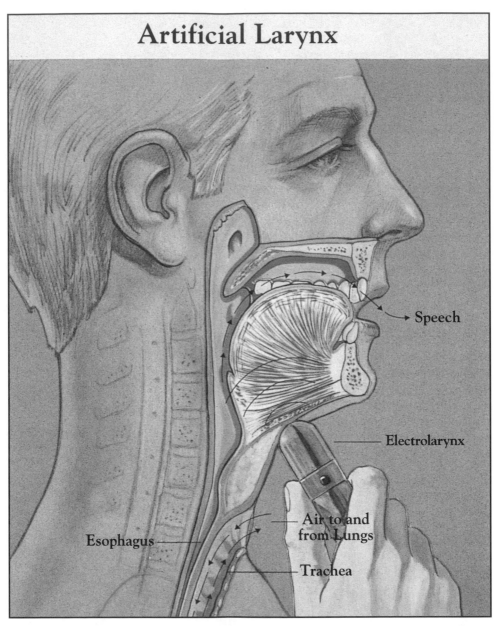

Figure 7.4. Sagittal view showing typical placement of electrolarynx after laryngectomy. (Illustration courtesy of International Healthcare Technologies.)

Pharyngeal phonation must be recognized by the speech–language pathologist as undesirable and should not be reinforced when it occurs. Once a client begins generating voice at a pharyngeal locus, it is difficult to correct, so it is better to avoid it at the outset. When a client does learn pharyngeal speech, an attempt should be made to change the locus of vibration to the esophagus.

Esophageal Speech

Most laryngectomized persons attempt to learn to speak again by using the upper musculature of the esophagus as a vibrating site for alaryngeal phonation. When this site becomes the source of sound vibration for speech, it is called esophageal phonation. It is called esophageal phonation for speech whether traditional methods of producing the voice are used or whether the patient uses some sort of prosthesis to provide air support for the process. Typical esophageal phonation is shown in Figure 7.5.

To produce esophageal phonation without TEP (tracheoesophageal puncture) support, the client moves air, which is present in the hypopharyngeal space above the esophagus, into the upper esophagus below its constrictive opening, then reverses the process so that air is forced out of the esophagus under pressure. This causes the tissue of the upper esophagus to vibrate to produce esophageal phonation. The sound is then resonated and articulated into human speech in the vocal tract by the structures of articulation.

ESOPHAGEAL SOUND MECHANISMS

To the laryngectomized person, producing speech by esophageal phonation is a simple process of using air to vibrate the tissues of the upper esophagus to produce sound that is then formed into human speech. To the scientist or clinician, this simple process becomes extremely complex and the subject of much debate and analysis in laboratory studies. Hundreds of articles have been written in an attempt to isolate the mechanisms involved in (a) air intake, (b) air reservoir (neolung), (c) air expulsion, and (d) nature of the vibrator. The following sections highlight those areas of investigation to provide the speech–language pathologist with the knowledge necessary to help laryngectomized persons learn to speak again.

METHODS OF AIR INTAKE

The schematic profile of the laryngectomized person shown in Figure 7.2 makes clear that surgical changes result in a trilevel configuration that is critical to understanding esophageal phonation: (a) the pharynx (the lower aspect, called the hypopharynx), (b) the pharyngoesophageal (P-E) junction or segment, and (c) the esophagus leading

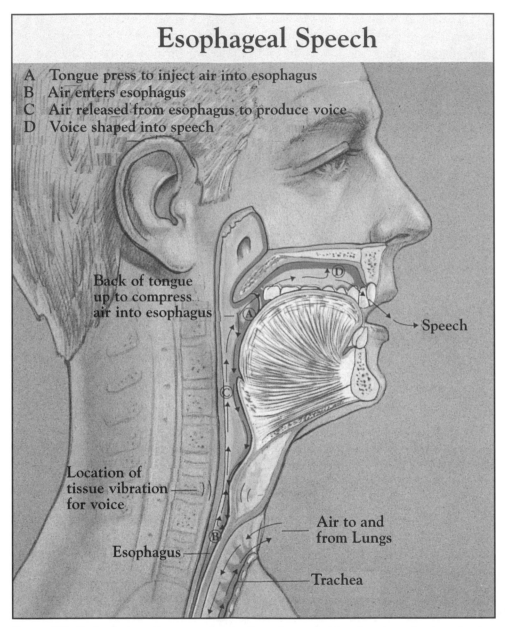

Esophageal Speech

A Tongue press to inject air into esophagus
B Air enters esophagus
C Air released from esophagus to produce voice
D Voice shaped into speech

Back of tongue
up to compress
air into esophagus — (A)

Speech

Location of
tissue vibration —
for voice

Air to and
from Lungs

Esophagus —

Trachea

Figure 7.5. Sagittal view of person using esophageal speech. Note location of voice vibration at the junction of the esophagus and pharynx. (Illustration courtesy of International Healthcare Technologies.)

to the stomach. Air intake for esophageal phonation involves somehow moving the air that is present in the hypopharynx through the P-E junction into the upper esophagus so that it then can be forced back through the junction to vibrate its tissues to produce sound. Two methods of accomplishing this air intake have been identified: injection and inhalation.

Injection

The injection method is divided into two forms, one occurring before the initiation of speech (glossopress) and the other simultaneously with speech (consonant injection).

Glossopress

The glossopress (also called glossopharyngeal press) method involves using the tongue (*glosso*) as a pumping mechanism for pushing or pressing (injecting) air into the esophagus. Although Diedrich and Youngstrom (1966) stated that this method involves either a glossopress or a glossopharyngeal press process, it is treated here as a single process and is described as a glossopress.

In this method, the laryngectomized person usually closes the lips and always closes the velopharyngeal mechanism to trap the air present in the oral and pharyngeal cavities, then uses the tongue to press or pump the air into the esophagus. The tongue essentially sweeps or squeezes the air along the hard and soft palates and then along the pharynx in a progressive wave to force the air back down into the esophagus. As air is pushed through the P-E junction, a "Klunking" sound can be heard as evidence that the esophagus has been loaded with air and is ready to be used to vibrate tissue to produce sound (Shanks, 1999).

Because this process involves movements similar to the tongue movements involved in swallowing, speech–language pathologists have used descriptions such as "half-swallow" or "swallow air" or "the beginning stage of swallow" in teaching clients. The use of such phrases should be discouraged for several reasons. It is counterproductive for the laryngectomized person to associate this injection process in any way with swallowing, because swallowing involves complex neuromuscular processes designed to move substances into the stomach. The air in esophageal phonation must not go into the stomach, and if the patient is attempting to duplicate in any fashion the process of swallowing when loading the esophagus with air, there is a great probability that air will be taken into the stomach.

Swallowing also involves a significant lag between occurrences, making it difficult for the movements involved to be repeated quickly, as is needed in esophageal phonation. This can be self-illustrated by dry swallowing, then as quickly as possible attempting to swallow again, then again, then again. It soon becomes apparent that several seconds pass between swallows. This latency is counter to efficient esophageal loading for alaryngeal phonation. I suggest that speech–language pathologists avoid comparing esophageal injection to swallowing, even semantically, and recommend teaching the client not to dry swallow to inject air, because of the vast differences between deglutition and the injection methods.

Consonant Injection

The second method of injecting air into the esophagus for alaryngeal phonation occurs simultaneously with consonant production. Inherent in the voicing of many consonants, particularly stops and fricatives, is intraoral breath pressure that builds behind the place of articulation. This breath pressure can be used to force or inject air into the esophagus during the articulation of the sound. The quick movement of air into and out of the esophagus provides tissue vibration for voice. Thus, esophageal voice is produced rather simultaneously with the articulation of the consonant.

To attempt voicing with this consonant injection method, the client is instructed to articulate sounds such as /pa/, /ta/, /ka/, /sta/, /tʃa/, /θa/. If the process works, esophageal voice is heard on the vowel sound following the consonant. The greater the air pressure on the consonant, the greater the probability that air will enter the esophagus. This method is effective for producing words that begin with the high-pressure consonants: *pie*, *tie*, *kite*, *stop*, *scotch*, *scratch*, *skips*, *paper*, and so on.

A word such as *toothpaste* has sufficient pressure consonants to load the esophagus for all the vowel sounds, and the client can say the word without much effort by merely articulating it as though a larynx existed. This also is true of such phrases as "pick it up" or "pass the salt." Unfortunately, most languages have many words and phrases that begin with vowels or low-pressure consonants, such as "I am here" or "roll your eyes." Consonant injection is not effective as a method of esophageal loading for such phrases, and other methods must be attempted (Duguay, 1999; Haroldson, 1999).

Inhalation

The injection methods described (glossopress and consonant injection) involve action of the tongue that increases the air pressure above the P-E junction to force air into the esophagus. The inhalation method is just the opposite: The person is instructed to inhale air into the esophagus simultaneously with the inhalation cycle of breathing air into the stoma. Just as negative pressure in the lungs draws air into them during inhalation, a similar negative pressure occurs in the esophagus, drawing air that is present in the hypopharynx into the esophagus.

Like the injection method, the inhalation method loads the esophagus with air to be used in producing esophageal vibration, but the method of loading is different. In the inhalation method, the tongue is passive and in a relaxed position in the oral cavity. The oral and nasal cavities are open, so air is free to move into the esophagus as negative pressure increases, which draws air in.

The normal relaxed (at rest) esophagus has a mean negative pressure of -4 to -7 mm Hg (mercury) below atmospheric pressure and may drop to as much as -15 mm Hg. During loading of the esophagus by inhalation, the negative pressure in the esophagus drops from -15 to -20 mm Hg. If the tonicity of the P-E junction is sufficiently relaxed, this drop in negative pressure is sufficient to draw air into the esophagus in a pressure-equalizing process. The more relaxed or devoid of tension the P-E junction is, the more efficiently air is drawn into it during inhalation (Casper & Colton, 1998; Diedrich, 1999; Duguay, 1999). After the esophagus is loaded, the process must be reversed to force the air out of the P-E junction under positive pressure. By this means, the tissues vibrate and produce alaryngeal phonation. Dey and Kirchner (1961), who did much of the primary work on esophageal pressures during respiration and esophageal voice, reported around 25 mm Hg to be sufficient to force the air out of the esophagus to vibrate the tissues.

Air Reservoir (Neolung) for Esophageal Voice

One reason esophageal speech is less efficient than normal laryngeal speech in communication is that the air reservoir for driving the vibrator is reduced significantly. In normal phonation with a larynx, the lung capacity is enormous—2,000 to 4,000 cc, depending on gender and size (Kent, 1994b). In comparison, the air capacity of the esophagus acting as a neolung to support alaryngeal phonation is generally around 80 cc (Diedrich, 1999), equal to about 5 tablespoons. Little wonder that the adult with a normal larynx can sustain phonation for as many as 30 seconds but the laryngectomized person does well to sustain it for 2 seconds.

The Neolarynx or Vibrator in Esophageal Voice

Diedrich and Youngstrom (1966) were the first to describe the nature of the tissue that vibrates in esophageal phonation, the typical laryngectomized neoglottis. This tissue is referred to in this text as the P-E junction. However, it is clear that the vibrator is more than simply a junction between two anatomical divisions of the gastrointestinal tract. Diedrich and Youngstrom, looking at the nature of the P-E junction, analyzed 27 laryngectomized patients (23 males) with cineradiography and still radiograms. They indicated that the level of the P-E junction was variable and located between cervical (C) vertebrae 3 through 7, with most around C_5 to C_{5-6}. They summarized the findings of several studies and reported general agreement that the P-E junction lies between C_4 and C_6.

Tremendous individual differences exist in the morphology of the P-E junction in both intersubject and intrasubject comparisons. Diedrich and Youngstrom (1966) described the morphology of the junction as involving constriction of tissue on the dorsal or ventral side of the pharyngoesophageal lumen, usually in some combination form. It must be kept in mind, however, that these views of the shape of the P-E junction were observed two-dimensionally from a lateral radiographic image. A three-dimensional perspective in endoscopic examination from a superior aspect revealed even more varied patterns of morphology as evidenced by Dworkin et al. (1999), who investigated the P-E junction in TEP speakers.

The length of the P-E junction responsible for alaryngeal phonation is as varied as intersubject and intrasubject comparisons, as is the morphology. Diedrich and Youngstrom (1966) found a range of 18 to 23 mm for different vowel phonemes. They also reported a mean P-E junction length of 21 mm when measured by cinefluorograms and 29 mm from spot films; however, during actual phonation, the length of the junction was at least 5 mm of contact tissue and as long as 15 mm. These length factors were not found to be significantly related in any way to proficiency of alaryngeal phonation. These variations in the P-E junction reported by Diedrich and Youngstrom have been verified more recently by endoscopic and radiographic inspection of the segment (Blom et al. 1998; Diedrich, 1999; Hirano, et al., 1999).

PERCEPTUAL AND ACOUSTIC CHARACTERISTICS

Now that the nature of mechanisms responsible for the production of phonation in alaryngeal speech has been reviewed, it is time to investigate the characteristics of the sound produced by these mechanisms and how they affect communication. The characteristics include pitch, loudness, voice quality, speaking rate, and intelligibility.

Pitch

The pitch, or frequency, of esophageal phonation has been studied thoroughly, as reviewed by Diedrich (1999). The studies in the early 1960s and 1970s reviewed by Diedrich revealed typical information regarding esophageal fundamental frequency: The average fundamental frequency for laryngectomized males is about 65 Hz, with a range of about four semitones. Superior esophageal speakers have a typical frequency on the higher end of the range, around 85 Hz.

The primary factors that determine fundamental frequency of esophageal vibration are tissue tonicity and vibrating mass, which differ slightly from person to person. Weinberg (1980) reviewed many studies reporting data that distinguish male from female esophageal speakers. Naive listeners were able to distinguish the sex of the speakers 98% of the time for males and 80% for females.

Data presented in semitone form for statistical comparison showed that female esophageal speakers averaged seven semitones higher for voice fundamental frequency than males. The F_0 for 15 female speakers ranged from 33 to 200 Hz. Strangely, the lowest fundamental frequency among 15 females and 18 males was produced by a female (33 Hz), but it should be kept in mind that 8 of the 15 females had F_0s exceeding the upper limit of the range of males.

Loudness

Loudness is the perceptual correlate of intensity. It stands to reason that esophageal speakers should have reduced loudness potential because their air support and airflow amounts are significantly less than those of normal speakers. Although Knox, Eccleston, Maurer, and Gordon (1987) reported that loudness is not highly correlated with esophageal speech proficiency, in my clinical experience reduced loudness makes communication difficult in noisy places and is one of the most distressing aspects of esophageal speech to these persons. Laryngectomized persons often complain of having difficulty being heard in restaurants; in traffic; in automobiles, as the driver or as a passenger; and even while watching television.

Esophageal speakers have less ability to generate a loud sound. A superior esophageal speaker might produce a spontaneous /a/ at 85 dB, compared with 95 to 100 dB by normal speakers. A normal speaker can make smooth loudness changes ranging up to 45 dB, whereas an esophageal speaker can manage only about 20 dB. Also, an ability to sustain an /a/ sound at 85 dB does not reflect an ability of the typical or even superior esophageal speaker to speak continuously at even close to that loudness level. Therefore, it is misleading to assume that a superior esophageal speaker should be able to communicate functionally at those levels.

Increased loudness of the esophageal voice can be produced, but usually at the expense of other dimensions, such as quality and durability. Increases in loudness should be managed clinically only after functional communication has been established and the speaker essentially has automatized the processes involved in esophageal phonation. Then loudness increases can be attempted for specific communication needs without significant sacrifice of control in other relevant dimensions.

Voice Quality

The voice quality of esophageal speech is described as perceptually raspy or hoarse. The variability in morphology of the P-E junction is responsible for the aperiodicity of vibration and vocal roughness heard. Of course, voice quality varies from person to person; there is considerable intrasubject variation as well.

One laryngectomized person with whom I worked put it best when he said, "You know, most people have good days and bad days. With regard to my voice quality,

I have good minutes and bad minutes." Another laryngectomized male said, "My voice quality is so bad that when someone who doesn't know me expresses concern about my bad cold, I feel I have been given a wonderful compliment." One female client expressed concern to her husband that she would never be able to sing. He said, "Hell, Betty, you never could sing, so why the concern?" All of these statements are testimony to the vocal quality that is typical of esophageal speech.

In a study on voice quality of esophageal speakers, Smith, Weinberg, Feth, and Horii (1978) tested earlier research findings that indicated that listener perception of the severity of vocal roughness was related to the degree or magnitude of spectral noise in the acoustic signal and that a strong, positive relationship existed between the magnitude of cycle-to-cycle frequency variation (jitter) and the degree of perceived roughness. Their findings indicated that jitter values of esophageal speakers were significantly greater than those of normal laryngeal speakers or persons with vocal or laryngeal pathologies. Dworkin et al. (1999) made similar findings for TEP speakers.

When trained listeners were asked to rate the severity of vocal toughness, they were able to do so reliably, and the esophageal speakers manifested varied degrees of vocal roughness. However, neither mean fundamental frequency nor mean jitter was a useful predictor of the perceived severity of vocal roughness; neither were jitter ratios. Therefore, it is not clear as to what physical variables form the basis for the perception of vocal roughness in esophageal speakers, other than assumed vibration aperiodicity. Diedrich (1999) also reported that a gurgling sound often is heard as one aspect of the voice quality of esophageal speakers, particularly when there is excessive mucus present above the P-E segment. Dairy products also increase this aspect of voice quality. Much of the esophageal speech data on these variables comes from earlier research, but the values remain the same. Most of the research on voice quality, pitch, loudness, and other dimensions of voice being done at this time include subjects who use TEP voice and speech, and more recent studies are reviewed later.

Speaking Rate

The esophageal voice speaking rate is slower than others because the process of loading the esophagus, then squeezing the air out to produce voice involves significant delays in number of words spoken per minute. Although the scientist or research clinician studies speaking rate in terms of words spoken per minute, data on words spoken per minute do not convey the problem as clearly as did a laryngectomized person with whom I worked: "By the time I tell my wife to go to hell, she has already died and gone there!"

Intelligibility

Regardless of speaking rate, pitch, loudness, and overall voice quality factors, if a laryngectomized person's speech is not intelligible, communication is thwarted and no other factors are important. Like the traveler in a foreign country unable to speak the language, the laryngectomized person can order filet of sole and end up with chicken soup if the speech is unintelligible. For this reason, several researchers have focused on the intelligibility and refinement of esophageal speech (Doyle, 1994; Doyle, Danhauer, & Reed, 1988; Hoops & Noll, 1969). Their findings seem to indicate that esophageal speakers are significantly less intelligible than normal speakers and vary more from individual to individual, although some speakers are very good at producing consonant distinctions for improved intelligibility. Much can be done to refine basic esophageal speech once the essentials have been developed (Haroldson, 1999).

Many of the studies on esophageal speech have focused more on acceptability than on direct measurements of intelligibility, but in either case effectiveness of communication was being analyzed. Factors found that significantly influenced intelligibility and acceptability included aperiodicity of the vocal signal (which is really a measure of quality), amount of respiration (stoma) noise during speech, amount of silence, vowel durations, rate of speech, and consonant error factors. This last factor refers to difficulty in distinguishing between voiced and voiceless cognates such as /p/ and /b/, /t/ and /d/, /k/ and /g/, and /s/ and /z/.

One interesting adjustment that esophageal speakers seem to make in providing cues for improved intelligibility is to increase the duration of their vowel sounds, particularly in consonant–vowel contexts in which the consonant is voiceless (Christensen & Weinberg, 1976). This finding led to an investigation as to whether esophageal speakers systematically varied voice onset time (VOT) to distinguish prevocalic stops (voiceless) /p/, /t/, and /k/ from the vocalic cognates /b/, /d/ and whether variance was dictated by place of articulation (Christensen, Weinberg, & Alfonso, 1978). These researchers found that average VOTs associated with the production of prevocalic voiceless stops of esophageal speakers are significantly shorter than those of normal speakers, and that esophageal speakers increase VOT as a function of moving place of articulation from labial /p/ to velar /k/. These results indicate that esophageal speakers are sensitive to the need for cognate distinction. Therefore, they attempt phonologically to modify articulation and phonation dimensions to accomplish these differences by varying VOT and increasing vowel duration in specific phonological contexts.

Esophageal Versus Artificial Larynx Phonation

Researchers have compared esophageal speech with artificial larynx speech in terms of intelligibility and other measures of preference. Kalb and Carpenter (1981) discerned significantly lower intelligibility scores for speakers who used only esophageal speech (78.5%), those who used only artificial larynx speech (61.8%), and those who used both methods (67.3% for esophageal sample and 70.7% for artificial larynx sample) compared to the scores for normal speakers (98.4%). Doyle (1994) reviewed many studies on the intelligibility of speakers using various electrolarynges and stated that both esophageal speech and speech with artificial devices can be very intelligible, depending on the speaker's skill and practice efforts. Watterson, Cox, and McFarlane (1998), however, provided data on speakers using four different types of electric-neck larynges and found on a scale from 1 to 5 (5 = *highly intelligible*) that the mean sentence intelligibility rating for all artificial larynges combined was only 2.98.

One of the major complaints against the use of electrolarynges is based on the difficulty individuals experience in directing all sound generated by the device into the vocal tract without having considerable amounts spill into the listening environment. Also, the acoustic spectrum that is produced sounds artificial and unlike human speech. Chenausky and MacAuslan (2000) reviewed efforts to mitigate these difficulties by using microprocessors and digital signal processing and filtering to bring electrolaryngeal spectra closer to those of normal larynges. The future looks bright for those individuals who use the electrolarynx for communication purposes as this work unfolds. Salmon (1999) also reviewed the advantages and disadvantages of electrolarynx usage. It is clear, in spite of whatever disadvantages there may be, that use of the artificial larynx in one form or another remains a significant aspect of alaryngeal rehabilitation.

REHABILITATION OF LARYNGECTOMIZED PERSONS

The rehabilitation of a laryngectomized person requires the efforts of many people. A medical team is responsible for the physical care of the patient before, during, and after the surgery. Other laryngectomized persons in social clubs organized under the auspices of the International Association of Laryngectomees, a branch of the American Cancer Society, are helpful. Friends and family can offer valuable support, and successful rehabilitation is almost impossible without them. Reeves (1999) provided an interesting history of the association and the support structure provided by this organization and the state organizations associated with it.

In addition, psychologists and psychiatrists usually are available for counseling service. Finally, the speech–language pathologist is the primary professional responsible for communication rehabilitation. Each of these persons, professionals, and loved ones must function as a team working toward the successful adjustment and rehabilitation of the laryngectomized individual. Strasser (1999) provided an insightful documentary of living with a spouse with laryngeal cancer and alaryngeal communication for more than 40 years. This is an excellent reference for any significant person in a patient's life who has been touched by these surgical and rehabilitation considerations.

Presurgery Visit by the Speech–Language Pathologist

The role of the speech–language pathologist in the rehabilitation process often begins before the surgery. Many physicians request that the speech–language pathologist visit the patient, perhaps accompanied by a trained laryngectomized person who can provide a model of successful general and communication adjustment. Doyle (1994) and Salmon (1999) provided clear suggestions for the laryngectomized person who is involved in patient visitation, and any speech–language pathologist who works with these individuals should be familiar with these references. Regardless of whether a laryngectomized individual is included, the visit must be planned carefully if it is to contribute successfully to the psychological well-being of the patient and family members.

The presurgery visit should start with advance notice to the client so that family members can be present if the patient desires. This visit usually occurs before the surgery when the patient is in the hospital for testing. The speech–language pathologist should realize that the patient may be in a state of shock, anxiety, denial, and confusion about the surgery and its implications for the future, even when the physician has spent time explaining in detail the procedures and likely results. In this visit, the speech–language pathologist should explain to the patient and family members the changes that will exist after surgery, particularly from a phonation and speech point of view. Following is a dialogue taken from a tape recording of a presurgery visit by a speech–language pathologist the day before patient R.A. had a total laryngectomy.

SLP: I know Dr. R. has gone over the specifics of the surgery but I wanted to review the implications of what the surgery will mean from a communication point of view. These diagrams [Figures 7.1 and 7.2 or similar diagrams] show the before-and-after surgery changes. The main point is that your larynx will be removed. Your larynx is important for two reasons: First, it is a valve that protects the airway to your lungs—your trachea—from food, liquid, saliva, and so on. Second, when air is forced through the valve during exhalation, the air vibrates the tissues of the valve and sound is produced. The tissues that vibrate are the vocal folds in the larynx. The sound of the vibration is what is known as the voice. You can feel the vibration of the larynx when you are talking by touching here. [Demonstration.]

R.A.: I think I understand about that.

SLP: Good. Now, since the larynx must be removed, the protective valve will be gone and the tissue that produces voice will also be gone. To protect your airway, the operation will include bringing your trachea forward and attaching it to an opening in your neck. You can see that in this diagram.

You will breathe through this opening in your neck for the rest of your life. It is called a stoma. Do you understand that?

R.A.: Yes, I knew that.

SLP: So, after your surgery you will breathe through the stoma and air will no longer go up through your mouth and nose, and you will no longer have a voice. You will not even be able to effectively whisper, because whispering requires air movement. [Demonstration.] And that is why I am here: To help you regain the ability to communicate, to help you find new ways of producing voice. Any questions so far?

R.A.: Dr. R. said I should be able to talk within a few weeks after surgery. Is that right?

SLP: My plan is to begin working with you as soon as possible. Dr. R. will have to tell me when you are ready. In the early days after surgery, you will likely spend much of your communication in writing simple requests on a pad. Then, when he gives me the green light, we will work as hard as possible to get you talking again. We have many options available to help you with communication. Some can be used immediately after your surgery. Some will be faster than others, and I want to go over some of those options now. First, many devices have been invented and are available to laryngectomized persons. Some of these devices are very effective in giving the laryngectomized person almost immediate communication. Let me demonstrate some of these. [The next few minutes were spent demonstrating the Cooper–Rand and Servox electrolarynges.]

R.A.: Do you sell these?

SLP: No, but I can tell you where you can get one, and loaners are available until you can get your own, should you decide to do that. Most laryngectomized persons try to learn what is called esophageal speech, even when they are using one of these devices. What this involves is taking air that is always present in your mouth and throat down into your esophagus—right here [shows diagram]. This air is then pushed gently up past this constriction and these tissues in the constriction are vibrated, very much like your vocal folds in the larynx are vibrated. This vibration produces a new sound, a new voice, and this sound is then resonated and articulated into the sounds of human speech. Because the esophagus is vibrating, it is called esophageal speech.

R.A.: You swallow air, and I heard someone say it is belched up, is that right?

SLP: Not quite. You won't swallow the air, because that would take it into the stomach, and we don't want it to go down that far; just a little way into the esophagus. Then it is brought back up to vibrate the tissue. There are many ways to get the air into the esophagus without swallowing it, and I will help you learn them when the time is right to begin. I want to play some tapes of people who have been laryngectomized and who speak with esophageal speech. Some of these people are very good, and others are more typical. Then later, after surgery, I will visit you again with a man who has been laryngectomized and speaks with esophageal voice. I think you will find his visit quite helpful. [Tapes are played and discussed.] I will leave these pamphlets [American Cancer Society] and this book [*Self-Help for Laryngectomees*, Lauder] with you. You and your family can look over the material. Here is my card with phone numbers. If you or any members of your family have questions, please call. Good luck on your surgery. Dr. R. is an excellent surgeon and you could not be in better hands. I'll be in touch.

This example shows how a presurgery visit should usually be handled. It is short, involves demonstrations and materials, involves the patient as well as family members, and is encouraging about the future of communication. It provides information but not in great detail. If the surgeon is planning on a primary and secondary TEP procedure, then details about that option should be included.

Doyle (1994) and Salmon (1999) provided an extensive listing of information that could be covered in the process of preoperative counseling. Preoperative counseling offers an opportunity for the patient to receive information and ask questions. Most important, it establishes the professional relationship necessary for good communication rehabilitation. This initial meeting, which should not occur until the physician requests it, will likely be the first of many, and additional information will unfold. The speech–language pathologist should be careful not to overwhelm the patient and significant others. It is most important to establish a relationship of trust and communication. I have found that going over the same information with a patient on several occasions is helpful, not repetitive and redundant. The first time the patient hears the physician explain about his or her cancer, what treatment options are available, and when such options will unfold, little information is retained or understood, because of the shock of hearing about the disease itself. Information provided after that initial consultation between the patient and physician is more likely to be understood and retained by the patient and family members.

The Artificial Larynx Controversy

The artificial larynx is not without controversy in the rehabilitation of laryngectomees. As reported by Lerman (1991), many laryngologists and laryngectomized persons have strong negative attitudes about the use of artificial devices for communication. Reasons for this attitude vary, but generally the objections are that the sound generated has an artificial nature and that using the devices prevents one from learning esophageal speech. A physician with a strong bias against the use of artificial devices can have such a significant influence on patients that they develop the same attitude.

This attitude is unfortunate because it is evident from the literature and clinical experience that for various reasons many laryngectomized persons do not learn functional and intelligible esophageal speech (Doyle, 1994; Gilmore, 1999). These individuals then have to turn to what has been described as a crutch or a backup system because they could not learn the "best" method. A more reasonable approach would be for all persons working with a laryngectomized person to have an open mind about all forms of alaryngeal phonation, expose the patient to each of them, and allow the individual to choose the form of communication after the surgery. The decision belongs to the patient, not to the physician, not to the speech–language pathologist, and not to another laryngectomized individual who might be in a position to offer advice.

The speech–language pathologist should mention early that, during the immediate period after surgery, much communication will likely occur by writing or by using an intraoral device. The speech–language pathologist might provide specific instructions on the use of an electrolarynx before surgery. The Cooper–Rand or some modification of another type of device that involves intraoral sound generation should be demonstrated and given to the patient to practice speaking. Then, after surgery, when the patient is out of intensive care and feeling stronger, the electrolarynx can be used in communication instead of writing. If an intraoral device is introduced, the speech–language pathologist should visit the patient after surgery to determine whether it is being used. Therapy can be given at that time to facilitate its use for immediate postsurgical communication. All of these instructions are modified when primary or secondary tracheoesophageal puncture (TEP) procedures are planned, as explained later in this chapter.

Because most hospitals in which laryngectomy surgery is performed have in-house speech–language pathology services, close patient contact is possible during pre- and postsurgical care. Each visit with the patient should be noted in the hospital record, detailing the essentials that the medical staff should be aware of (e.g., whether an electrolarynx has been presented, what questions were answered, and what specific instructions were given about communication). These notations also inform the physician that contact has been made (see Benninger & Grywalski, 1998; Doyle, 1994; Golper, 1998; Salmon, 1999).

Formal Alaryngeal Therapy

Although the speech–language pathologist's contacts with the patient occur before surgery and within a few days postsurgery, the time to initiate formal therapy directed toward esophageal voice depends on many factors, such as recovery progress, whether radiation is to occur before therapy, and physician attitudes. The speech–language pathologist should never begin esophageal speech therapy, however, until medical clearance has occurred.

Initial therapy efforts usually are directed at facilitating communication by means of artificial devices. Work with esophageal speech, assuming the patient has chosen that option, begins later. If the patient has been given an electrolarynx before surgery and wishes to continue using it, the speech–language pathologist should evaluate the effectiveness of mouth placement as well as articulation accuracy and intelligibility. If another device is desired, help should be provided in using it.

Some writing on paper or erasable marker boards will likely be a common means of communication in the early period after surgery. Many laryngectomized individuals who are given marker slates prefer those without children's themes. One man with whom I worked had been given Disney character slates. He said, "By the time I had an alternative means of communication, I went through Mickey Mouse, Donald Duck, and had started on Goofy. I was beginning to feel a little goofy myself."

If a neck device is chosen, the speech–language pathologist should provide direction, with the following recommendations:

• The nondominant hand is preferable for holding the device against the neck if the patient can handle the device without awkwardness. The placement is so critical, however, that it might be necessary to use the dominant hand. This, however, keeps the dominant hand from being used to write while talking, shake hands if right handed, or hold a phone.

• Neck placement is critical for proper transmission of sound into the vocal tract. The diaphragm of the device must be flat against the tissue of the neck, with enough pressure to transmit the sound into the vocal tract. Too little or too much pressure must be avoided. Trial and error will help determine the right amount of pressure and the best spot for placement.

• The patient must be able to move the device to the neck with accuracy and speed. Once the right spot is determined and proper placement pressure established, the patient must repeatedly practice moving the device to and from the neck. For example, the speech–language pathologist can have the patient (a) place the device, (b) say "1, 2, 3," and (c) move the device. After the patient repeats this process 10 times, the clinician can evaluate percentage of accuracy.

• Timing of switch activation must also be practiced. The patient must learn to depress the switch to turn on the vibration at the exact moment of speech initiation. Often the patient turns on the electrolarynx too early and it begins "talking" before the patient does, or, conversely, the patient says several sounds before the electrolarynx is turned on. With a larynx, timing of voicing and articulation is neurologically automatic. Without a larynx, the brain must be reprogrammed to establish timing.

• The patient must be trained not to continue electrolarynx vibration during speech pauses. This vibration causes unarticulated buzzing that can be most distracting. To eliminate this, a "magic thumb" must be established to turn the device off and on in concert with speech. Some patients have a difficult time accomplishing this process. Again, only practice and feedback from the speech–language pathologist will provide this accuracy of speech and electrolarynx voicing.

• The patient must be taught to clearly articulate the consonants of speech and to distinguish voiced from voiceless sounds, such as /t/ from /d/ and /k/ from /g/. This also requires much practice.

• It is important to establish that a patient can effectively use an electrolarynx on the phone. Should a patient need to contact someone over the phone, it is important that the patient have confidence in his or her ability. Developing this confidence must be part of the therapy process. (One man with whom I worked found his wife passed out on the floor one afternoon. He was able to telephone for help using his electrolarynx. His esophageal speech was not developed sufficiently at that time to communicate over the phone.)

• The patient should understand how to adjust the device in terms of loudness and pitch. The patient also must understand how to monitor the loudness in social settings such as restaurants so that more private conversations can occur.

To accomplish these goals, the speech–pathologist needs to incorporate electrolarynx use into many therapy sessions because it can be nearly as complex as esophageal speech (Salmon, 1999).

Teaching Esophageal Speech

In the event the TEP procedure is not being considered, the speech–language pathologist can use these instructions to help teach traditional esophageal speech. During the first session, the patient should be introduced to esophageal speech if this means of communication has been chosen by the patient. The speech–language pathologist should determine how technical the instructions should be. Most patients do not understand complex instructions regarding the anatomical and physiological bases of esophageal voice, so a behavioral approach is recommended.

My clinical experience indicates that a simple, rather direct approach is better during the first few sessions of teaching esophageal speech. It is better to tell the patient to say "ta" and determine whether esophageal voice occurs than to say something such as, "I would like you to put your tongue behind your upper teeth, build up some pressure, hold the pressure a little while until it has a chance to move down into your esophagus, then, when the air goes into your esophagus, bring it back up and that will cause the tissues of the P-E junction to vibrate. That vibration will be your new voice, and with it you can say /ta/." While the speech–language pathologist was giving all of those complex instructions (which more than likely would not be understood), the patient could have been practicing several /ta/ sounds.

With this concept of simplicity in mind, the following format for teaching a patient to produce esophageal voice is recommended. These steps are based on the work of many professionals already referenced, as well as on my clinical experience. The order of the following steps is not critical, but each procedure should be attempted until esophageal voice is elicited.

Step 1: Burp and Belch

I am always concerned that my instructions will lead to processes of voice production that might be counterproductive. This is certainly true when either of the terms *burp* or *belch* is used, because most people have experience with these bodily functions. However, if a laryngectomized person is able to produce voice quickly by attempting to burp or belch and it does not appear that the patient is attempting to bring up gas from the stomach to accomplish the task, it can be a quick method of teaching esophageal voice. The speech–language pathologist asks whether the patient has experienced a burp or belch since the surgery. If the answer is yes, the patient is asked whether this can be produced again. If the patient can do so, the professional asks for several repetitions. Next, the patient continues belching but with the mouth shaped for an open vowel sound, such as /ɑ/. The speech–language pathologist should demonstrate the process. The mouth then is shaped for an /o/, then a /u/, and so on, until all of the following vowels have been attempted: /i/, /ɪ/, /e/, /ɛ/, /æ/, /ɒ/, /o/, /u/, and /ɔ/.

Some vowels will be easier to produce than others. The patient should practice until each can be said intelligibly. Such quick belching generally does not involve air from the stomach. I would recommend eliminating the word *burp* or *belch* early in this process if sound is being generated by it. Merely encourage the patient to continue "making sounds."

Step 2: Consonant Injection

If the method in Step 1 is not successful in stimulating esophageal voice, elicitation with a consonant injection can be attempted. The patient is instructed to say /ta/, /pa/, /ka/, /sta/, and all other stop and fricative consonants followed by a vowel that is produced with the tongue low in the mouth, such as /a/ or /ɒ/.

By having the patient attempt all of the consonants, the speech–language pathologist can determine whether one is a better esophageal loader than another. If a specific one is, the patient should practice that consonant in combination with all of the vowels. For example, if the /t/ sound is found to stimulate a high incidence of esophageal voice when followed by an /i/ vowel, the patient should say the /t/ consonant with all of the vowels. It may be necessary to provide key words for each vowel, such as /ti/

as in *tea*. This drill can be practiced many times. The same process then can be attempted with another consonant until all stops and fricatives have been tried.

Step 3: Inhalation

If the first two steps have not facilitated esophageal voice, the inhalation method (explained earlier under "Methods of Air Intake") can be attempted. The patient is told to relax the throat muscles as much as possible, open the mouth as though about to yawn, then quickly inhale air into the stoma and attempt to sniff air into the nose at the same time. The speech–language pathologist should demonstrate this rather than describe it orally. If it works, as air is drawn into the stoma, it also will be drawn into the esophagus.

The patient then is instructed to say some open vowel such as /ɒ/. If sound is heard on the vowel, the process should be repeated until consistent voice is demonstrated. The patient then can shape the mouth for other vowel sounds as the esophagus is loaded by this inhalation method. Consonants can be added to the vowels to form simple words such as *pie, tie, kick, I,* and *above*. In the inhalation method, it does not matter whether the words begin with a consonant or a vowel.

Step 4: Glossopress

If all of the preceding steps fail to stimulate esophageal voice, the speech–language pathologist can attempt to elicit it with the glossopress method, explained earlier in this chapter. Essentially, this method involves using the tongue to press or inject air into the esophagus in a piston like fashion. The patient is told to put the tongue tip on the roof of the mouth just behind the incisor teeth, then pump it against the palate or pharynx to squeeze air into the esophagus. The movements are similar to the beginning stage of swallowing, except that air, rather than food or liquid, is being moved. (However, as explained earlier, the term *swallow* should be avoided.)

As air is moved into the esophagus with these pressing methods, a slight noise ("klunk") can be heard. This is the signal that the air has entered the esophagus and the patient should then push the air out of the esophagus to generate the voice sound. The voice then is shaped into sounds and words in the manner described in Steps 1, 2, and 3. The sequence is

▶ *Inject . . . say "/ɒ/"; inject . . . say "/i/"; inject . . . say "/o/."*

Later, after continued practice, the sequence is

▶ *Inject . . . say "above"; inject . . . say "drink it."*

With this method of loading the esophagus, the patient can say sounds or words in any consonant–vowel or vowel–consonant combination.

The result of these steps is that the patient learns to produce esophageal voice and speech. It is quite possible that the individual will learn to take air into the esophagus in a manner that does not exactly parallel any of those described. However voice is accomplished, if the patient can duplicate the process and there are no negative aspects, it should be reinforced. It also is quite possible that after the patient begins to put sounds and words together into functional speech, combinations of methods can be used to load the esophagus with air. There is no problem with this, and it is more typical than atypical. Combinations are likely to occur without the patient's awareness as a consequence of the dynamic movements involved in alaryngeal voice and articulation processes. An excellent reference on many of these processes of teaching esophageal speech in the initial stages was provided by Duguay (1999).

Alaryngeal Phrasing

Once alaryngeal voice is produced and used in monosyllabic words, the next task is to teach simple phrases. It is the speech–language pathologist's responsibility to select phrases that are rather easy to acquire early in training. The patient should practice words that are easy to say, such as *pack, tack, stack,* and *pick,* and put them into phrases such as "pack it, tack it, stack it" or "pack it up, tack it up, stack it up." The patient should articulate these phrases quickly. It is quite probable that esophageal voice, limited as it may be in this early stage, is sufficient to support the entire phrase.

Once a patient consistently and reliably produces esophageal voice and puts it into easy phrases, steady progress toward functional communication occurs. It is important for the speech–language pathologist to keep the patient functioning at a high percentage of success (80% or better) as task difficulty is increased. For example, if a patient is reading a list of phrases and 80% are intelligible, it is not necessary to be concerned about the 20% that are causing difficulty. The patient should pass over them after a single attempt. Often, on some future reading of the list, the difficult ones will be spoken clearly. It is counterproductive to become hung up on difficult tasks.

In addition to consistency and reliability of voice production, it is most important to work for esophageal speech that is intelligible. Strangers should listen as the patient speaks lists of words or phrases to determine whether the speech is intelligible. The speech–language pathologist often becomes too familiar with the practice lists and thus is not a good judge of intelligibility. It is of some help if the speech–language pathologist turns away from the patient as lists are read to determine whether they are intelligible without the conscious or unconscious help of lip reading. If a patient can be intelligible without the listener's having the benefit of lip reading, progress is being made toward functional alaryngeal speech.

Key:

/ = Patient's first pause.
// = Suggested target of pause.

Terry/took the/truck/up the/road to/the camp/site/.   *Inadequate*
We wan/ted a/truck/as/soon as/possible.

Terry//took the truck//up the road// to the campsite//.   *Improved pause and*
We wanted//the truck//as soon as//possible.   *phrasing*

Figure 7.6. Patterns of phrasing.

Esophageal Speech Phrasing

Early in the esophageal speech training of laryngectomized persons, it becomes obvious that careful attention to phrasing is necessary. The patient soon learns that the capability has not yet been developed to produce sufficient voice to complete some long phrases, so the esophagus must be loaded with air again to continue. This loading process should be done at breaks that are natural to the flow of the utterance and must be practiced repeatedly. Long phrases can be marked at suggested places:

▶ Open the door/and bring/the book to me./

▶ Stay awhile/but please/don't awaken me./

▶ Tell the doctor/I'm not/feeling well./

Another technique helpful in teaching phrasing is to record a speech sample as the patient is talking about some topic of interest. For example, the patient is discussing going hunting over the weekend. After a few sentences of esophageal speech about hunting, the recorder is stopped and rewound. The speech–language pathologist then writes on a piece of paper or chalkboard the patient's actual language and marks the junctures used in esophageal loading. Whether the break occurred appropriately can then be determined. If it did not, a predetermined pattern of more appropriate phrasing is practiced (see Figure 7.6).

Usually, patients can improve their speech flow by consciously attending to phrasing. There are no hard rules on this for the esophageal speaker. Rather, pauses should occur at natural breaks in the flow of the speech. It is best, for example, not to pause to load between an article and its noun. By emphasizing the noun and de-emphasizing the article, the patient usually can put them together with the same load of esophageal air. Careful attention to appropriate phrasing facilitates better intelligibility in the patient's speech by providing context cues.

Avoidance of Poor Speech Habits

Many aspects of a laryngectomized person's esophageal voice, such as articulation, speech rhythm, and resonance, remain relatively unaffected by the surgery. However, the structural changes resulting from the surgery can have a negative effect on general speech habits and processes. The speech–language pathologist must be aware of any potential bad habits that might become distracting and affect intelligibility. The patient should be helped to eliminate them. The following are common areas of concern.

Facial Distortion

The patient should practice speech tasks in front of a mirror to minimize abnormal facial tics and distortions that often are part of esophageal speaking. Eye blinks and lip grimaces during esophageal loading occur often and should be avoided from the beginning of training. This also is true of head jerks as air is taken into the esophagus. Some patients have also had radical neck dissection as part of their laryngeal surgery, which can have an effect on head position during speaking. The speech–language pathologist can help the patient become aware of these facial, lip, head, and neck positions and determine whether adjustment during speech training can help eliminate them.

Stoma Management and Stoma Noise

Breathing through the stoma presents many problems to the laryngectomized person. Mucus accumulates at the orifice and must be wiped away continually. Tissues crust and become dried by the breathing process, often resulting in coughing when pieces fall into the trachea. Most patients are also psychologically concerned about the appearance of the stoma and use neckwear to cover it. Patients become excessively "stoma conscious." This is understandable because difficulties are common.

One primary concern of stoma control involves excessive noise during breathing and speaking. The size of the stoma varies from patient to patient. Some stomas are so small that breathing is impeded to the degree that air rushing into and out of the stoma produces excessive noise. This sound is distracting to the quality of speech. If a patient is to experience difficulty with this stoma noise, it will be apparent from the first few utterances. Help the individual become aware of the noise and attempt to reduce it. This can be done by teaching the person to breathe with less effort and not to push so hard with abdominal muscles during speech attempts. Once again, it is important that the speech–language pathologist be aware of this noise from the first moment it occurs so that it will not develop into a bad speech habit.

Reduced Loudness of Voice

One of the most perplexing problems a laryngectomized person experiences when using esophageal speech is, as noted earlier, the reduced loudness potential of the voice. It is difficult to communicate in noisy places such as stores, restaurants, night-clubs, sporting events, and cocktail parties. Counseling is necessary to help the patient recognize the loudness limitation. It usually is impossible to compete with the noise of society. To attempt to do so results in reduced articulation control, unintelligibility, stoma noise, injection noise, and general speech ineffectiveness.

Increasing loudness should not be attempted until functional and proficient esophageal speech has been achieved. It is not an early priority in the therapy process. After speech proficiency has been attained, the patient can work to increase loudness by shortening the utterance, loading the esophagus more often, and pushing harder with the abdominal muscles as voice is attempted. However, these adjustments should occur only in unique circumstances. The laryngectomee should be aware that these adjustments for greater loudness diminish quality control.

Another technique that has helped some patients increase loudness is to apply slight digital pressure (one or two fingers) on the tissue of the neck where esophageal vibration can be felt. This can add constriction and tonicity to the vibrating tissue and help increase the loudness of vibration. The speech–language pathologist can experiment with the digital pressure to determine whether the technique is helpful.

A laryngectomee also can increase loudness by using an artificial device when going into a social situation with an expected high noise level. Use of a Servox or similar device can be more effective than an esophageal voice. If a patient has been trained properly to use all possible methods of alaryngeal communication and has no bias against artificial devices, a difficult communication situation can be improved.

The speech–language pathologist must understand fully how to help the laryngectomized person with these special problems. Many experienced clinicians provide tips on strategies to accomplish these clinical goals (Doyle, 1994; Duguay, 1999; Haroldson, 1999; Salmon, 1999; Shanks, 1999).

GOAL OF FUNCTIONAL ESOPHAGEAL SPEECH

When has the goal of proficient and functional esophageal speech been reached? The speech–language pathologist and the patient together must evaluate progress to determine when the goal has been attained. Aronson (1990) listed several criteria that can be used as a guide:

- Reliable phonation on demand
- Rapid air intake
- Short latency between air intake and phonation
- Four to nine syllables per air charge
- 2 to 3 seconds of voice duration per air intake
- Eighty-five to 129 words per minute
- Fundamental frequency of 52 to 82 Hz
- Average intensity of 6 to 7 dB below normal
- Good intelligibility

These criteria represent the goal of communication rehabilitation in laryngectomees when esophageal speech is the chosen form of alaryngeal voice.

The following case illustrates the difficulty, frustration, and satisfaction of working with laryngectomized patients.

CASE EXAMPLE OF ALARYNGEAL PHONATION

L. W., a 49-year-old man, was laryngectomized as a result of cancer of the upper esophagus. His surgery was rather atypical in that both his esophagus and larynx were removed. This required construction of a pseudoesophagus by displacing stomach tissue upward to connect it to his pharynx (gastric pull-up; Hartley et al., 1999). He also had radical neck dissection and extensive radiation to his jaw and neck area.

After an extended stay in the hospital, L. W. was released with little clinical help in restoring communication ability because he lived far from the facility where the surgery was performed. He went for several weeks attempting to communicate by writing on a pad. He was an executive with a major telephone company and had been introduced to the electrolarynx but rejected it. On his own he developed a pharyngeal voice by squeezing air between his tongue and the pharynx and became quite intelligible except on the telephone. He reported that his work required extensive long-distance communication and that operators and clients continually hung up on him, thinking he was a prank caller.

Six months after his surgery, with pharyngeal speech his only means of communication, I met L.W. Because of his extensive surgery and radiation, the prognosis for learning any other means of communication besides his present method was unclear. I introduced him to several artificial devices, which he rejected. We decided to attempt "esophageal" speech to determine whether his displaced stomach tissue could be vibrated in the typical sense.

After 3 weeks of this therapy, L. W. could produce short and rather choppy utterances with the locus of vibration in the pseudoesophagus. Although he was not satisfied with the quality of his voice, it seemed to him better than his pharyngeal voice. He was loading his pseudoesophagus primarily by means of consonant and glossopress injection.

On one occasion, L. W. was speaking with a group of student speech–language pathologists about his experiences with throat cancer, using esophageal voice in a rather slow and choppy manner but with complete intelligibility. During his speech he put his hand up to press gently on the necktie he was wearing as he attempted to produce voice. A dramatic change in voice quality occurred. Rather than choppy and low in pitch, he produced voice with smoother quality and with less effort. The pitch also was higher.

After his speech, an analysis of the bases of change in his voice indicated that L. W. had begun to take air into his esophagus by inhalation and that the digital pressure, evenly disbursed by the tie, applied just enough pressure to the vibrating site (P-E junction) to allow quality phonation. The goal immediately became to improve this newly found technique of alaryngeal phonation. After 2 weeks of therapy, he had developed a superior voice quality with the following characteristics: $F_0 = 120$ Hz (B_1); 15 syllables per inhalation maximum with a mean of 10 syllables; 120 words spoken per minute with 100% intelligibility.

Several times at work after developing his new voice quality, L. W. reported that when talking on the phone, clients who did not know him asked if he had a slight cold. He considered such remarks great compliments. He now enjoys addressing youth groups and is in great demand as a speaker. He is a totally rehabilitated person and an inspiration to people who meet him.

TRACHEOESOPHAGEAL PUNCTURE

For several decades, attempts have been made to overcome the significant disadvantage of esophageal speech from the point of view of limited air reserve to drive the tissues of the upper esophagus to produce esophageal phonation. As mentioned previously, the esophagus when inflated with air can hold fewer than 100 ml of air. Thus, a new charge of air is needed after only a few syllables of esophageal phonation. Surgeons and researchers have attempted, therefore, to somehow connect the vast capacity of the lungs to provide the airflow and air pressure to drive the P-E junction. The complication has always been centered on diverting the air into the esophagus while maintaining the safety of the respiratory tract during swallowing of saliva, liquids, and foods. Weinberg (1980) reviewed several of these surgical and prosthetic approaches to tapping the pulmonary capacity of the lungs to drive the P-E junction while protecting the airway. He reviewed the work of Conley, Calcaterra, Taub, Sisson, Miller, Serafini, Asai, and others. The road leading to the current status of the tracheoesophageal fistula or puncture (referred to here simply as TEP) is fascinating, and any speech–language pathologist who works with TEP patients should have a historical appreciation of the many steps leading to it.

Additional references to historical perspective were provided by Singer, Blom, and Hamaker (1989) and Blom (1998a), who reviewed the pioneering efforts to connect the lungs to the esophagus. The procedures reviewed met with mixed success but failed to gain generalized acceptance and use. Most of the reviewed procedures are no longer used. The attempt to shunt air from the lungs and the difficulties involved changed when Blom and Singer (1979) reported endoscopic techniques for shunting air from the trachea into the esophagus, allowing pulmonary air to vibrate the P-E junction after laryngectomy. The procedure involves inserting a prosthesis into the TEP.

TEP Procedure

The TEP procedure involves a surgically produced tracheoesophageal fistula that links the trachea and esophagus for prosthesis insertion. The TEP can be done as a primary procedure at the time of laryngectomy or as a secondary procedure at any time after primary laryngectomy (Blom & Hamaker, 1996; Blom et al., 1998; Meyerhoff & Rice, 1992). Several physicians have developed prostheses, including Panje, Groningen, Algaba, Staffieri, Traissac, Herrmann, and Provox (Blom, 1998a). Whether done as a primary or a secondary procedure, a catheter stint is inserted into the TEP and maintained until healing has occurred. The catheter is then removed and replaced by a silicone (Silastic) prosthesis. The prosthesis functions as a one-way valve that allows air to be shunted from the lungs into the esophagus but prevents liquids, including saliva, and food from passing from the esophagus into the trachea. The original Blom–Singer prosthesis is now distributed by InHealth Technologies (see "Resource Information and Materials" section at the end of this chapter).

Once in place, the prosthesis is stabilized by a retention flange or strap (see Figure 7.7). The prosthesis is also held in place by means of a retention collar. At the proximal (esophageal) end of the prosthesis is a razor-thin slit that resembles a duck's bill or flapper. This slit or flapper constitutes the one-way valve aspect of the prosthesis. Variations of the prosthesis include different lengths and resistances (from duckbill type to low pressure). Current Blom–Singer prostheses include duckbill (16 French), low-pressure (16 French), low-pressure (20 French), and indwelling (20 French; Blom, 1998a).

To shunt air from the trachea into the esophagus for voice, the laryngectomized person must either manually occlude the stoma or be fitted with an air pressure tracheostoma valve that automatically closes during breathing for speech. A kit is available for determining the resistance of the tracheostoma valve so that it does not close during normal breathing but only when speech is intended. The valve chosen must not close easily during normal breathing, even under some conditions of exertion, such as walking up stairs, but be able to withstand the necessary airflow and pressure to shunt air behind it through the prosthesis for voice. A universal housing mechanism accompanies the tracheostoma valve and is held in place within the stoma by tape and a special glue. During coughing, the patient can easily reach up and remove the tracheostoma valve from its housing.

Air shunted from the lungs into the prosthesis is diverted into the esophagus below the P-E segment. This air will vibrate the tissue of the P-E segment to produce esophageal voice. Theoretically, the sound of TEP-produced esophageal voice should not differ in quality from traditional esophageal voice, but many TEP speakers demonstrate superior quality to traditional esophageal speakers. Certainly, TEP

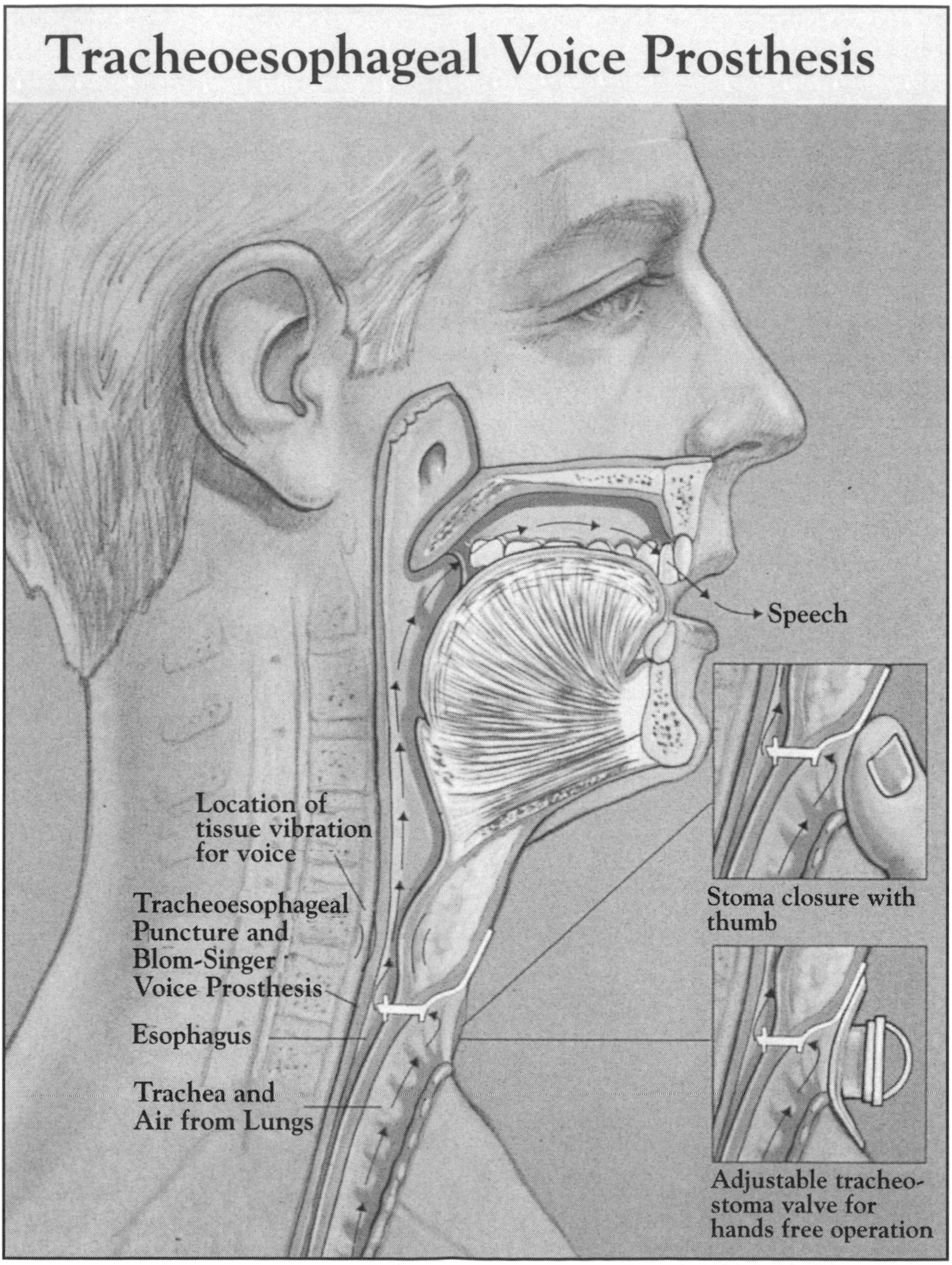

Tracheoesophageal Voice Prosthesis

Speech

Location of tissue vibration for voice

Tracheoesophageal Puncture and Blom-Singer Voice Prosthesis

Esophagus

Trachea and Air from Lungs

Stoma closure with thumb

Adjustable tracheo-stoma valve for hands free operation

Figure 7.7. Sagittal view of laryngectomized individual with Blom–Singer prosthesis in the tracheoesophageal puncture. Shown are two options for air diversion: thumb closure and tracheostomal valve. (Illustration courtesy of International Healthcare Technologies.)

speech differs in durability because it is driven by 3,000 ml of lung air, compared to less than 100 ml of air when the esophagus is the neolung. The esophageal voice produced is then resonated and articulated into speech in the vocal tract in the same manner as laryngeal or traditional esophageal speech after laryngectomy.

Choosing a Prosthesis After TEP

Juarbe et al. (1989) provided data to indicate that TEP can be used for voice restoration even after extended laryngopharyngectomy. Regardless of whether it is used after extended surgery or typical laryngectomy, several criteria have been established to guide clinicians in determining whether a patient would be a good candidate for TEP alaryngeal phonation. The TEP procedure may be used on many patients who fit the acceptance criteria that follow. The specific criteria to be met depend on whether the patient is being considered for primary (at the time of laryngectomy) or secondary TEP. However, there are some general principles that apply to both primary and secondary considerations. Secondary considerations are considered first (Perry, 1998).

• *Tonic pharyngoesophageal junction*. Postlaryngectomy, the patient must have a tonic or sufficiently patent junction between the pharynx and the esophagus (the P-E junction) to allow air to move in and out easily for alaryngeal voice. If the patient has attempted traditional esophageal speech and has been able to produce voice without difficulty, one can infer that the P-E junction is at least fairly adequate for TEP considerations. However, to determine directly the status of the PE junction for TEP consideration, Perry (1998) recommended a videofluoroscopic assessment with three components: modified barium swallow evaluation, attempted phonation, and esophageal insufflation test. The modified barium swallow consists of having the patient swallow liquid barium while the pharynx and upper esophagus are screened in the lateral position. This allows visualization of dilation potential of the PE junction. When the mucosa of the pharynx is outlined with barium, the patient is instructed to use esophageal speech by injecting air into the upper esophagus and counting from 1 to 10 or by repeating /pa/ three times. The esophageal insufflation test involves inserting transnasally a catheter to a distance of 25 cm in the P-E junction from the nares. The catheter is attached to an adapter for placement around the stoma. The patient occludes the adapter and diverts pulmonary air through the catheter into the esophagus or P-E junction while attempting to produce sustained voicing. Successful criteria include counting continuously from 1 to 15 and sustaining uninterrupted phonation of a vowel for 8 seconds.

• *Manual dexterity and visual acuity*. An additional criterion for TEP consideration involves the dexterity of the patient, who will have primary responsibility for management of the stoma and prosthesis, including placement on a regular basis when the indwelling prosthesis is not used. This dexterity allows proper cleaning, changeover, and maintenance of the prosthesis and stoma. To do these tasks, adequate visual acuity must be found in the patient. If the patient cannot fulfill these expectations for dexterity and visual acuity, a family member may be taught to assume these primary responsibilities, but this is considered a less satisfactory arrangement.

• *Tracheostoma size.* Stoma size has been a concern throughout the development of the TEP voice restoration history. In the past a stoma size of 2.0 cm in diameter was considered necessary, but now the stoma size can be managed by stomaplasty or use of a soft silicone laryngectomy tube. In secondary TEP processes, stomaplasty can be undertaken at the time of TEP surgery.

• *Psychological and familial considerations.* As in any medical procedure of change, it is important to consider the attitude and expectation of the patient and significant family members as one component in the decision-making process when considering TEP. If the patient and significant others expect the TEP to be an easy and quick solution to communication needs, disappointment is likely to result. The TEP procedure requires continual attention to many factors, some of which have already been described, and excellent information must be made available to patients about what is involved. Certainly, visits with other TEP users, as in laryngectomy support groups, would be helpful. A newsletter titled *Clinical Insights* is also available from the International Center for Post-Laryngectomy Voice Restoration, 7440 North Shadeland, Suite 200, Indianapolis, IN 42650; (800) 283-1056. This newsletter provides direction and suggestion on many problem-solving concerns. Additional concerns that must be considered in determining whether a patient would be a good candidate for secondary TEP include the following:

- The patient must be highly motivated to accomplish TEP communication and have a strong desire to establish excellent communication skill. A taciturn patient would not be a good candidate for TEP consideration.

- At least 6 weeks must pass after initial laryngectomy before secondary TEP surgery is performed.

- The patient must have adequate understanding of postsurgical anatomy and physiology.

- The patient must understand the basic function of TEP voice prosthesis processes.

- The patient must exhibit the ability to care for the prosthesis to maintain cleanliness and prevent bacterial and yeast strain (biofilm) formations on the prosthesis (Busscher & van der Mei, 1998).

- The patient should be healthy enough from a respiratory perspective to have adequate pulmonary support for prosthesis usage.

- The patient should meet another successful user of TEP to help evaluate whether the process would be desirable.

- The patient must have access to a speech–language pathologist or other professional with experience in the management of TEP processes.

- The patient should be mentally stable and have excellent mental health for rehabilitation (Doyle, 1994; Perry, 1998).

Videofluoroscopic Assessment Failure

One factor that will preclude successful use of the TEP procedure for alaryngeal voice is a pharyngoesophageal spasm. Some patients experience a spasm as pressure is increased in the esophagus. Effective voice must be produced for at least 8 seconds (counting audibly to 15) to pass the insufflation test. At least five trials are recommended. If there is pharyngoesophageal spasm, it will occur soon after voicing begins and the speech–language pathologist or laryngologist can visualize it on the fluoroscope.

If a patient fails the insufflation test but desires to proceed with TEP voice restoration, one of two clinical procedures will likely be necessary to eliminate a spasm (radiologically confirmed, see Hamaker & Cheesman, 1998; Singer et al., 1989): primary or secondary pharyngeal constrictor myotomy or pharyngeal plexus neurectomy. For the pharyngeal constrictor myotomy, the surgical intent is to identify and unilaterally cut (tunnel) the inferior (including cricopharyngeus) and middle pharyngeal constrictor muscles, thereby decreasing their sphincter to contractibility. In the pharyngeal plexus neurectomy, the surgeon identifies the nerves that provided innervation to the constrictor muscles, particularly the middle constrictor, and the nerve supply is sectioned when confirmed by stimulation and observation of muscles involved. The result of myotomy and neurectomy is to provide a P-E junction that is less likely to spasm under conditions of TEP and prosthetic voice use.

Since 1992, an additional means of establishing a more patent P-E junction for esophageal or TEP voice restoration has been BTX, discussed in Chapter 5. Hoffman and McCulloch (1998) described the basic techniques, which include use of EMG guidance for multiple-site injections. A trial lidocaine block may be administered as an initial indicator of likely success of BTX. Some patients require repeated injections after a few-month interval of successful patency, but others are able to maintain TEP use without repeated injections.

Steps in TEP Voice Restoration

Once the TEP has been surgically generated and maintained by means of a catheter, it often is the speech–language pathologist's responsibility to introduce to the patient the prosthesis that will be used and to train the laryngectomized person to use and maintain it. This requires training, skill, confidence, and tender hands. The patient can be fitted with a prosthesis about 3 to 4 days after the TEP surgery. The patient can begin speaking with the TEP as soon as it is inserted. General procedures involved in tracheoesophageal voice prosthesis fitting and training were provided by Leder and Blom (1998) and Bosone (1999). The following steps can serve as guidance, not as a recipe, for the procedure:

• The speech–language pathologist must wear sterile gloves during the entire procedure of catheter removal and prosthesis insertion and use. When the catheter is removed, the speech–language pathologist must be prepared to immediately insert the prosthesis. A voice prosthesis sizer is available so that the proper length of prosthesis can be used. Resizing routinely occurs during the first few weeks of prosthesis placement. The prosthesis sizer provides information for initial prosthesis length.

• When the catheter is removed, the patient should be instructed not to swallow until the prosthesis is in place. The patient can attempt to phonate by manually occluding the stoma prior to placement of the prosthesis.

• Next the prosthesis is inserted as determined by the sizing process. The catheter is removed, the prosthesis is placed on the inserter stick, the prosthesis strap is held against the inserter, the catheter is removed, and the prosthesis is inserted. As the prosthesis is inserted, a slight amount of pressure will be felt as the retention collar is pushed past the wall of the TEP. Once the prosthesis is securely in place, the difficult part of the procedure is over. The inserter is removed from the prosthesis by holding the strap against the patient's skin while twisting or twirling out the inserter. Before securing the strap with tape, voice can again be attempted. The retention strap can then be secured with tape. This procedure of prosthesis insertion is somewhat uncomfortable for the patient but does not hurt. Coughing may occur because the tissues around the stoma and TEP are sensitive to the touch. After prosthesis insertion and strap retention are completed, the patient should relax for a minute until any coughing is over.

• The patient is now ready to attempt voice usage. It is best for the speech–language pathologist to manually occlude the stoma for air shunting through the prosthesis during these initial voice trials. On instruction the patient takes a deep breath, exhales, and opens the mouth as if saying an /a/ sound. During exhalation the speech–language pathologist should occlude the stoma with as little pressure as necessary to stop all air from escaping from the stoma. If the prosthesis is working well, the patient will produce voice and a clear /a/ sound will be heard during the entire exhalation cycle. A little air escapement around the speech–language pathologist's thumb is not unusual at this point but should be minimal.

• After a few trials with the speech–language pathologist occluding the stoma, the patient should be allowed to occlude using the thumb of the nondominant hand. A large mirror will help the patient see what is happening. After a few trials of inhaling, occluding during exhaling while producing /a/, then removing the thumb for normal inhalation breathing, the patient should be comfortable with the procedure. Then the patient can be instructed to count, name the days of the week, and say simple phrases. This can be done with the patient occluding the stoma with his or her own thumb.

• Next the patient is taught to insert the prosthesis without help. The patient must learn to remove the catheter, refrain from swallowing while the TEP is open, then use the inserter stick to insert the prosthesis. The process for removing a prosthesis and inserting it again as would be done during cleaning should be followed. It is important that the patient understand that either a prosthesis or a catheter must be in the TEP at all times, even during the few minutes it takes to clean the prosthesis. Some patients like to remove the prosthesis for cleaning after a few days, whereas others can go a few weeks. This is an individual matter and depends on factors such as mucus secretions and general hygiene. International Healthcare Technologies also provides a silicon stent for placement in the TEP during cleaning or replacement of the prosthesis.

Tracheostomal Valve

With TEP alaryngeal voice, the patient has the option of manually occluding the stoma for voicing or using a tracheostomal valve (see Figure 7.7). The tracheostomal valve allows the patient to shunt lung air into the prosthesis for voicing without hand usage. There have been several design modifications to the original Blom–Singer Tracheostomal Valve as shown in Figure 7.7. The original design involved a latex flapper valve that was open for normal breathing but responded to respiratory pressure and closed for voicing. The current valve is made of silicone, rather than latex, giving it greater durability and sensitivity to closure pressures. The design also essentially eliminates the noise of closure, which sounded much like a tiny but audible thud. An alternative to the Blom–Singer valve is manufactured by Bivona and is spring-loaded for pressure closure. The Bivona design does not allow for quiet closure. Both devices require an attachment housing that fits over the stoma and into which the valve is inserted. According to Blom (1998b), approximately 35–65% of TEP users employ the Tracheostomal Valve for hands-free speech.

The most widely used method of tracheostoma valve attachment is by means of an adhesive-backed, flexible, polyvinylchloride housing that attaches to the skin surrounding the stoma and is held in place with a liquid adhesive. This is done after the skin has been cleaned with an alcohol swab. A circular disk of double-faced tape matching the valve housing in shape is applied to the valve housing. This allows positioning of the housing in the peristomal region. The closure valve can then be inserted into the housing and used for hands-free speech. The valve will be open for breathing and closed when gentle pressures of speech are applied to it. When excessive pressures occur, such as in a sudden cough, the valve allows breakthrough pressures. However, patients are encouraged to quickly remove the valve from the housing when a cough is expected. This prevents the mucus from accumulating on the valve, which would require cleaning. Many patients decide to merely use manual occlusion when speaking rather than deal with the many facets of tracheostomal valve usage. Patients can also select certain days on which the housing will be placed for use of the tracheostomal valve, for example, when giving a speech, having long conversations not normally experienced, or in other instances of prolonged voice use. Blom (1998b) discussed the reasons for failure of the tracheostomal valve and provided ways of overcoming the difficulties.

Currently, many surgeons perform the TEP as a primary procedure at the time of laryngectomy (Freeman & Hamaker, 1998), and the prosthesis is put into the TEP when sufficient healing has occurred, in about 7 to 10 days. The surgeon will decide when the patient is cleared for TEP placement. When the prosthesis is inserted after a primary TEP procedure, several days should pass with the prosthesis in place before the patient is asked to use it for voice. Leder and Blom (1998) recommended waiting at least 1 week. This caution is because of the remote possibility that the air pressure used in speech could produce a fistula on a healing suture line from the laryngectomy operation.

Another trend in TEP is use of the indwelling prosthesis. A kit is available from International Healthcare Technologies that includes a Blom–Singer Indwelling Low Pressure Voice Prosthesis, which must be inserted by a physician or trained speech–language pathologist. This indwelling prosthesis can remain in the patient for as long as 6 months and should be removed and replaced only by a trained clinician. It is recommended that an indwelling prosthesis be used only after tracheoesophageal wall tissues have stabilized (several weeks after the laryngectomy) and that replaceable prostheses be used until stabilization has occurred. The indwelling prosthesis is ideal for patients who are unable or unwilling to do the routine removing, cleaning, and reinsertion of the regular nonindwelling prosthesis (Leder & Blom, 1998).

The invention and manufacture of the various prostheses and tracheostomal valves for TEP speech constitute a remarkable advancement in voice restoration after laryngectomy. Duguay (1989) stated that, with the advent of TEP procedures and additional biotechnical developments, esophageal speech is being changed in a revolutionary manner. Lopez, Kraybill, McElroy, and Guena (1987) reported that 88% of surgeons (sample of 1,999) use TEP as a voice restoration procedure for an average of 30% of their patients. The younger the surgeon, the more likely it is that he or she will use the procedure.

A large body of literature compares the TEP to traditional esophageal speech and artificial devices and addresses general TEP concerns (Doyle, 1994; Gomyo & Doyle, 1989; Lewin, 1999; Pauloski, 1998; Pauloski, Fisher, Kempster, & Blom, 1989; Robbins, Christensen, & Kempster, 1986; Sedory, Hamlet, & Connor, 1989). The interested reader is encouraged to investigate these resources. In any regard, there is little question that the speech–language pathologist who works with laryngectomized individuals must be comfortable with TEP, the prostheses available, the tracheostomal valves, and management concerns.

CHALLENGES IN REHABILITATION OF LARYNGECTOMIZED PERSONS

The speech–language pathologist working with laryngectomized persons faces several challenges. The laryngectomized person often has difficulty accepting (a) the loss of communication; (b) the stoma and being a neck breather; (c) the feeling of being a whole person who still is desirable to others, particularly physically; (d) intimate physical contact; and (e) changes in the ability to smell, taste, swim, shower, and bathe. The person also may be unable to continue in a profession, have problems with alcohol or drug dependence, or live with the daily threat that all of the cancer was not removed and may return at any time. The speech–language pathologist must recognize that all of these factors can have an impact on progress. Instruction for management of these factors can be found in an excellent reference by Shanks (1999) titled "Consequences of Total Laryngectomy in Daily Living Activities." Shanks draws on his decades of experience working with laryngectomized individuals in his discussion of respiratory, protective, deglutitive, coughing, emotional, psychosocial, sexual, and many additional concerns and provides excellent recommendations to help the patient in these concerns of daily living.

Therapy for persons who have been laryngectomized can be provided individually or in group settings, regardless of the method of alaryngeal communication being used. When group settings are used, which is common, the guidance provided by Lerman (1999) is very helpful and highly recommended.

I once worked with a laryngectomized woman who taught me a great lesson about the importance of establishing alaryngeal communication. She had terminal cancer and was expected to die soon. Her physicians knew it, she knew it, her husband knew it, and her children knew it. I questioned whether she wanted to continue to work hard in her speech therapy. She rejected any attempt to discontinue her therapy, and she strived for improvement in her ability to communicate. She said, "I have to be able to plead my case with St. Peter very soon!"

To ignore the psychological state of this client or others like her would be tantamount to clinical faux pas. The laryngectomized person is not "a speech defect," or "a stoma," or "a missing larynx," or "a P-E segment," or "an esophageal speaker," or "a Blom–Singer prosthesis speaker," or "a terminal client," but rather is a person, a human being, and maybe a father or mother, a grandparent, a lover, a friend, and so on. All of these life roles that represent personhood transcend the significance of laryngeal amputation. I recently watched a television program in which a patient was dying from some disease. Her husband of many decades was pleading with the physician not to remove her life support. The physician clearly was not viewing this woman from the same perspective as her husband who reminded the physician, "I just want you to know that this woman has 14 grandchildren and 5 great-grandchildren." It is important for speech–language pathologists to look beyond patients' stomas and TEPS, P-E segments, and injection noises and remember the perspective of those who have lived with and loved those people.

LARYNGEAL TRANSPLANT

In January 1998 medical history was made when Dr. Marshall Strome of The Cleveland Clinic Foundation performed a successful human larynx transplant on Tim Heidler who had been laryngectomized after a tragic accident at age 21. This was a controversial procedure because there is significant risk with any organ transplant and the larynx is not a vital organ; thousands of individuals throughout the world live without a larynx. This chapter has been about those thousands. There were other risks, including a lifetime of having to take immunosuppressive drugs and the possibility of permanent dysphagia and compromised valving potential for respiration and voice. In addition to transplanting the entire larynx, Strome transplanted several rings of tracheal cartilage, a large portion of the pharynx, and the thyroid and parathyroid glands. The transplantation occurred with suturing of the main structures in place, reconnection of both superior laryngeal nerves and the right recurrent laryngeal nerve, and the establishment of a tracheostoma. All of this was done with the hope that function would be adequate for breathing, swallowing, and voice.

Heidler's voice and swallowing functions were evaluated carefully using a variety of acoustic and visual endoscopic and stroboscopic examinations at periodic intervals after transplant. His swallowing functions developed nicely without aspiration, and some voicing occurred. His vocal folds were found under visualization to be immobile, with the right vocal fold paralyzed in a median position and the left in a position off midline. Under conditions of attempted voice, both vocal folds interrupted the airstream and manifested vibratory potential. Heidler's voice was evaluated at various stages, and 16 months after transplant, his fundamental frequency was in the gender-appropriate range of 117–137 Hz, jitter values approached the normal range (.96–1.46%), sustained phonation duration was an excellent 20.3 seconds, and a near-normal mean laryngeal airflow of 157 ml/sec was manifested. Heidler's voice quality was judged as near normal with a somewhat softer, raspy voice quality. Speech–language patholgists who judged his voice expressed the opinion that vocal performance was not only better than expected but close enough to normal to be considered not clinically disordered. Heidler no longer uses any artificial larynx support for communication, maintains a full oral diet, and continues to breath uneventfully through a stoma. This is a fascinating and historical occurrence, and readers would enjoy Dr. Douglas Hicks's documentation of this journey from the perspective of human communication (Hicks, 2000).

RESOURCE INFORMATION AND MATERIALS

Laryngectomized individuals and speech–language pathologists may find the following addresses useful for learning more about equipment, materials, and services. Phone numbers are not listed because they change more often than addresses; please consult directory assistance for the phone numbers of these companies.

Association

American Cancer Society
International Association of Laryngectomees
1599 Clifton Road, NE
Atlanta, GA 30329-4251

Manufacturers

Bivona Medical Technologies, Inc.
5700 West 23rd Avenue
Gary, IN 46406

Blom–Singer Tracheoesophageal Voice Supplies

InHealth Technologies
110 Mark Avenue
Carpinteria, CA 93013-2918
www.inhealth.com

Suppliers

Bruce Medical Supply
Mail Order
411 Waverly Oaks Road
P.O. Box 9166
Waltham, MA 02254

Cooper–Rand Electronic Speech Aid

Luminaud, Inc.
8688 Tyler Boulevard
Mentor, OH 44060

Servox Inton Electro Larynx

Siemens Hearing Instruments
10 Constitution Avenue
P.O. Box 1397
Piscataway, NJ 08855

Publications

Lauder, E. *Self-Help for the Laryngectomee*. Available from Edmund Lauder, 1115 Whisper Hollow, San Antonio, TX 78230.

Clinical Insights

Eric Blom, Editor
International Center for Post-Laryngectomy Voice Restoration
7440 North Shadeland, Suite 200
Indianapolis, IN 42650

National Clearing House of Rehabilitation Training Materials (Videotapes)

Oklahoma State University
816 West Sixth Street
Stillwater, OK 74078-0435

SUMMARY

This chapter has provided the speech–language pathologist with background sufficient to understand the changes involved in laryngectomy and how they relate to rehabilitation of the laryngectomized person. General aspects of surgical alteration have been detailed. Considerable attention has been given to various forms of alaryngeal phonation, both extrinsic (electrolarynx, etc.) and intrinsic (esophageal and shunting procedures). Characteristics of esophageal speech have been discussed and specific instructions provided to the speech–language pathologist on how to teach the laryngectomized person to communicate again.

The main point this chapter was that the speech–language pathologist must provide information regarding all forms of alaryngeal phonation to the patient so that the patient can make appropriate decisions as to communication choice. The speech–language pathologist should feel confident and competent in facilitating alaryngeal communication regardless of what form a particular patient might choose, whether it is an electrolarynx, esophageal speech, tracheoesophageal voice restoration, or some combination.

Resonance and Miscellaneous Disorders

The chapter covers the resonance disorders of hypernasality, hyponasality, and those resulting from deafness or hearing impairment as well as miscellaneous disorders such as laryngeal papillomatosis, webs, cysts, polyps, sulcus vocalis, laryngomalacia, ventricular dysphonia, and trauma. Miscellaneous therapy techniques that can be applied to a variety of disorders are also covered. Thus, this chapter addresses a potpourri of disorders and therapies not covered earlier. One of the most significant areas of coverage is disorders of the velopharyngeal mechanism as it pertains to voice disorder only, not to articulation disorder related to orofacial clefting and craniofacial syndromes.

Following are some terms that will be used in the discussion of the velopharyngeal mechanism:

▶ **Velopharyngeal inadequacy:**

A generic term covering any type of abnormal velopharyngeal functioning, whether organically or structurally based.

▶ **Velopharyngeal insufficiency:**

Any structurally based malfunctioning that results in imperfect closure of the velopharyngeal mechanism.

▶ **Velopharyngeal incompetency:**

Imperfect closure of the velopharyngeal apparatus that is caused by a defect in neuromuscular functioning rather than a deficit of tissue.

▶ **Velopharyngeal misleading:**

Functionally based abnormal vetopharyngeal closure, such as in the case of phonological errors, poor modeling influence, deafness or hearing impairment, or any other nonstructural cause.

These definitions are somewhat consistent with those of Loney and Bloem (1987) and in complete accordance with Trost-Cardamone (1989), who recognized that the literature is filled with inconsistent use of these terms. I will hold to the above definitions except when quoting other researchers, in which case their terms will be maintained as written with added editorial clarification in parentheses. Peterson-Falzone et al. (2001) also discussed the use of these terms and noted a general agreement regarding the terminology and the definitions of the terms but recognized some disagreement among various clinicians and researchers about how the terms are used.

As explained in Chapter 1, many of the voice quality dimensions of human phonation result from resonance of the glottal sound in the vocal tract. Three types of vocal resonance abnormalities are hypernasality, hyponasality, and those resulting from deafness or hearing impairment.

HYPERNASALITY

Hypernasality is a general term with several synonyms in the literature: *nasality, hyperrhinolalia, hyperrhinophonia, rhinolalia aperta,* and *assimilated nasality*. The condition involves excessive resonance for vowels and vocalic consonants in the nasal cavity during voice production because of coupling of the oral and nasal cavities via the velopharyngeal port.

As mentioned, the speech articulation structure that regulates the extent of nasal cavity participation in the resonance of voice is the velopharyngeal mechanism (also called palatopharyngeal mechanism), composed of the velum (soft palate) and pharyngeal muscles at the same level (superior constrictor). In Chapter 1 the anatomical and physiological bases to velopharyngeal closure were reviewed. Figure 8.1 shows a lateral view of the velopharyngeal port in both open and closed states.

Under normal conditions, velopharyngeal closure is sufficient to completely separate the oral and nasal cavities so that no airflow is allowed to escape nasally during speech production of nonnasal consonants (Thompson & Hixon, 1979). With 112 typical persons ranging in age from 3 to 37, Thompson and Hixon reported nasal flow to be zero during all oral consonant and vowel utterances, suggesting airtight velopharyngeal closure. Flow occurred during all nasal consonants /m/, /n/, and /ŋ/ and during vowels adjacent to nasal consonants (assimilation). It is clear, therefore, that the normal velopharyngeal mechanism should be completely closed for nonnasal speech sounds and sufficiently open to allow resonance coupling and airflow for the nasal consonants and nasal breathing.

Before describing the various conditions that can affect the velopharyngeal port and produce speech phenomena that in the past were labeled *cleft palate speech* forms, I want to establish my philosophy regarding the role of the speech–language patholo-

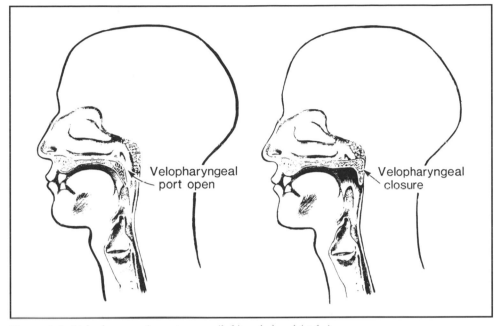

Figure 8.1. Velopharyngeal port in open (left) and closed (right) states.

gist in such cases. Because this chapter focuses on the resonance disorders surrounding velopharyngeal inadequacy and not the articulatory and non–voice-related aspects, it is appropriate to define the limits of voice therapy in cases of velopharyngeal difficulty.

When a child or adult has a hypernasal voice quality, the nasal cavity is participating as a resonator in the production of vowel sounds and voice consonants. Under normal conditions adequate velopharyngeal closure would prevent such resonance. In the majority of cases, such consistent nasal resonation on vowels and voiced consonants is evidence of velopharyngeal inadequacy. Depending on the extent of inadequacy, articulation processes are likely affected, and nasal air emission and reduced oral pressure would also occur consistently to some degree across all pressure sounds. In such cases the speech–language pathologist should direct efforts toward objective evaluation of the mechanism and not toward therapy to change speech or voice until organicity has been ruled out. When nasal air emission is heard on only isolated pressure sounds, such as the /s/ phoneme, therapy should be directed toward its elimination. This condition is a phoneme-specific velopharyngeal insufficiency. No hypernasality (consistent nasal quality on vowels and voiced consonants) will likely be heard.

One 10-year-old boy was seen in our clinic upon referral from his school speech–language pathologist, who assumed he had velopharyngeal inadequacy with a physical basis. Careful analysis, however, revealed that he only had nasal air emission on the /s/ phoneme. When I asked him to prolong an /s/ sound, he closed his lips and forced the air out of his nose. It was clear, phonologically, that he thought the /s/ phoneme should have air directed out of his nose. He did not do this for /v/, / θ/, /f/, or any other consonant sounds. His voice quality was devoid of hypernasality on vowels. Correction of this boy's speech difficulty was quick and phonological without any need for structural modification. Most of the children with craniofacial or clefting difficulty are not so easily managed.

Several clinical conditions can disrupt functioning of the velopharyngeal port, including (a) craniofacial anomalies with associated orofacial clefting; (b) structural abnormalities other than clefting, such as a deep pharynx, short soft palate, improper muscle attachment, as in a submucous cleft, or a short hard palate; (c) posttonsillectomy and postadenoidectomy unmasking some physical deficiency; (d) paresis from central or peripheral nerve damage; (e) maxillary advancement; and (f) miscellaneous factors.

Craniofacial Anomalies with Orofacial Clefting

Several researchers have provided data on the presence of speech and voice abnormalities secondary to craniofacial anomalies and orofacial clefting of the velum and other related structures (Bzoch, 1997; Moller & Starr, 1993; Peterson-Falzone et al., 2001; Shprintzen, 1997). Even after primary surgical correction of a craniofacial defect, including orofacial clefting, residual velopharyngeal insufficiency can remain to produce a deleterious effect on speech development.

When the velopharyngeal insufficiency is significant, articulation abnormalities occur on pressure consonants. If the insufficiency is slight or borderline, articulation of consonants is usually within normal parameters unless affected by some other etiology, such as dental malocclusion, hearing loss, or poor oral sensation. However, a slight or borderline insufficiency produces a nasal quality to the voice.

Perceptual judgments of hypernasality range from slight to severe. Often the nasality is assimilative when a vowel is adjacent to a nasal consonant. Sometimes it is intermittent. These variations must all be perceptually distinguished by the speech–language pathologist. Children born with orofacial clefts can also have normal speech when well managed surgically, or any one of these categories of hypernasality may be a residual.

Many excellent references exist to guide the speech–language pathologist in the management of clients born with craniofacial disorders associated with orofacial clefts, including the following:

- Etiological endogenesis factors of genetics and exogenous environmental factors (Jung, 1989; Shprintzen, 1997)

- Primary surgical considerations (Berkowitz, 1996; Shons, 1993; Williams, Ellenbogen, & Gruss, 1999)

- Dental, orthodontic, and prosthodontic concerns (Leeper, Sills, & Charles, 1993; R. E. Long, Semb, & Shaw, 2000; Peterson-Falzone et al., 2001; Mazaheri, 1996; Poyry, 1996; Reisberg, 2000)

- Audiological and otological problems (J. T. Jacobson & Northern, 1991; Kemker & Zarajczyk, 1989; Peterson-Falzone et al., 2001)

- Communication disorder associated with craniofacial anomalies and orofacial clefting (Bzoch, 1997; Moller & Starr, 1993; Peterson-Falzone et al., 2001)

The nature of the clinical problems resulting from craniofacial disorder with orofacial clefting is beyond the scope of this chapter, with the exception of the associated voice disorder, specifically the nasal resonance aspect. Only this aspect is covered in sufficient detail to provide management techniques for the speech–language pathologist working with a team of other professionals. Clinical management techniques are presented later, following the discussion of additional etiological considerations of hypernasality.

Other Structural Anomalies

Several oral anomalies other than orofacial clefting can have a deleterious effect on velopharyngeal closure and produce hypernasality. Some of these are described by Bradley (1989). Examples of palatopharyngeal (velopharyngeal) insufficiencies in the absence of overt cleft palate include (a) a short but intact hard palate; (b) a short but intact velum; (c) a deep pharynx, making closure difficult; (d) congenital palatal webbing of tissue that tethers the velum downward, impeding the movements of the velum during closure; and (e) abnormal muscle attachment in the velum, as in the submucous cleft (Stal & Hicks, 1998; Velasco, Ysunza, Hernandez, & Marquez, 1988). Any one of these conditions can alter velopharyngeal closure enough to allow coupling of the oral and nasal cavities to produce hypernasal resonance.

Posttonsillectomy and Postadenoidectomy

The most common surgical procedure on children is the removal of tonsils and adenoids. Although the numbers have decreased in recent years, many children still undergo this surgical procedure. The removal of this lymphatic tissue is done to control infection or chronic upper airway obstruction. In many cases both infection and airway obstruction are the bases for surgical decision.

Because velopharyngeal closure occurs in the nasopharynx where the adenoid tissue is located, hypernasality may result from the surgical removal of the pharyngeal tonsils (adenoids). Hypernasality also may be caused by the presence of hypertrophied and infected palatine tonsils, which can tether the velum during attempts at closure. The surgical removal of these tissues is called a tonsillectomy. Additional speech and voice considerations may result when both tonsillectomy and adenoidectomy are done. Clinicians are often confused about the interaction of the adenoids and tonsils on velopharyngeal closure. The following discussion regarding the contribution of these tissue masses to velopharyngeal function might clarify the issues involved.

The adenoid tissue is typically above the plane of the velum in the posterior nasopharynx both laterally and posteriorly. Therefore, as the velum moves to achieve closure, the adenoid pad is often involved in velar contact. In children closure is often veloadenoidal closure as much as velopharyngeal closure. Thus, removal of adenoid tissue requires modification and adjustment in closure processes, because the velum must move more extensively for contact against the pharyngeal wall rather than the pad of adenoid tissue.

In most cases adenoidectomy results in resonance change for a short period, during which time the adjustments are being made. When all structures are normal, the removal of the adenoid pad results in only temporary difficulties in velopharyngeal closure for a few days or weeks, but sometimes months (Chuma, Cacace, Rosen, Feustel, & Koltaii, 1999; Witzel, Rich, Margar-Bacal, & Cox, 1986).

Andreassen, Leeper, MacRae, and Nicholson (1994) reviewed many studies that document those children at risk for postadenoidectomy hypernasality who will not experience eventual normalization of velopharyngeal closure. These children include those with congenital cleft palate, congenital structural abnormalities such as those Bradley (1989) mentioned, submucous clefting, facial paralysis, Down syndrome, a history of nasal regurgitation in infancy, familial history of clefting or VPI, and anomalies of the upper cervical vertebrae and cranial base. When these factors are present, the physician would be wise to obtain surgical consent because persistent hypernasality will likely result from the operation. Although the risk is much lower, children without these factors and without presurgical evidence of nasality may have postsurgical hypernasality that is persistent. However, the majority of children who will have postsurgical hypernasality that is persistent and that likely will require further physical management will present with some degree of hypernasality prior to surgery and have one of the forementioned conditions.

The palatine tonsils are less likely to be involved in postsurgical hypernasality because of the location of these tissues. The tonsils are located between the faucial pillars below the level of velopharyngeal closure. When the velum moves to achieve closure, the direction of movement is upward away from the location of the tonsils, and unless the tonsils are significantly hypertrophied and extend into the nasopharynx, they will not be a significant factor in closure. However, as indicated previously, hypertrophied tonsils can be extensive and affect velar movement by tethering the velum downward. In such cases, removal of tonsils will likely facilitate improved velopharyngeal closure.

Hypertrophied tonsils and adenoids can result in increased nasal resistance for breathing and decreased resonatory space. When this occurs, a condition known as denasality or hyponasality occurs. Nasal resistance affects the patency of the nasal cavity for respiration (Hairfield, Warren, & Seaton, 1987; Warren, 1989; Warren, Hairfield, & Dalston, 1990; Warren, Odont, Drake, & Jefferson, 1996) and nasal resonation (Fox, Lynch, & Cronin, 1988). In addition to the tonsils and adenoids, several factors affect the patency of the nasal airway for these respiratory and resonatory phenomena, including nostril closure or restricted anterior nasal opening, collapsed liminal valve, hypertrophied turbinates, deviated nasal septum, nasal polypoid development or other growths such as cysts, and misplaced foreign objects such as beans or pencil erasers. Nasal airway resistance can also be affected by abnormalities at the velopharyngeal port itself in the case of pharyngeal flap pharyngoplasty, webbing, or large palatine tonsils. These factors can act singularly or in combination to decrease the patency of the nasal cavity for its intended purpose (Andreassen et al., 1994; Corey, Houser, & Ng, 2000).

Paresis from Nerve Damage

Several of the dysarthrias discussed in Chapter 5 involve dysfunction of the velopharyngeal mechanism, producing hypernasality and additional articulation disorder. Dysarthrias, for example, can produce palatal paresis, resulting in hypernasality (Duffy, 1995; Johns, 1985; McNeil, 1997).

HYPONASALITY

Hyponasality, also called denasality, is the opposite of hypernasality. It is a vocal quality that occurs when the nasal cavity has some condition that prevents it from participating normally as a resonance chamber. The English consonants /m/, /n/, and /ŋ/ require oral and nasal coupling for normal production. The velopharyngeal port is open to allow this to occur. Under coupling conditions, the chambers of the nasal cavity resonate these nasal consonants by allowing sound to enter. If some condition in the nasal cavity, such as an allergy, reduces resonance potential, the /m/ phoneme will be perceived more as a /b/, the /n/ phoneme as a /d/, and the /ŋ/ phoneme as a /g/.

Several conditions in the nasal cavity produce hyponasality (Corey et al., 2000; Lucente & Joseph, 1999b; Meyerhoff & Rice, 1992). The following can have a significant effect on the resonance potential of the nasal cavity to produce hyponasality:

• *Tonsils and adenoids.* The lymphatic tissue in the form of pharyngeal tonsils (adenoid) and palatine tonsil tissue can produce hyponasality and cause difficulty breathing through the nose. When the pharyngeal and palatine tonsilar masses become infected, a condition known as pharyngitis or tonsillitis is present, requiring medical and often surgical attention (tonsillectomy or adenoidectomy), as previously described.

• *Diseases of the turbinates.* Any disease caused by infection or allergy can cause the nasal turbinates (conchae) to become swollen or hypertrophied, thereby decreasing the space available in the nasal cavity for vocal resonance and nasal breathing.

• *Allergic rhinitis.* Many persons have severe allergies to environmental substances (smoke, grasses, pollen, dust, dairy products, etc.) and experience tissue reaction in the form of swelling and inflammation when exposed to them. Some individuals have acute experiences with intermittent effects; others have chronic difficulty, with nasal congestion almost constant. They can have persistent hyponasality as a voice quality and also become mouth breathers (Brody & Turk, 1999; Meyerhoff & Rice, 1992).

• *Nasal polyps.* Several types of nasal polyps can develop in the cavity and obstruct space for resonance and breathing. Nasal polyps are seen most often in patients with allergic rhinitis. They may be large or numerous enough to completely occlude the nasal cavity. The typical nasal polyp is soft, pale gray, nontender, and mobile and is attached by a pedlinculated base (Lucente & Joseph, 1999b).

• *Papillomas.* Papillomas are small wartlike growths that may develop in the squamous epithelium of the nasal cavity. Their cause is unknown, although a viral etiology is suspected. (More information is provided later.)

• *Foreign bodies.* Children enjoy putting objects into the cavities of the body, including the nasal orifice. These objects include buttons, beans, pebbles, and eraser tips. The object often is put into the nasal cavity inadvertently, then forgotten until some tissue reaction causes pain, swelling, or inflammation (Joseph & Goldsmith, 1999).

• *Neoplasm or malignant growth.* Although rare, malignant growths can develop in the nasal cavity, producing bloody discharge, pain or tenderness, difficulty in nasal breathing, and hyponasality.

• *Acute rhinitis (the common cold).* This high-incidence condition has afflicted most people. The plethora of over-the-counter medicines designed to eliminate or reduce the symptoms of acute rhinitis is evidence of its commonality. The symptoms of this condition include nasal discharge, nasal inflammation and edema, difficulty with nasal breathing, and hyponasality (Corey et al., 2000).

• *Deviated nasal septum.* The nasal septum, formed by the perpendicular plate of the ethmoid bone and the vomer, divides the nasal cavity into right and left chambers. Through birth injury, trauma, or aging, the septum can deviate to one side, causing nasal obstruction on the convex side of the deviation and occluding the passageway unilaterally, possibly producing a hyponasal voice quality.

• *Patulous eustachian tubes.* The eustachian tubes, leading from the posterior nasopharynx to the middle ear space normally are closed, opening only during the act of swallowing or yawning. Abnormal patency (openness) of the eustachian tubes can cause significant discomfort and anxiety because any change in acoustic or static pressure will be transmitted immediately to the ears. Some persons with patulous eustachian tubes have learned to eliminate some of the acoustic effect by maintaining constant velopharyngeal closure so that much of the acoustic energy is kept from the tubes. The effect is functional hyponasality because the velopharyngeal port remains closed for the nasal consonants (Batza & Parker, 1971).

• *Deafness.* Often deafness affects a person's ability to monitor the activity of the soft palate in velopharyngeal closure when attempting to communicate orally. Denasality might occur on sounds that should be nasal, and nasality might occur on sounds that should be nonnasal. (See case presentation on A.R. in this chapter.)

When hyponasality is detected, the only clinical course is medical. No therapy should be instituted to correct the hyponasality in the voice. The cause is organic in essentially every circumstance, with the exception of the patulous eustachian tube factor mentioned previously, and the treatment is entirely medical. When the factor responsible for the nasal congestion is eliminated, the voice will be normal.

Discrimination of Hypernasality and Hyponasality

A speech–language pathologist may listen to a person's voice and detect a nasal factor but have difficulty determining whether it is hypernasality, hyponasality, or a combination of both. This is not an easy decision in some cases, because of the possible combination of factors. For example, a person can have velopharyngeal insufficiency or incompetency that allows nasal resonance but, because of nasal congestion from an allergy, cold, or some other factor, also manifests decreased resonance on the nasal consonants. Another patient visiting the speech–language pathologist for an evaluation of velopharyngeal functioning might be upset and cry before the examination, causing nasal edema and congestion.

The best method for discriminating between hypernasality and hyponasality from a perceptual point of view is to have the client read words, phrases, or sentences that are either loaded with or lacking nasal consonants (see Table 8.1). By listening carefully to how these phrases sound, the speech–language pathologist can judge whether the voice quality heard is hypernasality or hyponasality. The person with a hypernasal voice quality will sound excessively nasal while reading nonnasal phrases and nearly normal on phrases loaded with nasal consonants. The hyponasal individual will manifest nearly normal voice quality on the nonnasal phrases and evidence the problem mainly on the nasally loaded phrases. In these phrases the person with hyponasality

TABLE 8.1
Nonnasal and Nasal Phrases

Nonnasal Phrases	Nasally Loaded Phrases
See what I do to it	My mom can be mean
If you see what I did	Mama made lemon jam
Carry it to the truck	Many men came home then
The cars are parked at the arcade	May I plan my menu?
Look at the truck over there	Ten times ten is one hundred
Be here at 6 o'clock	My time can never be turned back
Will you go to the store?	Ten men came when I sang

will distort the nasal consonants so that the /m/ will sound like a /b/, the /n/ like a /d/, and the /ŋ/ like a /g/.

The person with mixed hypernasality and hyponasality manifests these same differences, but the discrimination process usually is more difficult. Hypernasality is heard on the nonnasal phrases, but not very noticeably. Hyponasality is just as apparent in a mixed state as it is in its pure form; that is, the nasal consonants do not sound nasal.

Hyponasality and Nasal Breathing

It is important to determine how easily a person with resonance disorder can breathe through the nose. If sufficient nasal congestion is present to restrict airflow through the nose for respiration, it is likely that nasal resonance for the nasal consonants also will be dampened. It is a good idea to determine whether breathing is better through one nostril than the other. Congestion on only one side still is sufficient to generate hyponasal resonance.

Cul-de-Sac Resonance

The closed tube cul-de-sac resonance phenomenon can help the speech–language pathologist detect hypernasality. Cul-de-sac resonance occurs in humans when the nostrils are pinched together as a vowel sound is produced and prolonged if there is oral and nasal coupling through the velopharyngeal port. Under these conditions, the client emitting an /i/ as the nostrils are pinched experiences a sudden change in the nature of the sound. An extension of this is the nasal flutter test (Bzoch, 1997). It is performed by the client's alternately pinching and releasing the nostrils while prolonging the vowels /i/ or /u/. The rapidly alternated pattern makes the changes produced by cul-de-sac resonance more noticeable. If no such change is heard, there probably is no excessive or hypernasal resonance in the speech signal.

Enhanced Perception of Nasality Factors

One of the most helpful clinical devices available for detecting hypernasal or hyponasal resonance is the nasal listening tube (see Figure 8.2). It is a simple device constructed of rubber tubing with glass or plastic tips on each end that can be placed in either a nostril or an external auditory meatus. When one tip is placed in the client's nostril and the other tip in the speech–language pathologist's ear, amplified sound is heard when present in the nasal cavity. Hyponasality is detected by having the client alternate saying a /b/ and an /t-n/ sound in a consonant–vowel–consonant (CVC) phonemic relationship. For example, /bib/ and /mim/ do not sound significantly different through the listening tube when hyponasality is present—both essentially sound close to /bib/. Both CVCs would be dampened in intensity. However, with

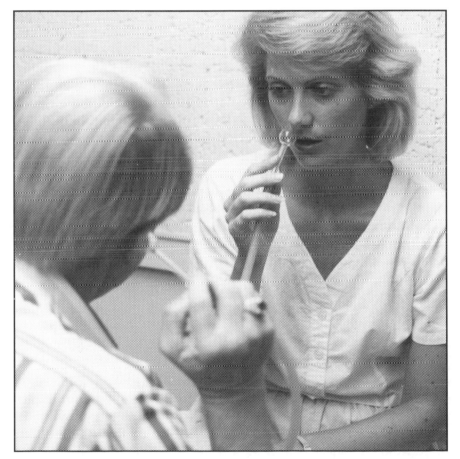

Figure 8.2. Nasal listening tube in action.

hypernasality, both /bib/ and /mim/ sound similar but closer to /mil-n/. Rather than the dampening of sound heard in hyponasality, the hypernasality productions through the listening tube seem quite loud. It also is possible to discern when air is escaping into the nasal cavity on the pressure consonants.

The nasal listening tube can be a helpful device in making some clinical perception judgments. The speech–language pathologist must remember that when the listening tube is used no objective information is obtained regarding the sufficiency or insufficiency of the velopharyngeal structures. However, the tube may help the speech–language pathologist in perceptual judgments of speech and resonance patterns that would be part of the administration of any test of articulation. It also may be of assistance in clinical judgments as to the presence or absence of hypernasality, hyponasality, or combinations. It may be useful in providing feedback in therapy to a client on articulation and voice productions that involve nasal airflow and resonance.

However, the tube should not be used by the speech–language pathologist to determine whether therapy or physical management is the procedure of choice. This decision should be based on information provided by more objective procedures, such as videofluoroscopy, aeromechanical data, and endoscopic examination coupled with clinical evaluations of oral examination, articulation, and voice testing. The use of the nasal listening tube is merely a means of enhancing clinical perceptions.

Maxillary Advancement

Many craniofacial anomalies are treated with various forms of surgery in which large segments of the facial skeleton are brought into harmony and balance. Common procedures used by oral surgeons are the LeFort I, II, and III maxillary advancement osteotomies. These are performed when there is maxillary hypoplasia resulting from childhood injury, cleft palate, specific craniofacial syndromes (Crouzen's, Apert's), and other miscellaneous anomalies (Gorlin, Cohen, & Levin, 1990). The basic technique is outlined by Deeb, Waite, and Curran (1993), Berkowitz, (1996), and Steinberg, Padwa, Boyne, and Kaban (1999). The entire maxillary segment is advanced in relation to the mandible, including the soft tissue of the velum. Because of the anteriorly directed velum relative to the pharynx, velopharyngeal insufficiency can result from this procedure, producing hypernasality.

Maxillary advancement is unlikely to cause a deterioration of velopharyngeal functioning in non–cleft palate patients or patients who have had excellent velopharyngeal closure. Patients who have denasality and articulation disorder often demonstrate significant improvement in resonance and articulation following maxillary advancement. However, patients with clefts or borderline velopharyngeal closure are likely to manifest deterioration of velopharyngeal valving after advancement, and their voice quality will increase in nasal resonation. Also, individual patient variation and surgical techniques in maxillary advancement make it difficult to predict whether advancement will produce velopharyngeal insufficiency. The report by Kummer, Strife, Grau, Creaghead, and Lee (1989) and the commentary by Witzel (1989) will help the speech–language pathologist appreciate the polemics of maxillary advancement as they pertain to speech and voice. Several additional references are recommended in the case of maxillary advancement as part of the LeFort procedures in the treatment of the craniofacial dysostoses seen in Crouzon's, Apert's, and other anomalies (Bachmayer & Ross, 1986; Kaban, Conover, & Mulliken, 1986; Kreiborg & Aduss, 1986; Shprintzen, 1997).

CASE STUDY OF NASALITY FACTORS

M. H. is a 35-year-old woman born with Pfeiffer syndrome, an Apert-like and Saethre-Chotzen-like syndrome (acrocephalosyndactyly). As a result of this autosomal dominant mutation, M. H. was born with craniosynostosis (premature closure of cranial sutures, producing significant head growth deformity); midfacial hypoplasia, which caused eye protrusions (exopthalmia); dental malocclusion (Class III with severe openbite); and syndactyly (fusion of fingers and toes). Her oral cavity configurations, besides the malocclusion, included an abnormal palatal vault. Her midfacial hypoplasia produced a small nasopharyngeal space, forcing an open-mouth breathing posture, and her voice quality was hyponasal or denasal. She also had articulation abnormalities, but her speech was quite intelligible.

Because of the severity of her craniofacial and general body differences, M. H. was thought to be significantly retarded at birth and was institutionalized as mentally retarded for 14 years. However, she was later discovered to have essentially normal intelligence and learned to live successfully as an adult outside the institution. Her significant craniofacial differences continued to make life difficult for her.

M. H. was evaluated by the Southwest Craniofacial Team (of which I am a member). It was determined that craniofacial surgery could be done on M. H., and a plan was generated that involved two major surgeries, one on her cranium and another on her mid-facial area. The surgeries significantly helped M. H.'s speech and voice. The LeFort III osteotomy provided the opportunity to improve nasal airway for respiration and nasal resonance and to correct her dental malocclusion and openbite. Her voice quality significantly improved as the hyponasality factor was reduced. M. H. continues to improve with time. In her case a highly specialized team of physicians and nonmedical specialists have worked harmoniously to reduce the impact of nature's often cruel effects in terms of her cosmetic appearance, her speech and voice, and her sense of hope and future. (For information on Apert's and similar craniofacial syndromes, see Gorlin et al., 1990; Jung, 1989; Peterson-Falzone et al., 2001.)

Miscellaneous Factors

Several additional factors can alter the functional relationships of the velum and pharynx to produce hypernasality:

- Cancer of the oral cavity resulting in ablative surgery of a critical part involved in velopharyngeal closure (Perry & Shaw, 2000; Tardy, Toriumi, & Broadway, 1989)

- Abnormal regional growth abnormalities affecting velopharyngeal closure (Bradley, 1989; Turvey, Vig, & Fonseca, 1996)

- The "occult" submucous cleft in which the classic triad associated with the traditional submucous cleft is missing (notching of the bony hard palate, midline separation of muscles in the velum, and bifid or split uvula) but that nevertheless involves abnormal muscle attachment of the velum (Bradley, 1989; Kaplan, 1977; Peterson-Falzone et al., 2001; Stal & Hicks, 1998)

Phoneme-specific nasal emission without velopharyngeal inadequacy can often be mistaken for nasality and nasal emission patterns that require physical management. Phoneme-specific nasal emission is a phonologically based disorder that can be managed with therapy and does not require physical management. It is important that the speech–language pathologist recognize the difference. Excellent references for helping in that discrimination have been provided by Peterson-Falzone and Graham (1990) and Peterson-Falzone et al. (2001).

Significant use of cocaine takes its toll on the noses and pharyngeal structures of those who use or abuse this drug. Deutsch and Millard (1989) reported cases in which cocaine use caused significant deterioration of nasal and pharyngeal structures, including a retracted and asymmetric velum, absent uvula, and ulceration on the superior border of the palate down to the pharyngeal wall involved in velopharyngeal closure.

TREATMENT OF
HYPERNASALITY DISORDERS

Treatment of hypernasality often involves both physical management of the velopharyngeal mechanism (pharyngeal flap surgery, prosthetic obturation, Teflon pharyngoplasty) and various forms of voice therapy. One of the most important clinical tasks facing the speech–language pathologist in management of the hypernasal client is to determine whether the velopharyngeal mechanism is adequate, incompetent, insufficient, or inadequate. Several techniques can help in this diagnostic process. Several surveys have sampled the attitudes of speech–language pathologists with regard to this evaluation process (Pannbacker et al., 1984; Pannbacker, Lass, &

Stout, 1990; Schneider & Shprintzen, 1980). Since the earlier survey of Schneider and Shprintzen, speech–language pathologists have turned more toward instrumentation to aid perceptual judgments. As Pannbacker et al. (1990) stated, however, the number of speech–language pathologists who do not use any sort of instrumentation is unknown.

Table 8.2 lists the significant perceptual and instrumentation processes that are currently used by speech–language pathologists in the evaluation process, as well as useful references. Techniques that have rather limited or merely experimental use are not listed.

The studies of Schneider and Shprintzen (1980), Pannbacker et al. (1984), Pannbacker et al. (1990), and Pannbacker, Lass, Scheuerle, and English (1992) indicate that speech–language pathologists have had many techniques available to assess the adequacy or inadequacy of the velopharyngeal mechanism for speech and voice. Clinicians continue to use techniques that require little instrumentation, such as

TABLE 8.2
Velopharyngeal Evaluation Techniques

Technique	Reference
Listener judgment of voice	Gerratt, Drelman, Antonanzas-Barroso, & Berke, 1993; Kent & Ball, 2000
Oral examination of orofacial structures	Pannbacker, 1985; St. Louis & Ruscello, 1987; Zemlin, 1998
Articulation testing	Broen & Moller, 1993; Bzoch, 1997
Radiological assessment	Bzoch, 1997; Berkowitz, 1996; Skolnick, 1996; Peterson-Falzone et al., 2001
Videofluoroscopy	Skolnick, 1996; Peterson-Falzone et al., 2001
Multiview	Skolnick, 1996
Base and Towne views	Skolnick, 1996
Endoscopy (oral and nasopharyngoscopy)	Karnell, 1994; Berkowitz, 1996; Peterson-Falzone et al., 2001
Aeromechanical (airflow and pressure)	Dalston, Warren, & Dalston, 1992; Baken & Orlikoff, 2000
Nasometer (Nasalance)	Dalston, 1992; Bressmann et al., 2000
Miscellaneous measurements (accelerometers, photodetection, rhinometry, etc.)	Peterson-Falzone et al., 2001

articulation testing and listener judgment, but a growing trend is to use objective assessment, as evidenced by Pannbacker et al. (1992). This was true in 1992 and also true to some degree in 2001, but certainly the trend toward more objective assessment of velopharyngeal processes is improving.

It is imperative that speech–language pathologists who are evaluating many children and adults with possible velopharyngeal insufficiency, and who often recommend surgery on the basis of measurement findings, obtain the necessary training to use objective measurements to complement their clinical judgments. Those who evaluate few such clients must be prepared to refer to centers where such objective assessment is available when the velopharyngeal mechanism is suspect in the client's speech or voice.

In evaluating velopharyngeal closure, the speech–language pathologist needs to know the meanings of the terms *competent, functionally incompetent,* and *insufficient. Competent* means the mechanism is performing normally in continuous speech. *Functionally incompetent* indicates that it is structurally capable of normal velopharyngeal closure for continuous speech but is not being used properly by the individual (i.e., there is a functional turnoff of velopharyngeal closure). *Insufficient* refers to structural inadequacy for closure.

When the speech–language pathologist determines that the mechanism is functionally incompetent, it is appropriate to engage the client in therapy designed to eliminate its functional misuse. Therapy is appropriate only when there is functional incompetency, because there is little evidence that voluntary effort is capable of overcoming a velopharyngeal insufficiency in continuous speech. Efforts to produce velopharyngeal closure with an insufficient mechanism can lead to abnormal compensations in laryngeal adjustment, leading to hoarseness and vocal nodules, glottal stops and velar and pharyngeal fricatives, and abnormal articulation placement. With regard to voice disorder, that many clients with velopharyngeal insufficiency also present with vocal hoarseness is of significant clinical concern to the voice specialist.

Often judgments are made that a client will respond to therapy to improve velopharyngeal function on the basis of isolated ability to produce oral rather than nasal voice or speech. The speech–language pathologist should not be deceived into thinking that a client who can close the mechanism for some isolated behavior also should be able to close it in continuous speech with some amount of training. Such a decision leads only to prolonged trial therapy that may last years without achieving functional closure during continuous speech. An appropriate analogy is that most people can take a "giant step," but it is impossible to functionally walk that way. Too often, clinicians expect clients with velopharyngeal insufficiency to take giant steps in attempting velopharyngeal closure.

The question remains as to what action is appropriate for professionals (speech–language pathologists, plastic surgeons, radiologists, oral surgeons, prosthodontists) in the management of clients with speech and voice disorders resulting from the velopharyngeal mechanism. The most appropriate step is to evaluate the mechanism thoroughly, using methodology that is as objective as possible, and recommend physical management of the mechanism when an insufficiency exists.

Three secondary physical management procedures are typically used to treat velopharyngeal insufficiency: (a) pharyngeal flap pharyngoplasty, sphincter pharyngoplasty, and augmentations; (b) speech appliances (bulb or obturator); and (c) palatal lift prostheses.

Pharyngeal Flap Pharyngoplasty

Pharyngeal flap pharyngoplasty is the most common form of physical management for velopharyngeal inadequacy (Moller & Starr, 1993; Shons, 1993). The basic procedure for pharyngeal flap has changed little since it was introduced in the late 1800s. It involves isolating a variable-width section of tissue from the posterior pharyngeal wall, maintaining either an inferior or a superior attachment, then connecting the sectioned end to the velum. The trend since the 1970s is for surgeons to perform a superiorly based flap even though the inferiorly based is easier to accomplish. The flap produces a midline bridge between the velum and the pharynx, leaving lateral portals for nasal respiration. These portals remain open for breathing but are closed by residual velopharyngeal closure for speech or swallowing. The size of these lateral portals is a critical factor in the success of the surgery. They must be large enough to accommodate nasal respiration when open and small enough that residual attempts at velopharyngeal closure, which were inadequate prior to surgery, will now be sufficient. Nasoendoscopy prior to surgery is critical for guiding the surgeon on the specifics of how the tissue is attached, width of the flap, and general positional concerns (Karling, Henningsson, Larson, & Isberg, 1999).

After a few weeks of healing, nasoendoscopy can be redone to evaluate the adequacy of the procedure. Speech and voice quality are the primary considerations in this evaluation process because the pharyngeal flap surgery is done only to improve speech and voice performance (Keuning, Wieneke, & Dejonckere, 1999). It is common for a patient to experience difficulty in nasal respiration and sound a little denasal right after pharyngeal flap surgery.

Sphincter Pharyngoplasty

One significant variation on pharyngoplasty is called the Orticochea flap (Orticochea, 1970), which involves the reverse of the midline flap in which tissue is modified to narrow the lateral pharyngeal walls, leaving a small central orifice. The posterior faucial pillars are dissected from their inferior attachments and the lateral pharyngeal wall musculature, then sutured to an inferiorly based pharyngeal flap. This leaves a small central opening for breathing and nasal sounds that is designed to close during nonnasal speech utterances. Since the inception of Orticochea's method of pharyngoplasty, several variations of muscle attachment have been generated with increased success for hypernasality management. Teams considering the use of sphincter pharyngoplasty evaluate the particular movement pattern of the velum and determine whether midline pharyngeal flap or sphincter pharyngoplasty would best ameliorate the velopharyngeal difficulty (Peterson-Falzone et al., 2001; Riski, Ruff, Georgiade, Barwick, & Edwards, 1992).

Pharyngeal flap pharyngoplasty and sphincter pharyngoplasty have been done as a primary procedure at the time of basic palatoplasty to close the cleft, usually when the patient is around 1 year of age. More typically, these procedures are done as secondary procedures following the determination that further surgery after palatoplasty is needed for improved velopharyngeal valving.

It seems clear that improved results can be obtained regardless of flap procedures when the flaps are tailor-made for each patient. Because flaps tend to become passive rather than dynamic tissue obturators, it is important that the surgeon construct them to manage the variety of closure patterns possible. Thus, the best procedure is to provide surgery that accommodates the closure patterns. Some closure patterns are sphincteric in nature, others are coronal with little mesial movement of the lateral pharyngeal walls, and others are sagittal with much mesial movement and little lifting of the velum (Shprintzen, 1989). Nasoendoscopy is again critical for the surgeon to see the pattern of closure and tailor the flap to the closure pattern observed.

Sloan (2000) wrote a "state-of-the-art" article on the use of standard pharyngeal flap versus sphincter pharyngoplasty and reviewed the studies comparing airway obstruction, speech, and voice results with the two procedures. His summary statement indicated that although there were several studies of these issues of comparison, there is not as yet a consensus regarding the better choice to manage velopharyngeal insufficiency.

Speech Appliances

Pannbacker et al. (1990) reported that the services of dental specialists (prosthodontists) are rarely used for the treatment of velopharyngeal inadequacy or insufficiency. Surveying 296 speech–language pathologists who were members of the American Cleft Palate Association (return rate of 58.4%), they found that only 4 (2.3%) indicated that they would treat velopharyngeal insufficiency with prosthesis followed by therapy. None indicated that they would treat with prosthesis alone, without therapy. Although these data indicate a growing trend toward surgical management followed by therapy (90 speech–language pathologists, or 52%) or surgery alone (12, or 6.9%), some patients are unable to be treated by surgery and are viable candidates for prosthetic management. Riski, Hoke, and Dolan (1989) reported on two cases in which

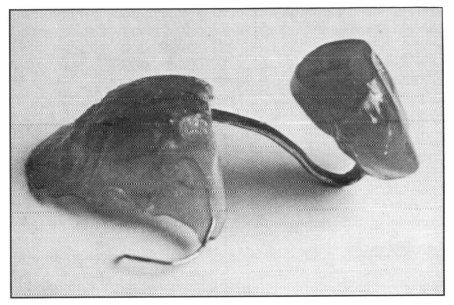

Figure 8.3. Example of a speech obturator.

obturators were used on patients who had significant velopharyngeal inadequacy and for whom surgery was contraindicated. Pressure and flow coupled with endoscopic examination of the velopharyngeal port aided in the proper fitting of the obturator. (Figure 8.3 shows a speech obturator.)

Palatal lifts are recommended for patients with neurologically based velopharyngeal insufficiency. They are typically constructed by dental prosthodontists and work very much like the obturators, except they function to push the velum toward the posterior pharyngeal wall for midline closure to facilitate improved speech and voice function. The lifting is necessary in neurologically based velopharyngeal insufficiency because in such patients little or no velar and pharyngeal movement occurs to allow closure around an obturator. Excellent references for dental and prosthodontic management of patients with neurologically based velopharyngeal insufficiency include Leeper et al. (1993), Peterson-Falzone et al. (2001), and Tachimura, Nohara, and Wada (2000).

VOICE THERAPY FOR HYPERNASALITY

This discussion focuses only on the clinical management of residual hypernasality (resonance) after any significant articulation disorders associated with the velopharyngeal valving difficulty have been controlled. Voice therapy for hypernasality can be done with simple feedback devices such as a nasal listening tube or with the objective feedback of instrumentation such as the Nasometer. I strongly recommend using objective feedback.

Whether the speech–language pathologist uses clinical techniques of simplicity, such as the nasal listening tube, or has access to instrumentation such as the Nasometer, the clinical process is much the same. Therapy must be structured to elicit voice behavior that is appropriate and that the client is able to accomplish and to provide feedback to him or her that the proper voice quality was produced.

Under conditions of feedback with the Nasometer or nasal listening tube, the speech–language pathologist should rate each of the following vowels: /i/, /I/, /e/, /ε/, /æ/, /ɔ/, /o/, /ʊ/, /u/, /ʌ/, and /ɚ/. The following ordinal scale can be used to rate each vowel if the listening tube is used: 0 = *normal, no nasality heard;* 1 = *slight nasality;* 2 = *moderate nasality;* 3 = *severe nasality.* When the vowels have been rated, the listening tube can be used to help clients identify their hypernasality. By inserting the listening tube into their own ear as they produce the vowels, they can differentiate between those that the speech–language pathologist judges to be normal or only slightly nasal and those that are more severe. When clients can discriminate the differences, it is appropriate to begin modification of the vowels judged to be moderately and severely nasal. If the Nasometer or similar instrument is used to determine nasal resonance, the nasalance score can be used for comparison as explained in the next section.

The following steps can be used in teaching the client to produce voice devoid of hypernasality:

1. The speech–language pathologist directs the client to say monosyllabic words in CVC relationships, beginning with vowels rated as normal (0) or only slightly nasal (1). The client listens to these sounds with the tube, then produces vowels rated as moderate (2) or severe (3) in the same CVC relationships so the contrast can be heard between the mildly nasal and the more severely nasal. The client then should be drilled to produce the severely nasal vowels in the CVC relationships until they are like the mild or normal vowels. This should be done by pairing the contrasting CVCs, such as /tat/ (1) with /tit/ (3).

2. Once the client can produce monosyllabic words or CVC relationships without nasality using the nasal listening tube to discriminate, the speech–language pathologist begins drilling on other words and phrases that do not contain nasal consonants while maintaining the normal or only slightly nasal rating of 0 or 1.

3. The speech–language pathologist introduces nasal consonants into the phrases by ending them on a nasal consonant (e.g., "see the ice cream," "put up the beam"). If the client can maintain voice without moderate or severe nasality even with the presence of a nasal consonant, the speech–language pathologist should begin

to scatter a few nasal consonants in other word positions in the phrases (e.g., "some of us care," "I am at my school"). The presence of the nasal consonants should not have a significant effect on the vowels in the phrase, which should remain nonnasal.

4. When the client is able to say these phrases without excessive nasality on the vowels while listening on the tube, the speech–language pathologist removes the tube to determine whether the client can tell when the voice is nasal or nonnasal without the tube. If the client can, and also can eliminate the excessive nasality, the clinician introduces consonants, then longer phrases, then context reading, and finally conversation. At each increase in task difficulty, the speech–language pathologist determines that proper discrimination and production of voice without nasality are occurring by spot-checking with the nasal listening tube rather than using it continually.

5. The speech–language pathologist may find negative practice to prove helpful at any of these steps. The client can be asked to speak the sound, word, phrase, or sentence with excessive and deliberate nasality. When the client learns to handle the resonance voluntarily in either a negative or positive manner, the carryover into everyday voice production is more likely to occur because the individual is in control of the process, instead of the reverse.

Nasometer Therapy for Hypernasality

The effectiveness of the preceding therapy steps is significantly enhanced by the use of instrumentation designed to detect nasal resonance, such as the Kay Elemetrics Nasometer (see Figure 3.8). The Nasometer provides excellent objective feedback on nasality. Using either the bar mode or time history mode from the main menu allows real-time feedback on oral versus nasal speech or voice productions. The Nasometer allows various threshold levels to be present on the screen, so a client can be shaped to produce less nasality from session to session until oral–nasal ratios (nasalance) are within the expected norms. Various practice sentences and norms are provided in the Nasometer manual under the treatment section. It is suggested that a 90% criterion level be established for each threshold level, and when the client reaches criterion, the threshold can be lowered 5%.

Starr (1993) extensively reviewed cases of patients who were treated for nasality using the Nasometer. In each case covered, the Nasometer provided excellent feedback and allowed progressive reduction of nasalance over a few sessions. In some instances, within one session the threshold of nasalance was lowered by over 50%. Clearly, a person with hypernasality from birth or early youth will not be aware of these subtle voice differences, and visual feedback is necessary to allow normal functioning of the velopharyngeal mechanism. Several authors have provided guidelines for the management of resonance disorders of hypernasality (Andrews, 1999; Boone & McFarlane, 2000; Rammage et al., 2001).

CASE EXAMPLE OF NASALITY TRAINING

A. R. was a 14-year-old girl who was deafened at the age of 2. She had received a cochlear implant and was orally trained. I received a call from her speech–language pathologist in the school system, who indicated that A. R. had excellent language, fairly good speech, and a nasal voice quality and wondered whether therapy with visual feedback potential would help.

From the beginning of therapy with A. R., I recognized that she did not know what she was doing to produce various sounds, and she was inconsistent in her productions. She did not produce her nasal consonants well, and her /m/, /n/, and /ŋ/ sounds were quite denasal and nearly all substitutions (e.g., /b/ for /m/ as in "baba" for "mama"). She was also hypernasal on all vowels, with voice quality that was typical of deaf individuals.

Our first task was to teach her how to produce the nasal sounds. Using the Nasometer, she was immediately able to increase nasalance on words with the nasal consonants. However, it took several sessions of practice speaking phrases typical of her language before she was able to control the soft palate consistently to produce nasals in connected speech.

The next task was to decrease the nasality factor in nonnasal sound combinations. To accomplish this, we began with words and phrases that did not contain nasal consonants and set her threshold level to 50%. Within one session, she was able to lower her nasalance to the 50% level, and we began the process of lowering the threshold level in 5% steps. She was able to achieve a 10% typical level on sentences without nasals within two sessions, and with nasals present in typical speech, her levels reached around the 30% level. We felt this was an acceptable level of nasalance, which she could likely carry over into daily speech activity without difficulty.

It was obvious that A. R. needed visual feedback on her speech productions, and the Nasometer was an excellent source of that feedback. A similar approach for the modification of hypernasality in young children was presented by Andrews, Tardy, and Pasternak (1984). This program, the *See-Scape* (available from PRO-ED, Inc., 8700 Shoal Creek Boulevard, Austin, TX 78757), is used as a feedback source indicating nasal resonance, but a nasal listening tube or the Nasometer could better be used. The program is divided into the following phases:

1. Discrimination between oral and nasal sounds in CVs and VCs

2. Spontaneous production of sentences produced with appropriate oral resonance (words composed only of vowels and oral consonants)

3. Production of oral and nasal sounds in structured phrases

4. Production of oral and nasal sounds in self-generated sentences

The program is designed to shape the child into appropriate production of self-generated sentences containing oral and nasal sounds with 90% accuracy. Although this program is designed to modify hypernasality in the young child, with minor modifications it is suitable for children of any age.

Hypernasality as a voice disorder can be modified clinically using available techniques and instruments. Two positive effects of such reduction are speaker intelligibility and improved social acceptability. Whether the etiology of the hypernasality is one of cleft palate, mental retardation, palate abnormalities, or hearing loss and deafness, the speech–language pathologist must consider hypernasality as a vocal parameter to be modified, particularly after any needed physical management of the velopharyngeal mechanisms of closure has been accomplished.

VOICES OF INDIVIDUALS WHO ARE HEARING IMPAIRED OR DEAF

Deafness or severe hearing loss has a direct impact on the voice, an effect that is determined by the degree of hearing loss and how early in speech development it occurs. The voice is affected in breath support; in control of pitch, stress, loudness, and general quality; and in particular subtle prosodic elements of speech.

Horii (1982b) compared the fundamental frequency of 12 hard-of-hearing young women with control subjects with normal hearing during reading and conversational speech. On average, the persons with hearing impairments had a higher mean F_0 (oral reading, 256.7; spontaneous speech, 264.1) than those with normal hearing (oral reading, 213.2; spontaneous speech, 203.5) and showed little difference in F_0. The subjects with normal hearing tended to increase their F_0 during oral reading. Smaller standard deviations also were observed for the subjects with hearing impairments regardless of speaking conditions. Similar findings were reported by Leder, Spitzer, and Kirchner (1987) for profoundly deaf adult men.

The typical voice quality of persons who are deaf or severely hearing impaired probably is a combination of poor respiratory control, inadequate laryngeal valving, and abnormal posturing of the tongue in the hypopharynx that produces a marked cul-de-sac resonance effect (Boone & McFarlane, 2000). These effects are coupled with the marked hypernasality also characteristic of deaf speakers on vowels and non-nasal consonants and the hyponasal quality heard when speech is loaded with nasal consonants (Fletcher & Hendarmin, 1999).

Subtelny, Li, Whitehead, and Subtelny (1989) studied the physiological basis for abnormal resonance in speakers with hearing impairments by means of cephalometric and cineradiographic analysis. They analyzed many vocal tract configurations, including postures of the lips, tongue, mandible, velum, hyoid bone, epiglottis, and laryngeal sinus. They found that speakers with hearing impairments, compared with normal speakers, manifested greater variation in basic tongue posture during vowel production, a significant retrusion of the tongue for front vowels, and consistent retrusion of the dorsum or root of the tongue during contextual speech. These postures affected the resonance of the speakers' voices and provided support for Boone and McFarlane's (2000) notions about the physiological bases for speech of persons with hearing impairments.

Voice Therapy in Hearing Loss

Several therapy techniques are recommended for modifying, under conditions of proper amplification, the voice quality of persons who are deaf or hearing impaired.

Pitch

Visual feedback of the F_0 produced by a speaker with a hearing impairment makes it rather easy to evaluate the pitch used and modify it when it is found to be aberrant. The Kay Visi-Pitch or similar instrumentation can provide easy modification of significantly high pitch patterns in these subjects. Because the visual display also provides feedback on pitch inflection patterns, the speech–language pathologist can use this instrument to demonstrate normal prosodic elements of speech. The split-screen potential of the Visi-Pitch allows the clinician to provide a model for clients with hearing impairments to use in attempting to produce a more normal inflection pattern.

Loudness

The intensity mode of the Visi-Pitch or a volume unit meter also can provide feedback on the appropriateness of voice loudness to the client who is hearing impaired. There are significant loudness factors in normal vocal prosody, and these can be taught more effectively with the visual feedback provided by this instrument. Wilson (1987) offered many techniques for modifying pitch and loudness in children with hearing impairments that can be used with the feedback potential of the Visi-Pitch or similar instrumentation. These techniques are more appropriate for children, but they can be modified for older clients.

Resonance

In attempting to modify nasality in subjects with hearing impairments, the speech–language pathologist should remember that such a characteristic as oral–nasal resonance is poorly perceived by persons with hearing impairments and that special amplification is needed. As Ling (1975) pointed out, amplification in the 300-Hz range is necessary to discriminate the acoustics of nasality. A high-quality group amplifier will be more effective for this problem than most individual systems, which often do not amplify low frequencies well. When an auditory training system is used to help the client discriminate nasality productions, the speech–language pathologist must remember that the person's own hearing aid eventually must be sufficient for these discriminations. The group trainer merely provides initial support for the training process.

Boone and McFarlane (2000) stated that much of the unusual voice quality heard in speakers who are deaf is cul-de-sac resonance resulting from a backward tongue placement. Voice quality can be improved by teaching persons who are hearing impaired to carry the tongue in a more forward position during speech. Drills on CV combinations that involve forward placement of the tongue, such as /ta/ and /da/, can help the client learn this forward placement. Boone and McFarlane added that such approaches as (a) chewing, (b) open mouth, (c) relaxation training, (d) yawn–sigh, and (e) negative practice can be helpful in contrasting voice quality that is more normally resonated in the oral cavity from hypernasal quality. When the voice quality of the client who is hearing impaired is hypernasal as a result of velopharyngeal dysfunction rather than the cul-de-sac resonance described by Boone and McFarlane, the speech–language pathologist can teach the client to monitor the nasality by resting a finger lightly on the side of the nose to feel the vibrations of nasal resonance or, more important, to use the Nasometer to provide visual feedback, as in the previous case example about A. R.

As stated previously, the speech–language pathologist must evaluate several factors—pitch, loudness, respiration, laryngeal tension, velopharyngeal closure, and tone focus—to determine which need modification to improve vocal quality. Several characteristics distinguish persons who are deaf and those who are profoundly hard-of-hearing from a voice and speech point of view, including the appearance of excessive speaking effort known as *over fortis*. Speech–language pathologists and teachers of persons who are hearing impaired are often called upon to modify many of these speaking and vocal characteristics (Morrison & Rammage, 1998; Wirz, 1992).

MISCELLANEOUS DISORDERS OF VOICE

Many miscellaneous conditions produce dysphonia. Some of these are treated only medically, and the speech–language pathologist generally is not involved in their management. However, the speech–language pathologist should be aware of all possible conditions to be effective in voice management.

Papillomatosis

The most common benign laryngeal tumor in children is the squamous cell juvenile papillomatosis or papillomas (multiple forms; MacArthur & Healy, 1995; Meyerhoff & Rice, 1992). Papillomas can develop at any age, but two thirds of the patients experience the onset between birth and 15 years of age (Suen & Stern, 1995). The etiology of papillomas has not been established conclusively, but there is strong evidence that the human papilloma virus (HPV) is the cause. A genetic basis is also being investigated by Niedzielska and Kocki (2000) directed toward identifying genes that dictate when cell apoptosis—the programmed death of a cell—occurs normally and abnormally in cases of neoplasm such as papilloma. Their theory is that a specific gene might be responsible for delaying the apoptosis of cells in the larynx, allowing papilloma to develop. Sun, Weatherly, Koopmann, and Carey (2000) reported that HPV could be detected by mucosal swab of the endolarynx and provided data showing transmission is not horizontal among family members but vertically from vaginal condylomas in the mother when the condition is detected congenitally.

Most of the cases of papilloma identified are benign lesions, but malignancy with papillomatosis is found in approximately 2% of the cases, with most of these cases occurring in adult patients. Most of the reported cases of papillomatosis changing into squamous cell carcinoma appear to correlate with a history of previous smoking or radiation therapy (Suen & Stern, 1995).

Papillomas take the form of fingers of connective tissue growths covered with squamous epithelium lying on a basement of intact membrane. These have a warty appearance in both single and multiple forms. Papillomas have a well-identifiable appearance under laryngoscopic inspection: white to pinkish-red glistening nodules with either sessile (broad-based) or pedunculated (stem) attachment.

The symptomatology of laryngeal papillomas depends on the site of lesion. The most common symptom is hoarseness in adults and symptoms of an abnormal or raspy cry, dyspnea, cough, and sometimes stridor in children. Most patients with laryngeal papillomas present with moderate hoarseness that progresses in severity. Airway obstruction, a critical and life-threatening concern, is common in many of the children who have this disorder.

Treatment of Papillomas

The management of juvenile respiratory papillomas involves maintaining the airway patency while awaiting spontaneous resolution of the condition, often around the time of puberty. Because childhood papillomas have a tendency to reappear after treatment, the most effective method of dealing with them has been meticulous surgical removal. Even so, some children have had numerous surgeries for removal. In reviewing the literature on childhood papillomas, most patients undergo from 30 to more than 230 surgical procedures (Harcourt, Worley, & Leighton, 1999).

Treatment consists of either cup forceps surgery or, more typically, CO_2 laser surgery (Harcourt et al., 1999; Meyerhoff & Rice, 1992). Zeitels and Sataloff (1999) reported on a process of phonomicrosurgical resection of glottal papillomatosis in adults that resulted in excellent management in 22 patients. Alpha-interferon therapy is often used as an adjuvant treatment to surgery (Benjamin et al., 1988; Suen & Stern, 1995) and has been shown to slow down the cycle of recurrence. Other medications, such as Cimetidine, used for the treatment of peptic ulcers and numerous wartlike conditions, are being tested in the hope that one will be discovered that is effective in the treatment of papillomas (Harcourt et al., 1999). Because many childhood cases seem to spontaneously remit at puberty, a hormone factor is thought to be etiologically related. However, some cases do not remit at puberty, confusing this issue.

The patient with childhood papillomas who is undergoing numerous surgeries and other therapies, and who likely has been tracheotomized, is just as likely to be without effective voice. He or she will need the services of a speech–language pathologist for help in some form of augmentative communication or help with a "speaking trach," such as a Passy-Muir valve, during periods of ventilator dependency (Andrews, 1999; Lieu, Muntz, Prater, & Stahl, 1999). Additional insight on treatment options for inspiratory support in stable adult patients with papilloma was provided by Sapienza, Brown, Martin, and Davenport (1999).

A case example will help explain the management difficulty caused by laryngeal papillomas. One child I saw many years ago had aphonia, chronic airway obstruction requiring trachcostomy, and repeated surgeries every 6 to 8 weeks to remove his laryngeal papillomas. They were diagnosed at around age 22 months and remained active until age 15. Because of the severity of his case and his aphonia, his communication disorder was treated with augmentative devices and processes. He also used sign language, which he was taught in the schools he attended around his family.

I observed one of his laryngeal surgeries and photographed the process. The image on the slides taken cannot be identified as a larynx until the end of the surgery, when the laser finally removed enough papilloma tissue to expose his fragile larynx. I could not imagine that his larynx could undergo this surgical procedure frequently for years and emerge with any degree of normalcy.

I saw him once again as a 15-year-old. His papillomas had dissipated and his tracheostomy had been closed (decannulated). After many years of aphonia and augmentative communication, he was somewhat reluctant to verbally communicate, even though his physician had indicated that his larynx was working properly and he should be able to phonate without difficulty. He spoke with a rough and weak voice. On inspection of his larynx with rigid endoscopy, the nature of his vocal difficulty was apparent. He was speaking with significant ventricular involvement. His true vocal folds could be visualized, but their potential for sufficient adduction to produce voice could not be determined because of the masking effect of the ventricular folds. A significant anterior laryngeal web had also developed in the anterior commissure, which is a common concern when multiple surgeries have occurred with focus in the anterior aspect of the larynx (Desloge & Zeitels, 2000). His therapy is now directed toward eliminating the hyperfunctional nature of vocal effort that has resulted in ventricular dysphonia. His laryngeal web must also be medically managed to improve his voice efficiency.

Papillomas also occur in adults, and the management considerations are similar. Lim and Chang (1986) presented a case of a 34-year-old male who was treated for severe laryngeal obstruction, including progressive dyspnea, stridor, and loss of voice, for 3 years. The tissues in his larynx were biopsied and found to be papillomatosis with atypical manifestations. Because of the extensiveness of his involvement, this man was laryngectomized. Histologic sectioning disclosed a diffused papillomatosis and the presence of a well-differentiated squamous cell carcinoma. Abitbol, Mathe, and Battista (1988) also reported data suggesting a relationship between adults with different types of HPV and malignant lesions. They suggested that even though gynecologic research has been more aggressive in determining the relationship between genital or venereal warts and uterine cervical carcinoma, laryngologists are only beginning to study the possible relationship of HPV and laryngeal carcinoma. These studies add support to the concept that speech–language pathologists should not work with patients, particularly adults, with hoarseness without a medical diagnosis and referral for therapy.

A physician evaluating a patient with laryngeal papilloma will prescribe a treatment (i.e., surgery or a medical application such as interferon) that might not involve a speech–language pathologist. However, speech–language pathologists must understand laryngeal papillomatosis clearly because, through screening or other referral processes, a patient might be evaluated as having hoarseness or other dysphonia prior to medical examination. For example, the speech–language pathologist might assume that the persistent hoarseness of a yelling, screaming, vocally aggressive student is caused by vocal abuse. Without medical referral safeguards, such a child might receive inappropriate therapy. Even physicians can make mistakes on diagnosis. The following example illustrates how this might happen.

A 10-year-old girl was referred to the Arizona State University Speech and Hearing Clinic by an otolaryngologist who had diagnosed severe vocal nodules. I evaluated her and found many instances of vocal abuse behavior to explain why she had vocal nodules. She was a verbally aggressive child who continually argued with her siblings. According to her mother, she also was loud and vocal on the playground, talked all the times, and loved to sing with the radio and records.

I accepted the physician's diagnosis because her behavior was typical of children who develop vocal nodules. Her voice was extremely hoarse and typical of the voice heard in persons with severe vocal nodules. However, after a few weeks of therapy to eliminate her vocal abuse behavior, which she followed carefully, I became suspicious that something else was occurring in her larynx because I heard no improvement in her voice. I recommended videoendoscopy to determine the status of her nodules.

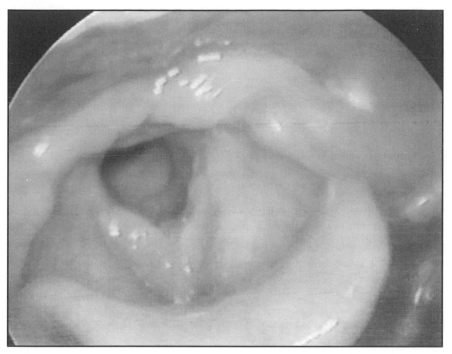

Figure 8.4. Laryngeal papillomas.

When I saw the girl's larynx endoscopically, I immediately knew we were not dealing with vocal nodules. I could see numerous growths all over her vocal folds and in the anterior commissure (see Figure 8.4). I mentioned to the mother that I did not believe that the girl had vocal nodules and that she should return to her physician for another opinion. I mentioned that I would send a copy of the video recording to him and perhaps that would help establish the diagnosis. Later the physician called and informed me that the girl had laryngeal papillomas and would undergo surgery and other medical treatments.

Even when the speech–language pathologist performs indirect laryngoscopy or videoendoscopy with stroboscopy, as many commonly do, it is inappropriate to start therapy with any child with persistent hoarseness without medical consultation. Laryngeal papillomatosis is one of the main reasons why this safeguard is critical. Vocal nodules are not responsible for juvenile death, but laryngeal papillomas can be. The misdiagnosis of the girl just discussed, even when the larynx was inspected medically, should alert the speech–language pathologist to be wary of diagnosing any person's voice solely on the basis of vocal symptoms and without adequate medical examination.

Laryngeal Polyps

Although vocal nodules are sometimes, perhaps inappropriately, classified as laryngeal polyps, many additional polyps develop in the laryngeal area that are unique, with different histological characteristics and etiology. They often are unilateral and can be found anywhere within the larynx (see Figure 8.5). They usually are attached to a sessile (broad) base but can be pedunculated (stem or small stalk). They may be blood filled and appear reddish, as in a hematoma; the term *angioma* often is used to describe blood-filled polyps. Meyerhoff and Rice (1992) and Sataloff (1998c) listed several precipitating and aggravating factors that have been related to the development of laryngeal polyps: allergies, thyroid imbalance, emotional imbalance, change of life, upper respiratory infections, sinus disease, cigarette smoking, alcohol consumption, and vocal abuse. Excellent photographs of various laryngeal pathologies, including polyps, can be found in Colton and Casper (1996), Shaw and Lancer (1987), Handler and Myer (1998), and Gulya and Wilson (1999).

The management of laryngeal polyps requires elimination of precipitating and aggravating factors and, usually, surgical removal or medical treatment. The

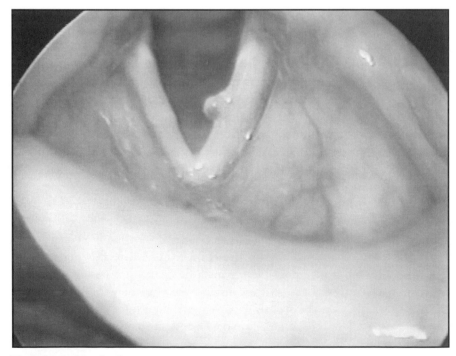

Figure 8.5. Vocal polyp.

speech–language pathologist may be called in on cases involving vocal abuse or mis-use or for postsurgical vocal hygiene therapy.

Ventricular Dysphonia

Ventricular dysphonia is the most common name of a disorder known by several other names, including dysphonia plicae ventricularis, dysphonia ventricularis, and false vocal fold phonation. This voice disorder results when the false or ventricular folds are involved in the generation of sound. The vocal symptoms heard in ventricular dysphonia include hoarseness, reduced intensity, aperiodicity, diplophonia, and hyperfunctional tension. It is a condition often associated with vocal abuse or misuse, and a review of Chapter 4 therapy techniques would also be helpful in the management of ventricular dysphonia.

In the case of a nonpathological larynx, the ventricular folds could not be respon-sible for phonation independent of the true folds; rather, both vibrating structures would be involved in ventricular dysphonia. However, in the case of laryngeal paraly-sis or dysphonia resulting from dysarthria, the ventricular folds might be responsible for a significant amount of the laryngeal tone. After cordectomy or hemilaryngectomy for cancer, the ventricular folds may contribute greatly to the sound generated in the larynx. Ventricular dysphonia probably is responsible for the vocal quality heard in many persons with Down syndrome (Aronson, 1990).

Most diagnoses of ventricular dysphonia result from indirect laryngoscopy. Typi-cally, the physician will see the overhanging ventricular folds meeting at midline dur-ing phonation and identify ventricular dysphonia. Technically, however, ventricular dysphonia should be diagnosed by means of frontal radiography (tomograms) to estab-lish the contribution of the ventricular as well as true vocal folds. There are several therapies for improving the voice quality in cases of ventricular dysphonia, as dis-cussed in the following sections.

Pitch Establishment

When the pitch of the voice is varied, a pitch often can be found that involves improved quality and vocal effort. This also is a means of eliminating any diplopho-nia. This attempt to establish a different vocal pitch range should be done in a con-text of overall improved vocal hygiene and musculoskeletal relaxation.

Relaxation Training

When ventricular phonation involves hyperfunctional effort, rather than paralysis or surgical ablation, training the client to phonate with less physical effort can reduce the involvement of the ventricular folds. After a more relaxed state has been achieved, the client should be recorded while producing vocal efforts, perhaps on a digital monograph such as the Kay Elemetrics CSL or 5500 Sonograph. As improved productions are heard, the recorded sample can be played back to the client for confirmation of improvement and stored for a comparison model. (See "Case Example of Voice Evaluation" presented at the end of Chapter 3.)

Digital Pressure

When the ventricular folds are used following surgical removal of tissue, a slight amount of pressure applied to the laryngeal area in various places during phonation can result in improved vocal quality without the effort that results in ventricular involvement. As this is done, the phonation effort should be recorded to document the effort and help establish a target voice quality. Once the client hears the improved voice under digital pressure and internalizes the feeling involved in producing it, the quality can be maintained by internal adjustment as the digital pressure is eliminated. Many of the case reports reviewed by Stemple (2000) apply to the management of ventricular dysphonia, including the ones by Glaze (2000), Casper (2000), Hufnagle (2000), and Lee (2000b). McFarlane and Von Berg (2000) reported on the use of the Facilitator 3100 (Kay Elemetrics), which would be helpful in providing feedback on voice production in any case of therapy, including ventricular dysphonia. Deem and Miller (2000) also provided helpful therapy techniques that can be used to manage cases of vocal hyperfunction. These studies apply various techniques described earlier, such as modifying the pitch of the voice, teaching relaxation in voice production, providing feedback on improvement, stabilizing the best voice productions, and teaching general principles of good vocal hygiene.

Laryngeal Webs

Several degrees of webbing across the glottal space can be responsible for laryngeal stenosis. These can range from a small web across the anterior commissure to complete agenesis of the glottis. Embryologically, the glottis is formed by tissue resorption that establishes the glottal lumen. Failure of this resorption results in a congenital web of some degree. When webbing is extensive in neonates, their lives are severely compromised and, unless emergency treatment (tracheotomy) is performed, there is a great chance the result will be another infant death statistic. An excellent review of clinical embryology and surgical management of congenital webs was provided by Milczuk, Smith, and Everts (2000).

The symptoms that should alert the attending physician that a neonate might have laryngeal stenosis from webbing or other malformation include cyanosis, stridor, restlessness, or other signs of respiratory distress. Direct laryngoscopy is necessary to confirm suspicions of laryngeal stenosis. A bronchoscope then can be passed into the laryngeal area to allow palpation of the web to determine its extent and thickness.

Severe stenosis or extensive webbing requires either cricothyrotomy or tracheostomy to provide an airway (Meyerhoff & Rice, 1992). Webs can also occur as a result of laryngeal trauma (Colton & Casper, 1996).

Surgical correction of a web requires the placement of a keel between the vocal folds to keep the web from re-forming during the reepithelialization stage of healing. Without the keel, the constant contact of the healing vocal folds regenerates the web. Casiano and Lundy (1998) provided a technique of web management involving a combination of transoral laser vaporization followed by transoral keel placement in patients with anterior webs. Although it would appear that a web could be corrected easily, the dynamic nature of vocal fold movement makes it difficult for easy management, and the client with a congenital laryngeal web may have to undergo several procedures of management, including dilations and surgical excision, the latter performed recently by means of the CO_2 laser. The surgical information provided by Zeitels and Sataloff (1999) on laryngeal papillomas would apply to any condition in which the tissues around the anterior commissure might require surgical treatment.

Congenital Chondromalacia or Laryngomalacia

Another congenital condition that can produce immediate symptoms of stridor, dyspnea, and cyanosis is congenital laryngomalacia, which involves flaccidity of the cartilaginous (chondro) structures of the larynx. Because of this flaccidity, the epiglottis and aryepiglottic folds are easily pulled down over the opening to the glottis, causing respiratory difficulty. Iyer, Pearman, and Raafat (1999) presented evidence of a relationship between gastroesophageal reflux disorder and the development of laryngomalacia.

This condition does not usually present such a problem that tracheostomy or intubation are required (Meyerhoff & Rice, 1992). It is also associated with many syndromes that are autosomal dominant in inheritance, including cri du chat, velocardiofacial, and Marshall-Smith, and numerous additional syndromes identified by Peterson-Falzone et al. (2001). This condition is usually managed medically without significant speech–language pathology involvement.

Cri du Chat Syndrome

Cri du chat (cry of the cat) syndrome was named because infants born with this condition have a high-pitched cry that sounds more like a kitten than a baby crying. It involves chromosome abnormality (partial deletion of a group B chromosome). Additional characteristics associated with the cri du chat syndrome include mental retardation, a rounded facies, a beaklike profile, microcephaly, hypotonia, hypertelorism, anti-Mongoloid palpebral fissures, epicanthal folds, strabismus, midline oral clefts, and generally poor development (A. E. Aronson, 1990; Gorlin et al., 1990).

Cysts and Miscellaneous Developments in the Larynx

A laryngeal cyst is a growth occurring in multifocal or singular form. It usually is found in the vocal folds as intracordal cysts of the mucous retention or epidermoid variety. They most often present unilaterally, but bilateral cysts are possible (Stemple, 2000). They appear typically as a whitish oval-form nodule just under the surface of the vocal fold. There are several hypotheses explaining the etiology of cysts, including (a) the occlusion of one or a few mucous gland ducts of the inferior part of the vocal fold, which causes the pressure of the ductal secretions to foster squamous metaplasia; (b) ingrowth of squamous elements from the free edge of the membranous vocal fold because of microtrauma from vocal abuse or misuse; and (c) some congenital anomaly (D. O. Smith, Callanan, Harcourt, & Albert, 2000). Even small cysts can be problematic to the professional voice user, particularly the singer (Sataloff, 1998c). Cysts generally do not respond to nonsurgical management, but when vocal abuse or misuse is considered an etiological factor, such behaviors must be eliminated for successful resolution of the cyst lesions. These cases need the services of a speech–language pathologist as an important aspect of vocal rehabilitation (Bais, Uppal, & Logani, 1989; Colton & Casper, 1996).

Laryngoceles

Another abnormality of the larynx is the laryngocele, an air sac connected to the laryngeal ventricle as well as to other locations. Sometimes laryngoceles contain fluid. Laryngoceles are dilatations of the laryngeal sacule within the ventricle of Morgagni, the space inferior to the false vocal folds and superior to the true vocal folds (see Figure 1.1). They are typically associated with behaviors that involve significant laryngeal air pressure use, such as glass blowing or playing a wind instrument. Recently they have been identifed with ventricular phonation because using the false vocal folds for voice requires greater effort (Dray, Waugh, & Hillel, 2000). Laryngoceles often are seen following laryngectomy in the area of the P-E junction. Laryngoceles differ from cysts in that they are typically filled with air, whereas cysts usually are filled with mucus. However, Dray et al. (2000) reported on a case in which a fluid-filled laryngocele developed in an adult patient who used ventricular phonation from extensive surgeries to manage persistent papillomas.

Laryngeal Trauma

Some persons have become dysphonic as a result of an automobile accident, a blow to the larynx in a fight, or a penetrating wound (e.g., from a bullet or knife). Each such form of laryngeal trauma is different, and the speech–language pathologist must evaluate every case on the basis of residual status of the larynx following all medical and reconstructive treatment.

When laryngeal trauma has occurred, there may be several consequences that affect laryngeal functioning for voice and biological protection. There may be a significant neurological component involving paralysis or paresis of one or both of the vocal folds. Significant edema usually occurs, and the remaining vocal impact from the trauma might not be apparent until the edema has been resolved. Some traumas involve heat from fire, smoke inhalation, or chemical ingestion, common occurrences, among children and firefighters (Prater & Deskin, 1998). Firefighters are often involved in rescues that challenge the respiratory support provided by their equipment. When this happens, they run out of provided oxygen and begin inhaling smoke surrounding the fire. If not rescued soon, they will die. If rescued, they will likely have a significant dysphonia from the heat and smoke inhalation (*Phoenix Fire Department Operations Manual*, 2000).

Cartilages of the larynx can also be damaged, fractured, or altered at normal cartilaginous connections, such as the cricoarytenoid or cricothyroid joints when laryngeal trauma occurs. Webs or adhesions can develop in the healing process (Andrews, 1999). Laryngeal injuries also occur from intubation and can occur with short- or long-term placement. Short-term endotracheal intubation is more likely to present with a vocal fold immobility or an anterior glottic web, whereas long-term intubation more likely presents with subglottic stenosis and granulomas (Lundy, Casiano, Shatz, Reisberg, & Xue, 1998).

The principles of evaluation and treatment for many of the disorders covered in this book apply to the person with dysphonia following laryngeal trauma. When the patient with trauma has been medically stabilized, videoendoscopy, stroboscopy, and other acoustic measurements can be used to determine residual consequences of the trauma. Effective strategies can then be generated to modify the voice to maximize vocal potential. Schaefer and Close (1989), in their excellent general reference for vocal trauma, provided medical and vocal rehabilitation guidelines for medical management of patients with laryngeal trauma (see also Brosch & Johannsen, 1999; Kurien & Zachariah, 1999; Sataloff, 1998c; Sataloff et al., 1988).

Airway Foreign Bodies

Aspiration of foreign bodies into the airway is a common occurrence, particularly in children. The array of materials and substances that can be aspirated is overwhelming, but certain items appear more commonly. Various foods are often aspirated. Some are large enough to present immediate threat to life, such as a piece of steak. The Heimlich maneuver has been widely taught to assist individuals in this aspiration difficulty. Other episodes of aspiration are more subtle because they involve smaller objects that irritate the tissues of the airway but are not sufficiently large to completely obstruct it, for example, peanuts, sunflower seeds, or tiny toy parts. An episode of aspiration is usually accompanied by immediate choking, coughing, stridor, wheezing, and respiratory distress. Most of these difficulties are managed by acute medical care and present no long-term voice difficulty, but some instances of aspiration result in prolonged respiratory difficulty, including pulmonary lobectomy (Oguz, Citak, Unuvar, & Sidal, 2000). If a residual dysphonia persists after aspiration trauma, the patient might require the assistance of a speech–language pathologist to restore vocal potential.

Acquired Immunodeficiency Syndrome

The speech–language pathologist is often involved in the evaluation and treatment of patients with acquired immunodeficiency syndrome (AIDS). It is therefore imperative that universal precautions be instituted when treating these and all patients. There must be concern about infection and the possible spreading of any virus, including the human immunodeficiency virus (HIV) of AIDS. Infection control must be instituted to protect the speech–language pathologist and the patient.

Hadderingh, Tange, Danner, and Schattenkerk (1987) reported that 43 of 63 (68%) cases of AIDS had otolaryngological manifestations, including neck masses, a greater incidence of shortness of breath, and chronic cough. Marelli, Biddinger, and Gluckman (1992) presented a case of a 40-year-old HIV-positive homosexual man who was seen in an emergency room with a 2-week history of progressive cough, hoarseness, night sweats, and fever. Flexible fiber-optic laryngoscopy confirmed a yellowish-white ulceration of the right false vocal cord with surrounding erythema and edema. The lesion was found to be cytomegalovirus (CMV), which is a member of the herpes virus family. Medical treatment was able to resolve the lesion and the symptoms. The authors indicated that nearly 100% of HIV-positive homosexual males are CMV seropositive (i.e., possess antibodies indicating infection or ongoing immunizing exposure to the organism). Although evidence is present in most HIV-positive patients, the overall incidence of serious CMV disease in AIDS patients is 7.4% (5.7% retinitis and 2.2% gastrointestinal disease). This patient with laryngeal manifestation provides a warning to those professionals who examine the larynx routinely and provides reinforcement for the application of universal precautions.

Roland, Rothstein, Khushbakhat, and Perksy (1993) reported on eight cases of squamous cell carcinoma in HIV-positive patients under 45 years of age, indicating that HIV can manifest itself in many ways, including squamous cell carcinoma. In these patients, the carcinoma occurred in the nasopharynx, oral cavity, oropharynx, or larynx. The authors indicated that HIV perhaps establishes a vulnerability factor that increases the risk from smoking and alcohol consumption in patients under age 45 who normally are not vulnerable to squamous cell carcinoma.

Care should be taken by speech–language pathologists to use gloves and other universal precautions whenever an exchange of body fluids is possible, such as during orolaryngeal and endoscopic examinations. Golper (1998) and Johnson and Jacobson (1998) provided excellent references containing guidelines for speech–language pathologists practicing in hospitals and clinics in which there is a greater probability of such examinations occurring.

Sulcus Vocalis

Hirano and Bless (1993) described sulcus vocalis as a condition in which a furrow along the edge of the vocal folds is related to dysphonia. Several etiologies are possible, including a congenital condition or chronic episodes of laryngeal inflammation and vocal abuse. It is usually bilateral and involves the superficial layer of the lamina propria. Histologically, the sulcus creates a blind sac with the epithelial walls thickened as stratified squamous epithelium. The sulcus extends to adhere to the vocal ligament. Because of its presence, the glottis is incompetent and bowed along the entire length of the vibrating vocal folds. This spindle-shaped gap also affects the amplitude of horizontal excursion of the vocal fold and the mucosal wave function, which stops at the furrow. The effect on vocal fold vibration is that the mass is reduced and the stiffness of the tissue is increased, and under stroboscopic examination a defect is often noted in the closure phase as a function of increased vocal fold stiffness. The lesions can be congenital or acquired, unilateral or bilateral. When bilateral, the effect on vocal dynamics is increased. The conservative approach to management is voice therapy, and if that is not successful in ameliorating the condition, surgery to excise the involved mucosa is recommend (Courey & Ossoff, 1995; Gould, Rubin, & Yanagisawa, 1995; Sataloff, 1998c).

A surgical treatment method was proposed by Pontes and Behlau (1993) in which the sulcus is surgically manipulated directly. A cranial incision is placed superior to the sulcus, and the sulcus mucosa is detached without disturbing the vocal ligament or deep layers of the lamina propria. Four or five vertical incisions of different lengths are made in the detached mucosa perpendicular to the sulcus. The purpose of this surgical approach is to free the mucosal tissue to vibrate independently from the vocal ligament. Following the surgery, intense vocal rehabilitation is recommended, ranging from 4 to 8 months. Ten patients were reported who had excellent results from this treatment technique. Various vocal parameters were carefully documented before and after the surgery and vocal rehabilitation.

Lindestad and Hertegard (1994) reported that, of 186 patients with spindle-shaped glottal insufficiency, at least 94, or 51%, had sulcus vocalis. This was a retrospective study, however, and the authors expressed concern that many of the patients had not been examined by stroboscopy. Had all patients been stroboscopically examined, the percentage with sulcus vocalis might have been higher.

Although this disorder is fairly rare, it is difficult to treat. Some of the glottal insufficiency effect can be reduced by intracordal injections or thyroplasty for medialization. These procedures do not eliminate the sulcus but can improve the airflow characteristics of the voice resulting from the glottal insufficiency (Colton & Casper, 1996).

MISCELLANEOUS THERAPY TECHNIQUES

The following sections describe therapy techniques that have not been discussed in previous chapters and can be applied to a variety of clinical disorders of voice.

Accent Method of Therapy

In 1976 Smith and Thyme introduced a method of therapy called the Accent Method, often referred to as the Smith Accent Method, which has continued to receive attention for voice management. It is based on the notion that human speech is a holistic process involving the integration of respiration, phonation, resonation, and articulation in a gestalt. Rather than separating these components in therapeutic focus, the goal is to integrate them.

Physiologically, the Accent Method purports to do the following:

• *Increase pulmonary output.* The speech–language pathologist teaches the patient proper abdominal–diaphragmatic breathing. The patient is taught about proper breathing as the driving force in human speech. Generally, a recumbent position is used first in clinics that have a means for lying down. The patient learns to monitor movements of the lower abdomen as respiratory effort is increased. These same strategies are used as the patient moves to the sitting position, the position that most clinicians use as the starting position.

• *Reduce excessive muscular tension.* No specific attention is directed toward relaxation, because increasing respiratory support for phonation allows the patient to produce voice with decreased effort and therefore less muscular tension. However, muscular tension is monitored and modified as necessary.

• *Normalize the vibratory pattern of the vocal folds during phonation.* Increasing respiratory effort and generally relaxing the body increases subglottal air pressure and laryngeal flow naturally, which will maximize the vibratory pattern of vocal fold vibration. The tone of the voice that emerges will be "natural" and "optimal." No attention is needed toward a specific vocal pitch or loudness. The result will also be an increased energy of the fundamental frequency, increased energy of the F_2 and F_3 formant regions, increased frequency and intensity (dynamic) ranges, and improved resonance filtering.

- *Use rhythmic vocal play.* Using various sounds in repeated fashion, the speech–language pathologist demonstrates the accents of speech in rhythms with single sounds. Perhaps a simple process is first introduced, such as "zzzz" "ZZZ" "ZZZ" or "vv" "VVV" "VVV" (underlines indicate accent). Vowels are also used as an important aspect of this vocal play.

- *Stress respiratory support for each accent.* As the various rhythms are introduced, the patient monitors breathing by noting a proper movement of the abdominal wall with each accented attempt. Throughout the stages of therapy, changes in body positioning (sitting, standing, walking, swinging the arms) are used. Using the newly trained method of breathing, the patient is encouraged to sing various vowels at slow and progressively faster rhythms, aiming at the production of repeated short phonations and developing to increased utterance length.

During the training sessions, the patient is led to increase pulmonary support and phonatory effort and to modify the phonatory characteristic (from breathiness to normal phonation). The goal is to teach the patient to control all aspects of speech and voice in this holistic manner. As control in nonspeech tasks is achieved, simple articulated speech utterances are introduced, modeled, and then copied by the patient. The Accent Method can be given in sessions twice weekly to twice daily and usually requires 20 to 25 sessions. Documentation is encouraged (Kotby, 1995). Researchers and writers who have documented the positive results of the Smith Accent Method of therapy include Koschkee and Carlson (1993), Kotby, El-Sady, Basiouny, Abou-Ross, and Hegazi (1991), Kotby, Shiromoto, and Hirano (1993), Kotby (1995), and Harris (2000).

Yawn–Sigh Technique

Many of the disorders discussed in this book have involved vocal hyperfunction or vocal tension, called musculoskeletal tension by Aronson (1990). Boone and McFarlane (2000) discussed the yawn–sigh technique, which has been widely used in the treatment of any dysphonia involving increased musculoskeletal tension. Boone and McFarlane (1993) used computerized tomographic scanning and flexible fiber-endoscopy to document changes in the vocal tract dimensions and larynx positioning in normal subjects during a yawn followed by a sigh of /i/. The subjects in this study generally were able to voluntarily approximate a yawn and follow it with a sign under inspection conditions. In most cases this technique produced a lowering of the laryngeal position, improved vocal acoustics, retracted elevation of the tongue, and resulted in a widened pharynx, all desirable voice traits. Boone and McFarlane's (1993) research and my clinical experience both indicate that this simple technique is valuable for decreasing musculoskeletal tension and vocal hyperfunction and for improving the vibratory and resonatory characteristics of voice. This technique is advocated for discriminate use by numerous authorities in voice management, including Andrews (1999), Deem and Miller (2000), and Awan (2001).

Facilitator

The Facilitator is a unique clinical tool that can provide five distinct modes of auditory feedback. It was developed by Kay Elemetrics in collaboration with Daniel Boone, and it is widely used in voice, articulation therapy, motor speech disorder management, fluency, accent reduction, and professional voice training and with children and adults who have learning disability. My focus in this chapter is to describe how the Facilitator can be used in voice management.

The methods of using the Facilitator depend on the voice signal that needs to be fed back to the patient for self-adjusting modifications. The patient wears a headset and lapel microphone. The sample of voice is then obtained and the patient is able to hear immediately the voice produced. With the help of the speech–language pathologist, the client can then be reinforced for improved voice production or instructed as to how modification of some vocal parameter might improve it. The client can be asked to repeat several utterances in up to 6 seconds of recording.

The five modes of auditory feedback provided by the Facilitator include (a) speech–voice amplification, (b) looping playback, (c) delayed auditory feedback with delay settings from 50 to 500 msec in 10 msec steps, (d) speech noise masking , and (e) metronomic pacing for use in dysarthric speech. I have used the Facilitator to mask a patient's voice during voicing to overcome the tendency of the patient to self-discriminate in attempting to maintain the voice we were trying to improve. This was done because the man had spoken with functional dysphonia for so many years that it had become the normal sound to him. When that sound was masked, he was able to improve the quality of his voice, which was then shaped and maintained even when he could hear it. Boone and McFarlane (2000) have discussed the Facilitator with several patients.

Therapy Outcomes: Does Any of This Work?

One reason I have enjoyed my 32 years of experience in evaluating and treating many clients with communication disorder is the success I have enjoyed in the voice disorder arena. It is not an expected outcome to treat a child with delayed language and expect significant change in one or two sessions of therapy. This is also true with clients who have neurological impairment producing aphasia or dysarthria or with children with phonological disorder or fluency difficulty. However, my experience with clients who have voice disorder is different. Many times I have seen clients with significant dysphonia modify voice production under instruction and leave the first or second therapy session with a normal voice. My secretary has often said, "Well, Dr. Case, I think this is going to be one of your miracle cures today." Sometimes she has been correct in her prediction. But it is no miracle when it happens. And when it happens, it is not because of a "golden touch" of management. It happens because experience allows judgment of what is wrong with the phonatory system, including instrumental analysis or perceptual analysis of specific parameters. After a judgment is made as to what is wrong, a decision must be made as to how to fix abnormal parameters, starting with the most critical factor. Is there an algorithm available to tell a clinician how to proceed from step to step? Not really, although Leonard (1999) has provided logical steps of evaluation and treatment for several types of voice disorder. These steps are greatly enhanced when followed by clinicians with many years of experience, years that have taught what is likely to generate failure or success. Sometimes the road less traveled *can* make all the difference, but usually a well-worn trail whose pathway has been deeply entrenched by experienced travelers with very large feet is the better choice.

Pannbacker (1998) reviewed numerous voice therapy techniques and identified treatment outcomes or directions needed to establish clinical efficacy for desirable outcomes. Her voice in this article was similar to that of many, including Ramig and Verdolini (1998) and Verdolini, Ramig, and Jacobson (1998), who have called for improved clinical outcome data. This is needed in the voice arena. Certainly, there is much to gain from the vast clinical experience of those who have been responsible for developing many of the voice therapy techniques used today. These techniques are communicated in articles written by these experts, who tell how they do it (Case, 1999; Casper, 1999; McFarlane & Von Berg, 1998; Poburka, 1999b). However, "how I do it" articles are often only helpful in the context of clinical applications done by experienced clinicians. What is needed in voice management is a concentrated effort to establish effective clinical processes and provide data showing that such processes are effective, whether the processes are applied by an experienced or novice clinician. This is the message of those who call for clinical outcome data. Furthermore, this must be accomplished in the context of diminished resources and funding for treatment in most health care systems.

Leonard (1999) has provided therapy models for the treatment of hyperfunctional disorders with or without lesions, psychogenic dysphonia, and neurogenic voice disorder. She provided decision steps the clinician can take depending on certain factors pertaining to the client's dysphonia. Her paradigm for each type of disorder is helpful to any clinician working with such patients, and this article is recommended. One helpful concept pertains to breaking down the client's voice into the categories of perturbation, harmonic-to-noise ratio, frequency, vital capacity and respiratory support, laryngeal resistance, phonatory airflow, and vocal intensity and then determining whether each of these parameters should be established as "higher, faster, or louder" or "lower, slower, or softer." For example, the judgment must be made on the basis of objective measurement and perceptual evaluation as to whether a client's respiratory support (vital capacity in Leonard's paradigm) needs to be made higher or lower in the context of other parameters.

Leonard presented a concept of targeting a "normal vocal space," which, for example, compares phonatory range from 0% to 100% on the y-axis with respiratory range from 0% to 100% on the x-axis. Between these axis variables, the parameters of vocal frequency (pitch), phonatory airflow, and vocal intensity (loudness) can be evaluated for effective range. The "normal vocal space" for a normal or typical speaker would be in the general area of 30% (low end) to 70% (high end) of each variable potential. No one speaks in the 90% range, for example, of pitch or loudness potential. People have that capacity, but it is rarely used in everyday vocal activity. Leonard's various paradigms for treatment are helpful in making clinical decisions in logical steps.

There are excellent references that outline therapy steps for various disorders of voice, including Andrews (1999), Awan (2001), Stemple (2000), Boone and McFarlane (2000), and Deem and Miller (2000). The steps outlined in these references for the modification of voice have been established as helpful by these experienced clinicians. They do not provide cookbook approaches to voice management. Rather, they provide logical steps to be taken when certain aspects of voice need care and attention.

Vocal Function Exercises

One of the most significant contributions in voice management has been provided by Stemple et al. (2000) in the establishment of Vocal Function Exercises (VFE). These exercises are based on the notion that when any part of the body is injured, such as a knee, there is a period of immobilization and rest, followed by acute treatment, which is then followed by efforts to *strengthen* the injured body part with physical therapy. This is true when the larynx has been injured. Often there is a period of vocal rest, particularly when a lesion or surgical management exists, followed by modification of factors responsible for the disorder, and then when healing has occurred, the muscles of voice must be strengthened. This strengthening aspect is the most unusual focus of VFE.

In VFE, the patient is taught the following series of four exercises to be done at home, two times each, twice per day, preferably morning and evening:

1. Sustain the vowel /i/ for as long as possible on an appropriate musical note (F above middle C for females and boys, F below middle C for men) or a note close to this level. The goal of this duration is marked by the duration of an /s/ sound production. The /s/ sound is voiceless and marks respiratory support for such an effort. Therefore, if a client is able to sustain an /s/ sound for 22 seconds, this should be the target goal for sustaining the /i/ vowel. Each time the client attempts this effort, the minimal goal should be reached and surpassed if possible.

2. Glide the voice from the lowest note to the highest note the client is able to produce while using the word *knoll*. The word *knoll* is used to establish a forward place-

ment of the voice as well as expand the pharynx for open resonation. This is considered a vocal stretching exercise. It should be done with no voice breaks occurring.

3. Glide the voice from the highest note to the lowest note on the word *knoll*. This is a reverse of Exercise 2. The client is instructed to feel a half-yawn in the throat throughout this exercise, which keeps the pharynx more opened and relaxed. This downward glide encourages a slow, systematic engagement of the thyroarytenoid (vocalis muscles or muscles of the vocal fold) without the presence of a back-focused growl sound. This is considered a contracting exercise.

4. Sustain the musical notes (C-D-E-F-G) in the appropriate gender octave for as long as possible on the word *knoll* minus the *kn* consonants. The *oll* vowel and liquid sounds are once again produced with an open pharynx and lips that are somewhat constricted so that they can sympathetically vibrate. This helps the client know that the sound is being produced in a forward manner.

These exercises should be done initially in the presence of the voice clinician to ensure that they are done correctly. The vocal effort must be done with soft but not breathy voice production. Clients are provided with a graph on which to mark their progress. When the client has reached the predetermined goal and the voice quality and other vocal symptoms have improved, the VFE protocol provides an opportunity for tapering of the exercises to maintain the vocal strengthening that has occurred.

FINAL SUGGESTIONS

Although voice therapy is complex, in many cases it provides great satisfaction because change is often dramatic and immediate. Many authors have provided the student of voice, from the beginning graduate student to the seasoned clinician, marvelous suggestions to help patients and clients improve vocal performance. Throughout this book I have drawn from the excellent writings of Andrews (1999), A. E. Aronson (1990), Boone and McFarlane (2000), Colton and Casper (1996), Deem and Miller (2000), Dworkin and Meleca (1997), Morrison and Rammage (2001), Stemple (2000), Stemple et al. (2000), Awan (2001), and Sataloff (1998c), and I recommend all of them for excellent coverage in voice evaluation and treatment.

Following is a list of general principles of management for speech–language pathologists to keep in mind when working with individuals who have voice disorders:

- Teach clients the importance of good vocal hygiene—taking care of the vocal instrument—by avoiding throat clearing, vocal abuse forms, speaking with competing noise, speaking or singing at the edges of pitch and loudness, speaking much during strenuous physical exercise, speaking to large groups without amplification, speaking without sufficient breath support, speaking too long without taking a fresh breath, or speaking with a tight throat and excessive jaw closure.

- Teach clients not to speak more than necessary when they are sick, tired, dehydrated, or emotionally upset; when they have had too much alcohol to drink; or when they have been around smoke or atmospheric irritants (Sataloff, 1998c).

- Teach clients to avoid excessive alcohol, any form of tobacco, excessive caffeine, eating just before bedtime (they should wait 2 to 3 hours after eating), and environmental pollutants or chemical agents (Sataloff, Castell, et al., 1999).

- Teach clients to increase rest, sleep, and water consumption (remember the suggestion "Speak and sing wet, pee pale") and to spend much time with good friends who encourage smiles and laughter (Brodnitz, 1988).

- Teach clients to speak or sing with proper body alignment for good respiratory support (Thorpe, Cala, Chapman, & Davis, 2001).

- Teach clients to warm the voice before using it extensively. It is not wise to start a car's engine in the extreme cold and immediately race down the highway; it also is damaging to vocal folds to vocally perform without proper warm-up and preparation. (See Vintturi et al., 2001.)

- Teach clients about the anatomy and physiology of voice production. Avoid being too technical or too condescending. Knowledge will help clients improve their vocal abilities.

- Be willing to try many techniques, even those that might seem too artistic and not scientifically based. Recently, a music professor and I put on shorts and visited the theater lab of a colleague who taught us how to increase respiratory control while assuming various odd positions on a mat. I was mildly uncomfortable but at the end was invigorated by the process. The next day, I ordered a voice clinic mat.

- Enter the world of technology—master it, use it, learn a new computer fact or program each day—but keep a listening and sensitive attitude. Don't let technology force you away from being a caring human being. Most of us will never do great things, but, as someone has said, each of us can do small and little things in a great way. Helping a person change his or her voice, even a little, can be one of those small things done in a great way. Finally, smile and enjoy the process.

SUMMARY

The main focus of this chapter has been a description of resonance disorders of the voice, including degrees of hypernasality, mixed nasality, and hearing impairment. The nature of these disorders and their etiology, along with evaluation procedures, medical and rehabilitation therapies, and general management considerations for them, have been discussed. Several miscellaneous laryngeal disorders, including papillomas, polyps, ventricular dysphonia, laryngeal webs, laryngomalacia, cysts, laryngoceles, trauma, and sulcus vocalis, also have been described.

REFERENCES

Abitbol, J. (1995). *Atlas of laser voice surgery*. San Diego, CA: Singular.

Abitbol, J., de Brux, J., Millot, G., Masson, M.-F., Mimoun, O. L., Pau, H., & Abitbol, B. (1989). Does a hormonal vocal cord cycle exist in women? Study of vocal premenstrual syndrome in voice performers by videostroboscopy-glottography and cytology on 38 women. *Journal of Voice, 3*, 157–162.

Abitbol, J., Mathe, G., & Battista, C. (1988). Preliminary report on detection of papillomaviruses types 6, 11, 16, and 18 in laryngeal benign and malignant lesions. *Journal of Voice, 2*, 334–337.

Adams, S. G. (1997). Hypokinetic dysarthria in Parkinson's disease. In M. R. McNeil (Ed.), *Clinical management of sensorimotor speech disorders*. New York: Thieme.

Alipour, F., & Scherer, R. C. (2000). Vocal fold bulging effects on phonation using a biophysical computer model. *Journal of Voice, 14*, 470–483.

Altman, J. S., & Benninger, M. S. (1997). The evaluation of unilateral vocal fold immobility: Is chest X-ray enough? *Journal of Voice, 11*, 364–367.

American Cancer Society. (2001). *Statistics on cancer facts and figures: Secondhand smoke* [Online]. Available: www.cancer.org

American Joint Committee for Cancer Staging and End-Results Reporting. (1988). *Manual for stages of cancer* (2nd ed.). Philadelphia: Lippincott.

American Medical Association. (2000). *Graduate medical education directory*. Chicago: Author.

American Psychiatric Association. (2000). *Diagnostic and statistical manual of mental disorders—Fourth edition—Text revision*. Washington, DC: Author.

American Speech-Language-Hearing Association. (1998). Roles of otolaryngologists and speech-language pathologists in the performance and intrepretation of strobovideolaryngoscopy. *ASHA, 40*(Suppl. 18), 2–10.

Andrade, D. F., Heuer, R., Hockstein, N. E., Castro, E., Spiegel, J. R., & Sataloff, R. T. (1999). The frequency of hard glottal attacks in patients with muscle tension dysphonia, unilateral benign masses and bilateral benign masses. *Journal of Voice, 14*, 240–246.

Andreassen, M. L., Leeper, H. A., MacRae, D. L., & Nicholson, I. R. (1994). Aerodynamic, acoustic, and perceptual changes following adenoidectomy. *Cleft Palate—Craniofacial Journal, 31*, 263–270.

Andrews, M., Tardy, S., & Pasternak, L. (1984). The modification of hypernasality in young children: A programming approach. *Language, Speech & Hearing Services in Schools, 15*, 37–43.

Andrews, M. L. (1986). *Voice therapy for children*. New York: Longman.

Andrews, M. L. (1999). *Manual of voice treatment: Pediatrics through geriatrics* (2nd ed.). San Diego, CA: Singular.

Andrianopoulos, M. V. (2000). A case of the young athlete with associated psychosocial contributions. In J. C. Stemple (Ed.), *Voice therapy clinical studies*. San Diego, CA: Singular.

Arnold, G. E. (1980). Disorders in laryngeal function. In M. M. Paparella & D. A. Shumrick (Eds.), *Otolaryngology* (Vol. 3). Philadelphia: Saunders.

Aronson, A. E. (1990). *Clinical voice disorders: An interdisciplinary approach* (3rd ed.). New York: Thieme-Stratton.

Aronson, A. E. (1998). Dysarthria, crying, and laughing in pseudobulbar palsy from right middle cerebral artery CVA: Overview and personal account. *Journal of Medical Speech-Language Pathology, 6*, 111–114.

Aronson, A. E., & DeSanto, L. W. (1983). Adductor spastic dysphonia: Three years after recurrent laryngeal nerve resection. *Laryngoscope, 93*, 1–8.

Aronson, A. E., & Lagerlund, T. D. (1991). Neuroimaging studies do not prove the existence of brain abnormalities in spastic (spasmodic) dysphonia. *Journal of Speech and Hearing Research, 34*, 801–805.

351

Aronson, L. R., & Cooper, M. L. (1979). Amygdaloid hypersexuality in male rats reexamined. *Physiology and Behavior, 22*, 257–265.

Askenfelt, A. G., & Hammarberg, B. (1986). Speech waveform perturbation analysis: A perceptual-acoustical comparison of seven measures. *Journal of Speech and Hearing Research, 29*, 50–64.

Awan, S. N. (1997). Analysis of nasalance: NasalView. In W. Ziegler & K. Deger (Eds.), *Clinical phonetics and linguistics*. London: Whurr-Publishers.

Awan, S. N. (2001). *The Voice Diagnostic Protocol*. Gaithersburg, MD: Aspen.

Azuma, T., Cruz, R. F., Bayles, K. A., Tomoeda, C. K., Wood, J. A., & Montgomery, E. B. (2000). Incidental learning and verbal memory in individuals with Parkinson's disease. *Journal of Medical Speech-Language Pathology, 8*, 163–174.

Bachmayer, D., & Ross, R. B. (1986). Stability of Le Fort III advancement surgery in children with Crouzon's, Apert's, and Pfeiffer's syndromes. *Cleft Palate Journal, 23*(Suppl. 1), 69–74.

Bais, A. S., Uppal, K., & Logani, K. B. (1989). Congenital cysts of the larynx. *Journal of Laryngology and Otology, 103*, 966–967.

Baken, R. J., & Daniloff, R. G. (1991). *Readings in clinical spectrography of speech*. San Diego, CA and Pine Brook, NJ: Singular and Kay Elemetrics.

Baken, R. J., & Orlikoff, R. F. (2000). *Clinical measurement of speech and voice* (2nd ed.). San Diego, CA: Singular.

Barkmeier, J. M., & Case, J. L. (2000). Differential diagnosis of adductor-type spasmodic dysphonia, vocal tremor, and muscle tension dysphonia. *Current Opinion in Otolaryngology & Head and Neck Surgery, 8*, 174–179.

Barkmeier, J. M., Case, J. L., & Ludlow, C. L. (2001). Identification of symptoms for spasmodic dysphonia and vocal tremor: A comparison of expert and nonexpert judges. *Journal of Communication Disorders, 34*, 21–37.

Bassich, C. J., & Ludlow, C. L. (1986). The use of perceptual methods by new clinicians for assessing voice quality. *Journal of Speech and Hearing Disorders, 51*, 125–133.

Bastian, R. W. (1999, September/October). *Why do patients continue or discontinue botulinum toxin therapy for spasmodic dysphonia? Are there newer, better methods?* International Dystonia Symposium Summary, 12–13.

Bastian, R. W. (2001, January). When BOTOX doesn't work. *National Spasmodic Dysphonia Association Newsletter*, pp. 10–11.

Bastian, R. W., & Delsupehe, K. (1998). Indirect procedures of the larynx and pharynx. In A. Blitzer, H. C. Pillsbury, A. F. Jahn, & W. J. Binder (Eds.), *Office-based surgery in otolaryngology*. New York: Thieme.

Batza, E. M., & Parker, W. (1971). Hyponasality associated with patulous eustachian tubes: Report of a case. *Journal of Speech and Hearing Disorders, 36*, 410– 413.

Bear, M. F., Connors, B. W., & Paradiso, M. A. (1996). *Neuroscience exploring the brain*. Baltimore: Williams & Wilkins.

Bell-Berti, F. (1976). Electromyographic study of velopharyngeal function in speech. *Journal of Speech and Hearing Research, 19*, 225–240.

Benjamin, B. N., Gatenby, P. A., Kitchen, R., Harrison, H., Cameron, K., & D'Phil, A. B. (1988). Alpha-interferon (wellferon) as an adjunct to standard surgical therapy in the management of recurrent respiratory papillomatosis. *Annals of Otology, Rhinology, and Laryngology, 97*, 376–380.

Bennett, S., & Netsell, R. W. (1999). Possible roles of the insula in speech and language processing: Directions for research. *Journal of Medical Speech-Language Pathology, 7*, 255–272.

Benninger, M. S., & Gardner, G. M. (1998). Medical and surgical management in otolaryngology. In A. F. Johnson & B. H. Jacobson (Eds.), *Medical speech-language pathology: A practitioner's guide*. New York: Thieme.

Benninger, M. S., & Grywalski, C. (1998). Rehabilitation of the head and neck cancer patient. In A. F. Johnson & B. H. Jacobson (Eds.), *Medical speech-language pathology: A practitioner's guide*. New York: Thieme.

Benninger, M. S., & Schwimmer, C. (1996). Functional neurophysiology and vocal fold paralysis. In J. S. Rubin, R. T. Sataloff, G. S. Korovin, & W. J. Gould (Eds.), *Diagnosis and treatment of voice disorders*. New York: IGAKU-SHOIN.

Berke, G. (1999, September/October). *Spasmodic dysphonia*. International Dystonia Symposium Summary, 23, 30.

Berkowitz, S. (1996). *Cleft lip and palate: Perspectives in management with an introduction to other craniofacial anomalies* (Vol. 1). San Diego, CA: Singular.

Berry, D. A., Moon, J. B., & Kuehn, D. P. (1999). A finite element model of the soft palate. *Cleft Palate—Craniofacial Journal, 36*, 217–223.

Beukelman, D. R., Yorkston, K. M., & Reichle, J. (2000). *Augmentative and alternative communication for adults with acquired neurological disorders*. Baltimore: Brookes.

Bevan, K., Griffiths, M. V., & Morgan, M. H. (1989). Cricothyroid muscle paralysis: Its recognition and diagnosis. *Journal of Laryngology and Otology, 103*, 191–195.

Bielamowicz, S., & Ludlow, C. L. (2000). Effects of botulinum toxin on pathophysiology in spasmodic dysphonia. *Annals of Otology, Rhinology, and Laryngology, 109*, 194–203.

Blager, F. B. (2000). Paradoxical vocal fold movement: Diagnosis and management. *Current Opinion in Otolaryngology & Head and Neck Surgery, 8*, 180–183.

Blaugrund, S. M. (1995). Laryngeal framework surgery. In J. S. Rubin, R. T. Sataloff, G. S. Korovin, & W. J. Gould (Eds.), *Diagnosis and treatment of voice disorders*. New York: IGAKU-SHOIN.

Blaugrund, S. M., Isshiki, N., & Taira, T. (1992). Phonosurgery. In A. Blitzer, M. E. Brin, C. T. Sasaki, S. Fahn, & K. S. Harris (Eds.), *Neurologic disorders of the larynx*. New York: Thieme Medical.

Bless, D., & Poburka, B. (2001). *Video laryngeal stroboscopy multimedia tutorial* [CD-ROM]. San Diego, CA: Singular.

Blitzer, A., & Brin, M. E. (1992a). The dystonic larynx. *Journal of Voice, 6*, 294–297.

Blitzer, A., & Brin, M. E. (1992b). Treatment of spasmodic dysphonia (laryngeal dystonia) with local injections of botulinum toxin. *Journal of Voice, 6*, 365–369.

Blitzer, A., & Brin, M. E. (1998). Laryngeal electromyography and injection of botulinum toxin. In A. Blitzer, H. C. Pillsbury, A. F. Jahn, & W. J. Binder (Eds.), *Office-based surgery in otolaryngology*. New York: Thieme.

Blitzer, A., Brin, M. E., Green, P. E., & Fahn, S. (1989). Botulinum toxin injection for the treatment of oromandibular dystonia. *Annals of Otology, Rhinology, and Laryngology, 98*, 93–97.

Blitzer, A., Brin, M. E., Sasaki, C. T., Fahn, S., & Harris, K. S. (1992). *Neurologic disorders of the larynx*. New York: Thieme Medical.

Blitzer, A., Pillsbury, H. C., Jahn, A. F., & Binder, W. J. (Eds.). (1998). *Office-based surgery in otolaryngology*. New York: Thieme.

Blom, E. D. (1998a). Evolution of tracheoesophageal voice prostheses. In E. D. Blom, M. I. Singer, & R. C. Hamaker (Eds.), *Tracheoesophageal voice restoration following total laryngectomy*. San Diego, CA: Singular.

Blom, E. D. (1998b). Tracheostoma valve fitting and instruction. In E. D. Blom, M. I. Singer, & R. C. Hamaker (Eds.), *Tracheoesophageal voice restoration following total laryngectomy*. San Diego, CA: Singular.

Blom, E. D., & Hamaker, R. C. (1996). Tracheoesophageal voice restoration following total laryngectomy. In E. N. Myers & J. Suen (Eds.), *Cancer of the head and neck*. Philadelphia: Saunders.

Blom, E. D., & Singer, M. I. (1979). Surgical-prosthetic approaches for postlaryngectomy voice restoration. In R. L. Keith & E. L. Darley (Eds.), *Laryngectomee rehabilitation*. Austin, TX: PRO-ED.

Blom, E. D., Singer, M. I., & Hamaker, R. C. (1998). *Tracheoesophageal voice restoration following total laryngectomy*. San Diego, CA: Singular.

Boone, D. R. (1966). Treatment of functional aphonia in a child and an adult. *Journal of Speech and Hearing Disorders, 31*, 69–74.

Boone, D. R. (1982). *The Boone voice program for adults.* Austin, TX: PRO-ED.

Boone, D. R. (1988). Respiratory training in voice therapy. *Journal of Voice, 2,* 20–25.

Boone, D. R. (1991). *Is your voice telling on you?* San Diego, CA: Singular.

Boone, D. R. (1993). *The Boone voice program for children* (2nd ed.). Austin, TX: PRO-ED.

Boone, D. R., & McFarlane, S. (1988). *The voice and voice therapy* (4th ed.). Englewood Cliffs, NJ: Prentice Hall.

Boone, D. R., & McFarlane, S. C. (1993). A critical view of the yawn-sigh as a voice therapy technique. *Journal of Voice, 7,* 75–80.

Boone, D. R., & McFarlane, S. C. (2000). *The voice and voice therapy* (6th ed.). Boston: Allyn & Bacon.

Bosone, Z. T. (1999). Tracheoesophageal speech: Treatment considerations before and after surgery. In S. J. Salmon (Ed.), *Alaryngeal speech rehabilitation—by clinicians for clinicians* (2nd ed.). Austin, TX: PRO-ED.

Bradley, D. P. (1989). Congenital and acquired velopharyngeal inadequacy. In K. R. Bzoch (Ed.), *Communicative disorders related to cleft lip and palate.* Austin, TX: PRO-ED.

Bressman, S. (1999, September/October). *What is the most important thing you can tell a newly diagnosed patient about prognosis?* International Dystonia Symposium Summary, 9–10.

Bressmann, T., Sader, R., Whitehill, T. L., Awan, S. N., Zeilhofer, H.-F., & Horch, H. H. (2000). Nasalance distance and ratio: Two new measures. *Cleft Palate—Craniofacial Journal, 37,* 248–256.

Brin, M. E., Blitzer, A., Stewart, C., & Fahn, S. (1992). Treatment of spasmodic dysphonia (laryngeal dystonia) with local injections of botulinum toxin: Review and technical aspects. In A. Blitzer, M. E. Brin, C. T. Sasaki, S. Fahn, & K. S. Harris (Eds.), *Neurologic disorders of the larynx.* New York: Thieme Medical.

Brin, M. E., Fahn, S., Blitzer, A., Ramig, L. O., & Stewart, C. (1992). Movement disorders of the larynx. In A. Blitzer, M. E. Brin, C. T. Sasaki, S. Fahn, & K. D. Harris (Eds.), *Neurologic disorders of the larynx.* New York: Thieme Medical.

Brodnitz, E. S. (1988). *Keep your voice healthy: A guide to the intelligent use and care of the speaking and singing voice* (2nd ed.). Austin, TX: PRO-ED.

Brody, R., & Turk, J. B. (1999). Allergic disorders. In F. E. Lucente & G. Har-El (Eds.), *Essentials of otolaryngology* (4th ed.). Philadelphia: Lippincott-Williams & Wilkins.

Broen, P. A., & Moller, K. T. (1993). Early phonological development and the child with cleft palate. In K. T. Moller & C. D. Starr (Eds.), *Cleft palate interdisciplinary issues and treatment—for clinicians by clinicians.* Austin, TX: PRO-ED.

Brosch, S., & Johannsen, H. S. (1999). Clinical course of acute laryngeal trauma and associated effects on phonation. *Journal of Laryngology and Otology, 113,* 58–61.

Brown, W. S., Morris, R. J., Hicks, D. M., & Howell, E. (1993). Phonational profiles of female professional singers and nonsingers. *Journal of Voice, 3,* 219–226.

Brown, W. S., Morris, R. J., & Michel, J. E. (1989). Vocal jitter in young adult and aged female voices. *Journal of Voice, 3,* 113–119.

Buder, E. H. (2000). Acoustic analysis of voice quality: A tabulation of algorithms 1902–1900. In R. D. Kent & M. J. Ball (Eds.), *Voice quality measurement.* San Diego, CA: Singular.

Burns, P. (1991). Clinical management of country and western singers. *Journal of Voice, 5,* 349–353.

Busscher, H. J., & van der Mei, H. C. (1998). Biofilm formation and its prevention on silicone rubber voice prostheses. In E. D. Blom, M. I. Singer, & R. C. Hamaker (Eds.), *Tracheoesophageal voice restoration following total laryngectomy.* San Diego, CA: Singular.

Bzoch, K. R. (Ed.). (1997). *Communicative disorders related to cleft lip and palate* (4th ed.). Austin, TX: PRO-ED.

Campbell, S. L., Reich, A. R., Klockars, A. J., & McHenry, M. A. (1988). Factors associated with dysphonia in high school cheerleaders. *Journal of Speech and Hearing Disorders, 53,* 175–185.

Cannon, C. R., & McLean, W. C. (1982). Laryngectomy for chronic aspiration. *American Journal of Otolaryngology, 3,* 145–149.

Case, J. L. (1987, November). *Puberphonia: Before and after therapy. Acoustic analysis of pitch.* Paper presented at the annual meeting of the American Speech-Language-Hearing Association, New Orleans.

Case, J. L. (1993). The voice: Across the age-span. In R. Kastenbatim (Ed.), *Encyclopedia of adult development.* Phoenix, AZ: Oyx Press.

Case, J. L. (1994, November). *Clinical grand rounds: Ventricular dysphonia.* Paper presented at the meeting of the American Speech-Language-Hearing Association, New Orleans.

Case, J. L. (1998). *Videostroboscopy and the clinical management of voice* (Telerounds #40). Tucson: University of Arizona, National Center for Neurogenic Communication Disorders.

Case, J. L. (1999). Clinical management of psychogenic aphonia. *Phonoscope, 2,* 109–112.

Case, J. L. (2000). A Case of PVFM and functional dysphonia. In J. C. Stemple (Ed.), *Voice therapy clinical studies.* San Diego, CA: Singular.

Case, J. L., Beaver, V. L., & Nenaber, P. J. (1978, November). *A longitudinal study of a high-risk population for vocal abuse—university cheerleaders.* Paper presented at the meeting of the American Speech-Language-Hearing Association, San Francisco.

Case, J. L., LaPointe, L. L., & Duane, D. D. (1990, July). *Speech and voice characteristics in spasmodic torticollis.* Paper presented at the International Congress of Movement Disorders, Washington, DC.

Case, J. L., LaPointe, L. L., & Duane, D. D. (1993, November). *The dystonias: Speech and voice characteristics.* Miniseminar at the annual meeting of the American Speech-Language-Hearing Association, Los Angeles.

Case, J. L., Thome, J., & Kohler, S. (1979, November). *A longitudinal study of vocal abuse among cheerleaders.* Paper presented at the meeting of the American Speech-Language-Hearing Association, Atlanta.

Casiano, R. R., & Lundy, D. S. (1998). Outpatient transoral laser vaporization of anterior glottic webs and keel placement: Risks of airway compromise. *Journal of Voice, 12,* 536–539.

Casper, J. K. (1999). Voice treatment for psychogenic dysphonia. *Phonoscope, 2,* 51–55.

Casper, J. K. (2000). Confidential voice. In J. C. Stemple (Ed.), *Voice therapy clinical studies.* San Diego: Singular.

Casper, J. K., Brewer, D. W., & Colton, R. H. (1987). Variations in normal human laryngeal anatomy and physiology as viewed fiberscopically. *Journal of Voice, 1,* 180–185.

Casper, J. K., Brewer, D. W., & Colton, R. H. (1988). Pitfalls and problems in flexible fiberoptic videolaryngoscopy. *Journal of Voice, 1,* 347–352.

Casper, J. K., & Colton, R. H. (1998). *Clinical manual for laryngectomy and head and neck cancer rehabilitation* (2nd ed.). San Diego, CA: Singular.

Cassell, M. D., & Elkudi, H. (1995). Anatomy and physiology of the palate and velopharyngeal structures. In R. J. Shprintzen & J. Bardach (Eds.), *Cleft palate speech management.* St. Louis, MO: Mosby.

Cavalli, L., & Hirson, A. (1999). Diplophonia reappraised. *Journal of Voice, 13,* 542–556.

Chenausky, K., & MacAuslan, J. (2000). Utilization of microprocessors in voice quality improvement: The electrolarynx. *Current Opinion in Otolaryngology & Head and Neck Surgery, 8,* 138–142.

Christensen, J. M., Weinberg, B., & Alfonso, P. J. (1978). Productive voice onset time characteristics of esophageal speech. *Journal of Speech and Hearing Research, 21,* 56–62.

Christensen, J. M., & Weinberg, B. (1976). Vowel duration characteristics of esophageal speech. *Journal of Speech and Hearing Research, 19,* 678–689.

Christopher, K. L., Wood, R. P., Eckert, R. C., Blager, F. B., Raney, R. A., & Souhrada, D. E. (1983). Vocal cord dysfunction presenting as asthma. *New England Journal of Medicine, 308,* 1566–1570.

Chuma, A. V., Cacace, A. T., Rosen, R., Feustel, P., & Koltaii, P. J. (1999). Effects of tonsillectomy and/or adenoidectomy on vocal function: Laryngeal, supralaryngeal and perceptual characteristics. *International Journal of Pediatric Otorhinolaryngology, 47,* 1–9.

Citardi, M. J., Gracco, C. L., & Sasaki, C. T. (1995). The anatomy of the human larynx. In J. S. Rubin, R. T. Sataloff, G. S. Korovin, & W. J. Gould (Eds.), *Diagnosis and treatment of voice disorders.* New York: IGAKU-SHOIN.

Cleveland, T. F. (1994). A clearer view of singing voice production: 25 years of progress. *Journal of Voice, 8*, 18–23.

Cohen, S. R., Geller, K. A., Birns, J. W., & Thompson, J. W. (1982). Laryngeal paralysis in children: A long-term retrospective study. *Annals of Otology, Rhinology, and Laryngology, 91*, 417–424.

Cohn, J. R., Spiegel, J. R., Hawkshaw, M., & Sataloff, R. T. (1998). Allergy. In R. T. Sataloff (Ed.), *Vocal health and pedagogy*. San Diego, CA: Singular.

Coleman, R. F. (1987). Performance demands and the performer's vocal capabilities. *Journal of Voice, 1*, 209–216.

Colton, R. H., & Casper, J. K. (1996). *Understanding voice problems: A physiological perspective for diagnosis and treatment* (2nd ed.). Baltimore: Williams & Wilkins.

Colton, R. H., & Conture, E. G. (1990). Problems and pitfalls of electroglottography. *Journal of Voice, 4*, 10–24.

Comella, C. (1999, September/October). *How is dystonia diagnosed? What tests are used?* International Dystonia Symposium Summary, 10.

Compston, A. (1997). Genetic epidemiology of multiple sclerosis. *Journal of Neurology, Neurosurgery, and Psychiatry, 62*, 553–561.

Cooper, D. S., & Lawson, W. (1992). Laryngeal sensory receptors. In A. Blitzer, M. F. Brin, C. T. Sasaki, S. Fahn, & K. S. Harris (Eds.), *Neurologic disorders of the larynx*. New York: Thieme Medical.

Cooper, D. S., & Titze, I. R. (1985). Generation and dissipation of heat in vocal fold tissue. *Journal of Speech and Hearing Research, 28*, 207–215.

Cordero, O. (1999). Speech-language pathology. In F. E. Lucente & G. Har-El (Eds.), *Essentials of otolaryngology*. Philadelphia: Lippincott-Williams & Wilkins.

Corey, J. P., Houser, S. M., & Ng, B. A. (2000). Nasal congestion: A review of its etiology, evaluation, and treatment. *ENT—Ear, Nose & Throat Journal, 79*, 690–702.

Countryman, S., Ramig, L. O., & Pawlas, A. A. (1994). Speech and voice deficits in Parkinsonian plus syndromes: Can they be treated? *Journal of Medical Speech-Language Pathology, 2*, 211–225.

Courey, M. S., Garrett, C. G., Billante, C. R., Stone, E. R., Portell, M. D., Smith, T. L., & Netterville, J. L. (2000). Outcomes assessment following treatment of spasmodic dysphonia with botulinum toxin. *Annals of Otology, Rhinology, and Laryngology, 109*, 819–822.

Courey, M. S., & Ossoff, R. H. (1995). Surgical management of benign voice disorders. In J. S. Rubin, R. T. Sataloff, G. S. Korovin, & W. J. Gould (Eds.), *Diagnosis and treatment of voice disorders*. New York: IGAKU-SHOIN.

Cranen, B., & de Jong, F. (2000). Laryngostroboscopy. In R. D. Kent & M. J. Ball (Eds.), *Voice quality measurement*. San Diego, CA: Singular.

Crary, M. A. (1993). Developmental motor speech disorders. In L. L. LaPointe (Series Ed.), *Neurogenic communication disorders series*. San Diego, CA: Singular.

Crevier-Buchman, L., Laccourreye, O., Papon, J.-F., Nurit, D., & Brasnu, D. (1997). Adductor spasmodic dysphonia: Case reports with acoustic analysis following botulinum toxin injection and acupuncture. *Journal of Voice, 11*, 232–237.

Crumley, R. L. (1994). Unilateral recurrent laryngeal nerve paralysis. *Journal of Voice, 8*, 79–83.

Crysdale, W. S., Feldman, R. I., & Naito, K. (1988). Tracheotomies: A 10-year experience in 319 children. *Annals of Otology, Rhinology, and Laryngology, 97*, 439–443.

Dalston, R. M. (1992). Acoustic assessment of the nasal airway. *Cleft Palate—Craniofacial Journal, 29*, 520–526.

Dalston, R. M., & Keefe, M. J. (1988). Digital, labial, and velopharyngeal reaction times in normal speakers. *Cleft Palate Journal, 25*, 203–209.

Dalston, R. M., Warren, D. W., & Dalston, E. T. (1991). Use of nasometry as a diagnostic tool for identifying patients with velopharyngeal impairment. *Cleft Palate—Craniofacial Journal, 28*, 184–189.

Dalston, R. M., Warren, D. W., & Dalston, E. T. (1992). A preliminary study of nasal airway patency and its potential effect on speech performance. *Cleft Palate—Craniofacial Journal, 29*, 330–335.

Daniloff, R., Schuckers, G., & Feth, L. (1980). *The physiology of speech and hearing: An introduction*. Englewood Cliffs, NJ: Prentice Hall.

Darley, F. L., Aronson, A. E., & Brown, J. R. (1969a). Clusters of deviant speech dimensions in the dysarthrias. *Journal of Speech and Hearing Research, 12,* 462–496.

Darley, F. L., Aronson, A. E., & Brown, J. R. (1969b). Differential diagnostic patterns of dysarthria. *Journal of Speech and Hearing Research, 12,* 246–269.

Darley, F. L., Aronson, A. E., & Brown, J. R. (1975a). *Audio seminars in speech pathology: Motor speech disorders*. Philadelphia: Saunders.

Darley, F. L., Aronson, A. E., & Brown, J. R. (1975b). *Motor-speech disorders*. Philadelphia: Saunders.

Darley, F. L., Brown, J. R., & Goldstein, N. P. (1972). Dysarthria in multiple sclerosis. *Journal of Speech and Hearing Research, 15,* 229–245.

Davis, C. B., & Davis, M. L. (1993). The effects of premenstrual syndrome (PMS) on the female singer. *Journal of Voice, 7,* 337–353.

Debruyne, F., Ostyn, F., Delaere, P., & Wellens, W. (1991). Acoustic analysis of the speaking voice after thyroidectomy. *Journal of Voice, II,* 479–482.

Dedo, H. H. (1976). Recurrent laryngeal nerve section for spastic dysphonia. *Annals of Otology, Rhinology, and Laryngology, 85,* 1–9.

Dedo, H. H., & Izdebski, K. (1983). Intermediate results of 306 recurrent laryngeal nerve sections for spastic dysphonia. *Laryngoscope, 93,* 9–15.

Dedo, H. H., & Izdebski, K. (1999). Indirect teflon injection in unilateral vocal fold paralysis: A response to criticisms and discussion of essentials to successful outcome. *Phonoscope, 2,* 15–22.

Dedo, H. H., Izdebski, K., & Behlau, M. (1993, October). *Treatment of adductor spasmodic dysphonia with RLN section: 16 years of experience*. Paper presented at the Sixth Annual Pacific Voice Conference, San Francisco.

Deeb, M. E., Waite, D. E., & Curran, J. (1993). Oral and maxillofacial surgery and the management of cleft lip and palate. In K. T. Moller & C. D. Starr (Eds.), *Cleft palate: Interdisciplinary issues and treatment—for clinicians by clinicians*. Austin, TX: PRO-ED.

Deem, J. F., & Miller, L. (2000). *Manual of voice therapy* (2nd ed.). Austin, TX: PRO-ED.

Delorey, R., Leeper, H. A., & Hudson, A. J. (1999). Measures of velopharyngeal functioning in subgroups of individuals with amyotrophic lateral sclerosis. *Journal of Medical Speech-Language Pathology, 7,* 19–31.

Denny, D. (1994). *Gender dysphoria: A guide to research*. New York: Garland.

DePaul, R., & Kent, R. D. (2000). A longitudinal case study of ALS: Effects of listener familiarity and proficiency on intelligibility judgments. *American Journal of Speech-Language Pathology, 9,* 230–240.

Descartes, R. (1968). *Discourse on method and the meditations* (F. E. Sutcliffe, Trans.). London: Penguin. (Original work published 1637)

Desloge, R. B., & Zeitels, S. M. (2000). Endolaryngeal microsurgery at the anterior glottal commissure: Controversies and observations. *Annals of Otology, Rhinology, and Laryngology, 109,* 385–392.

Deutsch, H. L., & Millard, D. R. (1989). A new cocaine abuse complex: Involvement in the nose, septum, palate, and pharynx. *Archives of Otolaryngology: Head & Neck Surgery, 115,* 235–237.

Dey, F. L., & Kirchner, J. A. (1961). The upper esophageal sphincter after laryngectomy. *Laryngoscope, 71,* 99–115.

Dickson, D. R., & Dickson, W. M. (1982). *Anatomical and physiological bases of speech*. Austin, TX: PRO-ED.

Diedrich, W. M. (1999). Anatomy and physiology of esophageal speech. In S. J. Salmon (Ed.), *Alaryngeal speech rehabilitation—for clinicians by clinicians* (2nd ed.). Austin, TX: PRO-ED.

Diedrich, W. M., & Youngstrom, K. A. (1966). *Alaryngeal speech*. Springfield, IL: Charles C Thomas.

Doherty, T. E., & Shipp, T. (1988). Tape recorder effects on jitter and shimmer extraction. *Journal of Speech and Hearing Research, 31,* 485–490.

Doorn, J. V., & Purcell, A. (1998). Nasalance levels in the speech of normal Australian children. *Cleft Palate— Craniofacial Journal, 35*, 287–292.

Doyle, P. C. (1994). *Foundations of voice and speech rehabilitation following laryngeal cancer.* San Diego, CA: Singular.

Doyle, P. C., Danhauer, J. L., & Reed, C. G. (1988). Listeners' perception of consonants produced by esophageal and tracheoesophageal talkers. *Journal of Speech and Hearing Disorders, 53*, 400–407.

Dray, T. G., Waugh, P. F., & Hillel, A. D. (2000). The association of laryngoceles with ventricular phonation. *Journal of Voice, 14*, 278–281.

Drudge, M. K. M., & Philips, B. J. (1976). Shaping behavior in voice therapy. *Journal of Speech and Hearing Disorders, 41*, 398–411.

Duane, D. D. (1988). Spasmodic torticollis: Clinical and biologic features and their implications for focal dystonia. In S. Fahn, C. D. Marsden, & D. B. Caine (Eds.), *Advances in neurology: Vol. 50, Dystonia 2.* New York: Raven.

Duffy, J. R. (1995). *Motor speech disorders: Substrates, differential diagnosis, and management.* St. Louis, MO: Mosby.

Duguay, M. J. (1989). Esophageal voice: An historical review. *Journal of Voice, 3*, 264–268.

Duguay, M. J. (1998). Esophageal speech training: The initial phase. In S. J. Salmon (Ed.), *Alaryngeal speech rehabilitation—for clinicians by clinicians* (2nd ed.). Austin, TX: PRO-ED.

Durden-Smith, J., & Desimone, D. (1984). *Sex and the brain.* New York: Arbor House.

Dworkin, J. P. (1996). Bite-block therapy for oromandibular dystonia. *Journal of Medical Speech-Language Pathology, 4*, 47–56.

Dworkin, J. P., & Meleca, R. J. (1997). *Vocal pathologies: Diagnosis, treatment, and case studies.* San Diego, CA: Singular.

Dworkin, J. P., Meleca, R. J., & Abkarian, G. G. (2000). Muscle tension dysphonia. *Current Opinion in Otolaryngology & Head and Neck Surgery, 8*, 169–173.

Dworkin, J. P., Meleca, R. J., Simpson, M. L., Zormeier, M., Garfield, I., Jacobs, J., & Mathog, R. H. (1999). Vibratory characteristics of the pharyngoesophageal segment in total laryngectomees. *Journal of Medical Speech-Language Pathology, 7*, 1–18.

Ebers, G. C., & Sadovnick, A. D. (1998). Epidemiology. In D. W. Paty & G. C. Ebers (Eds.), *Multiple sclerosis.* Philadelphia: Davis.

Eckel, F. C., & Boone, D. R. (1981). The s/z ratio as an indicator of laryngeal pathology. *Journal of Speech and Hearing Disorders, 46*, 147–149.

Eckley, C. A., Sataloff, R. T., Hawkshaw, M., Spiegel, J. R., & Mandel, S. (1998). Voice range in superior laryngeal nerve paresis and paralysis. *Journal of Voice, 12*, 340–348.

Emami, A. J., Morrison, M., Rammage, L., & Bosch, D. (1999). Treatment of laryngeal contact ulcers and granulomas: A 12-year retrospective analysis. *Journal of Voice, 13*, 612–617.

Emerick, L. L., & Hatten, J. T. (1974). *Diagnosis and evaluation in speech pathology.* Englewood Cliffs, NJ: Prentice Hall.

Esposito, S. J., Mitsumoto, H., & Shanks, M. (2000). Use of palatal life and palatal augmentation prostheses to improve dysarthria in patients with amyotrophic lateral sclerosis: A case report. *Journal of Prosthetic Dentistry, 83*, 90–98.

Fahn, S. (1999, September/October). *How has the definition of dystonia changed over the years? Do you expect new definitions?* International Dystonia Symposium Summary, 9–10.

Fahn, S., Marsden, C. D., & DeLong, M. R. (Eds.). (1998). *Advances in neurology: Vol. 50, Dystonia 3.* Philadelphia: Lippincott-Raven.

Fairbanks, G. (1960). *Voice and articulation drillbook* (2nd ed.). New York: Harper & Brothers.

Fendler, M., & Shearer, W. M. (1988). Reliability of the s/z ratio in normal children's voices. *Language Speech and Hearing Services in Schools, 19*, 2.

Ferlito, A., & Rinaldo, A. (1998). Selective lateral neck dissection for laryngeal cancer in the clinically negative neck: Is it justified? *Journal of Laryngology and Otology, 112*, 921–924.

Ferlito, A., Rinaldo, A., & Marioni, G. (1999). Laryngeal malignant neoplasms in children and adolescents. *International Journal of Pediatric Otorhinolaryngology, 49*, 1–14.

Ferrand, C. T. (2000). Harmonic-to-noise ratios in normally speaking prepubescent girls and boys. *Journal of Voice, 14*, 17–21.

Finitzo, T., & Freeman, F. (1989). Spasmodic dysphonia, whether and where: Results of seven years of research. *Journal of Speech and Hearing Research, 32*, 541–555.

Finitzo, T., Freeman, F., Devous, M. D., & Watson, B. C. (1991). Whether and wherefore: A response to Aronson & Lagerlund. *Journal of Speech and Hearing Research, 32*, 806–811.

Finnegan, E. M., Luschei, E. S., Gordon, J. D., Barkmeier, J. M., & Hoffman, H. T. (1999). Increased stability of airflow following botulinum toxin injection. *Laryngoscope, 109*, 1300–1306.

Fisher, K. V., Xu, D., & Parish, T. (1999). Magnetic resonance imaging to assess the water environment of laryngeal tissues. *Phonoscope, 2*, 79–86.

Fletcher, S. G. (1978). *Diagnosing speech disorders from cleft palate*. New York: Grune & Stratton.

Fletcher, S. G., Adams, L. E., & McCutcheon, M. J. (1989). Cleft palate speech assessment through oral-nasal acoustic measures. In K. R. Bzoch (Ed.), *Communicative disorders related to cleft palate speech* (3rd ed.). Austin, TX: PRO-ED.

Fletcher, S. G., & Hendarmin, F. M. H. (1999). Nasalance in the speech of children with normal hearing and children with hearing loss. *American Journal of Speech-Language Pathology, 8*, 241–248.

Ford, C. N., Bless, D. M., & Prehn, R. B. (1992). Thyroplasty as primary and adjunctive treatment of glottic insufficiency. *Journal of Voice, 6*, 277–285.

Fourcin, A. (2000). Voice quality and electrolaryngography. In R. D. Kent & M. J. Ball (Eds.), *Voice quality measurement*. San Diego, CA: Singular.

Fox, D. R., Lynch, J. I., & Cronin, T. D. (1988). Change in nasal resonance over time: A clinical study. *Cleft Palate Journal, 25*, 245–247.

Franco, R. A., & Har-El, G. (1999). Cancer of the head and neck. In F. E. Lucente & G. Har-El (Eds.), *Essentials of otolaryngology* (4th ed.). Philadelphia: Lippincott-Williams & Wilkins.

Freeman, S. B., & Hamaker, R. C. (1998). Tracheoesophageal voice restoration at the time of laryngectomy. In E. D. Blom, M. I. Singer, & R. C. Hamaker (Eds.), *Tracheoesophageal voice restoration following total laryngectomy*. San Diego, CA: Singular.

Fritzell, B., Hammarberg, B., Schiratzki, H., Haglund, S., Knutsson, E., & Martensson, A. (1993). Long-term results of recurrent laryngeal nerve resection for adductor spasmodic dysphonia. *Journal of Voice, 7*, 172–178.

Fritzell, B., & Hertegard, S. (1986). A retrospective study of treatment for vocal fold edema: A preliminary report. In J. A. Kirchner (Ed.), *Vocal fold histopathology: A symposium*. Austin, TX: PRO-ED.

Gacek, R. R., & Malmgren, L. T. (1992). Laryngeal motor innervation-central. In A. Blitzer, M. F. Brin, C. T. Sasaki, S. Fahn, & K. S. Harris (Eds.), *Neurologic disorders of the larynx*. New York: Thieme Medical.

Garfinkle, T. J., & Kimmelman, C. P. (1982). Neurological disorders: Amyotrophic lateral sclerosis, myasthenia gravis, multiple sclerosis, and poliomyelitis. *American Journal of Otolaryngology, 3*, 204–212.

Gates, G. A., & Montalbo, P. J. (1987). The effects of low-dose beta-blockade on performance anxiety in singers. *Journal of Voice, 1*, 105–108.

Gay, T., & Hirose, H. (1972). Electromyography of the intrinsic laryngeal muscles during phonation. *Annals of Otology, Rhinology, and Laryngology, 81*, 401–409.

Gelfer, M. P. (1988). Perceptual attributes of voice: Development and use of rating scales. *Journal of Voice, 2*, 320–326.

Gelfer, M. P. (1999). Voice treatment for the male-to-female transgendered client. *American Journal of Speech-Language Pathology, 8,* 201–208.

Gelfer, M. P., & Schofield, K. J. (2000). Comparison of acoustic and perceptual measures of voice in male-to-female transsexuals perceived as female versus those perceived as male. *Journal of Voice, 14,* 22–33.

George, K. P., Vikingstad, E. M., & Cao, Y. (1999). Brain imaging in neurocommunicative disorders. In A. F. Johnson & B. H. Jacobson (Eds.), *Medical speech-language pathology: A practitioner's guide.* New York: Thieme.

Gerratt, B. R., Drelman, J., Antonanzas-Barroso, N., & Berke, G. S. (1993). Comparing internal and external standards in voice quality judgments. *Journal of Speech and Hearing Research, 36,* 14–20.

Gerratt, B. R., Till, J. A., Rosenbek, J. C., Wertz, R. T., & Boysen, A. E. (1991). Use and perceived value of perceptual and instrumental measures in dysarthria management. In C. A. Moore, K. M. Yorkston, & D. R. Beukelman (Eds.), *Dysarthria and apraxia of speech.* Baltimore: Brookes.

Gilbert, H. R., & Weismer, G. G. (1974). The effects of smoking on the speaking fundamental frequency of adult women. *Journal of Psycholinguistic Research, 3,* 225–231.

Gillespie, M., Bielamowicz, S., Yamashita, T., & Ludlow, C. L. (1999). Laryngeal long latency response conditioning in abductor spasmodic dysphonia. *Annals of Otology, Rhinology, and Laryngology, 108,* 612–619.

Gilmore, S. I. (1999). Failure in acquiring esophageal speech. In S. J. Salmon (Ed.), *Alaryngeal speech rehabilitation* (2nd ed.). Austin, TX: PRO-ED.

Glaze, L. E. (2000). Use of patient and family education and behavior modification in the treatment of vocal hyperfunction. In J. C. Stemple (Ed.), *Voice therapy clinical studies* (2nd ed.). San Diego, CA: Singular.

Gluckman, J. L. (1998). Ultrasonography. In A. Blitzer, H. C. Pillsbury, A. F. Jahn, & W. J. Finder (Eds.), *Office-based surgery in otolaryngology.* New York: Thieme.

Golper, L. C. (1998). *Sourcebook for medical speech pathology* (2nd ed.). San Diego, CA: Singular.

Golub, S. (1992). *Periods.* Newbury Park, CA: Sage.

Gomyo, Y., & Doyle, P. C. (1989). Perception of stop consonants produced by esophageal and tracheoesophageal speakers. *Journal of Otolaryngology, 18,* 184–188.

Gordon, T. (1994). Mechanisms for functional recovery of the larynx after surgical repair of injured nerves. *Journal of Voice, 8,* 70–78.

Gorenflo, C. W., & Gorenflo, D. W. (1991). The effects of information and augmentative communication technique on attitudes toward nonspeaking individuals. *Journal of Speech and Hearing Research, 34,* 19–26.

Gorlin, R. J., Cohen, M. M., & Levin, S. L. (1990). *Syndromes of the head and neck* (3rd ed.). New York: Oxford University Press.

Gosselink, R., Kovacs, L., & Decramer, M. (1999). Respiratory muscle involvement in multiple sclerosis. *European Respiratory Journal, 13,* 449–454.

Gould, W. J. (1987). The clinical voice laboratory: Clinical application of voice research. *Journal of Voice, 1,* 305–309.

Gould, W. J., Rubin, J. S., & Yanagisawa, E. (1995). Benign vocal fold pathology through the eyes of the laryngologist. In J. S. Rubin, R. T. Sataloff, G. S. Korovin, & W. J. Gould (Eds.), *Diagnosis and treatment of voice disorders.* New York: IGAKU-SHOIN.

Gramming, P., Sundberg, J., Ternstrom, S., Leanderson, R., & Perkins, W. H. (1988). *Journal of Voice, 2,* 118–126.

Gregg, J. W. (1997). The three ages of voice: The singing/acting mature adult—singing instruction perspective. *Journal of Voice, 11,* 165–170.

Griffiths, C., & Bough, I. D., Jr. (1989). Neurological diseases and their effect on voice. *Journal of Voice, 3,* 148–156.

Gross, M. (1999). Pitch-raising surgery in male-to-female transsexuals. *Journal of Voice, 13,* 246–250.

Guberman, A. (1994). *An introduction to clinical neurology: Pathophysiology, diagnosis, and treatment.* Boston: Little, Brown.

Gulya, A. J., & Wilson, W. R. (1999). *An atlas of ear, nose and throat disorders.* New York: Parthenon.

Hadderingh, R. J., Tange, R. A., Danner, S. A., & Schattenkerk, J. K. M. E. (1987). Otorhinolaryngological findings in AIDS patients: A study of 63 cases. *Archives of Otorhinolaryngology, 244,* 11–14.

Hairfield, W. M., Warren, D. W., & Seaton, D. L. (1987). Prevalence of mouth-breathing in cleft lip and palate. *Cleft Palate Journal, 24,* 135–138.

Hamaker, R. C., & Cheesman, A. D. (1998). Surgical management of pharyngeal constrictor muscle hypertrophy. In E. D. Blom, M. I. Singer, & R. C. Hamaker (Eds.), *Tracheoesophageal voice restoration following laryngectomy.* San Diego, CA: Singular.

Handler, S. D., & Myer, C. M. (1998). *An atlas of ear, nose and throat disorders in children.* Hamilton Toronto, Ontario, Canada: Decker.

Hanson, D. G., Gerratt, B. R., & Ward, P. H. (1984). Cinegraphic observations of laryngeal function in Parkinson's disease. *Laryngoscope, 90,* 348–353.

Harcourt, J. P., Worley, G., & Leighton, S. E. J. (1999). Cimetidine treatment for recurrent respiratory papillomatosis. *International Journal of Pediatric Otorhinolaryngology, 51,* 109–113.

Hardin, M. A., Van Demark, D. R., Morris, H. L., & Payne, M. M. (1992). Correspondence between nasalance scores and listener judgments of hypernasality and hyponasality. *Cleft Palate—Craniofacial Journal, 29,* 346–351.

Hardy, J. C. (1994). Cerebral palsy. In G. H. Shames, E. H. Wiig, & W. A. Secord (Eds.), *Human communication disorders: An introduction* (4th ed.). New York: Merrill.

Haroldson, S. K. (1999). Toward advancing esophageal communication. In S. J. Salmon (Ed.), *Alaryngeal speech rehabilitation* (2nd ed.). Austin, TX: PRO-ED

Harris, S. (2000). The accent method in clinical practice. In J. C. Stemple (Ed.), *Voice therapy clinical studies.* San Diego, CA: Singular.

Hartelius, L., Buder, E. H., & Strand, E. A. (1997). Long-term phonatory instability in individuals with multiple sclerosis. *Journal of Speech, Language, and Hearing Research, 40,* 1056–1072.

Hartelius, L., Wising, C., & Nord, L. (1997). Speech modification in dysarthria associated with multiple sclerosis: An intervention based on vocal efficiency, contrastive stress, and verbal repair strategies. *Journal of Medical Speech-Language Pathology, 5,* 113–140.

Hartley, B. E. J., Bottrill, I. D., & Howard, D. J. (1999). A third decade's experience with the gastric pull-up operation for hypopharyngeal carcinoma: Changing patterns of use. *Journal of Laryngology and Otology, 113,* 241–243.

Hartman, D. E., & Aronson, A. E. (1983). Psychogenic aphonia masking mutational falsetto. *Archives of Otolaryngology, 109,* 415–416.

Hartman, D. E., Daily, W. W., & Morin, K. N. (1989). A case of superior laryngeal nerve paresis and psychogenic dysphonia. *Journal of Speech and Hearing Disorders, 54,* 526–529.

Hausman, B. L. (1995). *Changing sex.* Durham, NC: Duke University Press.

Heidel, S. E., & Torgerson, J. K. (1993). Vocal problems among aerobic instructors and aerobic participants. *Journal of Communicative Disorders, 26,* 179–191.

Hertegard, S., Granqvist, S., & Lindestad, P. A. (2000). Botulinum toxin injections for essential tremor. *Annals of Otology, Rhinology, and Laryngology, 109,* 204–209.

Hess, M., Verdolini, K., Bierhals, W., Mansmann, U., & Gross, M. (1998). Endolaryngeal contact pressures. *Journal of Voice, 12,* 50–67.

Hicks, D. H. (2000). The human larynx transplant. In J. C. Stemple (Ed.), *Voice therapy clinical studies* (2nd ed.). San Diego, CA: Singular.

Hicks, D. H., & Teas, E. (1987). An electroglottographic study of vocal vibrato. *Journal of Voice, 1,* 142–147.

Higgins, M. B., Carney, A. E., & Schulte, L. (1994). Physiological assessment of speech and voice production of adults with hearing loss. *Journal of Speech and Hearing Research, 37,* 510–521.

Higgins, M. B., & Saxman, J. H. (1989). Variations in vocal frequency perturbation across the menstrual cycle. *Journal of Voice, 3,* 233–243.

Hillenbrand, J., Cleveland, R. A., & Erickson, R. L. (1994). Acoustic correlates of breathy vocal quality. *Journal of Speech and Hearing Research, 37,* 769–778.

Hillman, R. E., Holmberg, E. B., Perkell, J. S., Walsh, M., & Vaughan, C. (1989). Objective assessment of vocal hyperfunction: An experimental framework and initial results. *Journal of Speech and Hearing Research, 32,* 373–392.

Hillman, R. E., & Kobler, J. B. (2000). Aerodynamic measures of voice production. In R. D. Kent & M. J. Ball (Eds.), *Voice quality measurement.* San Diego, CA: Singular.

Hirano, M. (1996). Surgical and medical management of voice disorders. In R. H. Colton & J. K. Casper (Eds.), *Understanding voice problems: A physiological perspective for diagnosis and treatment* (2nd ed.). Baltimore: Williams & Wilkins.

Hirano, M., & Bless, D. (1993). *Videostroboscopic examination of the larynx.* San Diego, CA: Singular.

Hirano, M., Kurita, S., & Nakashima, T. (1981). The structure of the vocal cords. In K. N. Stevens & M. Hirano (Eds.), *Vocal fold physiology.* Tokyo: Tokyo University Press.

Hirano, M., Kurita, S., & Sakaguchi, S. (1989). Aging of the vibratory tissue of human vocal folds. *Acta Otolaryngology, 107,* 428–433.

Hirano, S., Kojima, H., Shoji, K., Kaneko, K., Tateya, I., Asoto, R., & Omori, K. (1999). Vibratory analysis of the neoglottis after surgical intervention of cricopharyngeal myotomy and implantation of tracheal cartilage. *Archives of Otolaryngology Head and Neck Surgery, 125,* 1335–1340.

Hixon, T. J., Hawley, J. L., & Wilson, K. J. (1982). An around-the-house device for the clinical determination of respiratory driving pressure: A note on making simple even simpler. *Journal of Speech and Hearing Disorders, 47,* 413–415.

Hixon, T., Watson, P., Harris, E. P., & Pearl, N. B. (1988). Relative volume changes of the rib cage and abdomen during prephonatory chest wall posturing. *Journal of Voice, 2,* 13–19.

Hixon, T., Watson, P., & Maher, M. (1987). To breathe or not to breathe—that is the question: An investigation of speech breathing kinematics in world class Shakespearean actors. *Journal of Voice, 1,* 269–272.

Hixon, T. J., & Hoit, J. (1998). Physical examination of the diaphragm by the speech-language pathologist. *American Journal of Speech-Language Pathology, 7,* 37–45.

Hixon, T. J., & Hoit, J. (1999). Physical examination of the abdominal wall the speech-language pathologist. *American Journal of Speech-Language Pathology, 8,* 35–46.

Hixon, T. J., & Hoit, J. D. (2000). Physical examination of the rib cage wall by the speech-language pathologist. *American Journal of Speech-Language Pathology, 9,* 179–196.

Hodge, M. M., & Rochet, A. P. (1989). Characteristics of speech breathing in young women. *Journal of Speech and Hearing Research, 32,* 466–480.

Hoffman, H. T., Karnell, L. H., Funk, G. F., Robinson, R. A., & Menck, H. R. (1998). The national cancer database report on cancer of the head and neck. *Archives of Otolaryngology Head and Neck Surgery, 124,* 951–962.

Hoffman, H. T., & McCulloch, T. M. (1998). Botulinum neurotoxin for tracheoesophageal voice failure. In E. D. Blom, M. I. Singer, & R. C. Hamaker (Eds.), *Tracheoesophageal voice restoration following total laryngectomy.* San Diego, CA: Singular.

Hoit, J., & Hixon, T. (1987). Age and speech breathing. *Journal of Speech and Hearing Research, 30,* 351–366.

Hoit, J., Hixon, T., Altman, M., & Morgan, W. (1989). Speech breathing in women. *Journal of Speech and Hearing Research, 32,* 353–365.

Hoit, J., Hixon, T., Watson, P., & Morgan, W. (1990). Speech breathing in children and adolescents. *Journal of Speech and Hearing Research, 33*, 51–69.

Hoit, J., Watson, P. J., Hixon, K. E., McMahon, P., & Johnson, C. L. (1994). Age and velopharyngeal function during speech production. *Journal of Speech and Hearing Research, 37*, 295–302.

Hoit, J. D., & Hixon, T. J. (1992). Age and laryngeal airway resistance during vowel production in women. *Journal of Speech and Hearing Research, 35*, 309–313.

Hollien, H. (1987). Old voices: What do we really know about them? *Journal of Voice, 1*, 2–17.

Honocodeevar-Boltezar, I., & Zargi, M. (2000). Voice quality after radiation therapy for early glottic cancer. *Archives of Otolaryngology: Head and Neck Surgery, 126*, 1097–1100.

Hooper, C. R. (2000). Voice treatment for the male-to-female transsexual. In J. C. Stemple (Ed.), *Voice therapy clinical studies* (2nd ed.). San Diego, CA: Singular.

Hoops, H. R., & Noll, J. D. (1969). Relationship of selected acoustic variables to judgments of esophageal speech. *Journal of Communication Disorders, 2*, 1–13.

Hoover, L. A., Wortham, D. G., Lufkin, R. B., & Hanafee, W. N. (1987). Magnetic resonance imaging of the larynx and tongue base: Clinical applications. *Otolaryngology: Head and Neck Surgery, 97*, 245–256.

Horii, Y. (1982a). Jitter and shimmer differences among sustained vowel phonations. *Journal of Speech and Hearing Research, 25*, 12–14.

Horii, Y. (1982b). Some voice fundamental frequency characteristics of oral reading and spontaneous speech by hard-of-hearing young women. *Journal of Speech and Hearing Research, 25*, 608–610.

Horii, Y. (1989). Frequency modulation characteristics of sustained /á/ sung in vocal vibrato. *Journal of Speech and Hearing Research, 32*, 829–836.

Hufnagle, J. (2000). "Soft whisper" technique. In J. C. Stemple (Ed.), *Voice therapy clinical studies* (2nd ed.). San Diego, CA: Singular.

Hufnagle, J., & Hufnagle, K. K. (1988). S/Z ratio in dysphonic children with and without vocal cord nodules. *Language Speech and Hearing Services in Schools, 19*, 418–422.

Hutchinson, B. B., Hanson, M. L., & Mecham, M. J. (1979). *Diagnostic handbook of speech pathology*. Baltimore: Williams & Wilkins.

Isshiki, N. (1998). Mechanical and dynamic aspects of voice production as related to voice therapy and phonosurgery. *Journal of Voice, 12*, 125–137.

Isshiki, N., Taira, T., & Tanabe, M. (1983). Surgical alteration of the vocal pitch. *Journal of Otolaryngology, 12*, 335–340.

Iversen-Thoburn, S. K., & Hayden, P. A. (2000). Alaryngeal speech utilization: A survey. *Journal of Medical Speech-Language Pathology, 8*, 85–99.

Iyer, V. K., Pearman, K., & Raafat, F. (1999). Laryngeal mucosal histology in laryngomalacia: The evidence for gastroesophageal reflux laryngitis. *International Journal of Pediatric Otorhinolaryngology, 49*, 225–230.

Izdebski, K., Ross, J. C., & Klein, J. C. (1990). Transoral rigid laryngovideostroboscopy (phonoscopy). In S. C. McFarlane (Ed.), *Seminars in speech and language, 11*. New York: Thieme Medical.

Izdebski, K., Ward, R. R., & Dedo, H. H. (1999). Voice therapy following surgical (or chemical) treatment for adductor spasmodic dysphonia. *Phonoscope, 2*, 149–158.

Jackson-Menaldi, C. A., Dzul, A. I., & Holland, W. R. (1999). Allergies and vocal fold edema: A preliminary report. *Journal of Voice, 13*, 113–122.

Jacobson, E. (1978). *You must relax* (5th ed.). New York: McGraw-Hill.

Jacobson, J. T., & Northern, J. L. (1991). *Diagnostic audiology*. Austin, TX: PRO-ED.

Janas, J. D., Waugh, P., Swenson, E. R., & Hillel, A. (1999). Effect of thyroplasty on laryngeal airflow. *Annals of Otology, Rhinology, and Laryngology, 108*, 286–291.

Jiang, J. J., O'Mara, T. O., Chen, H. J., Stern, J. I., Vlagos, D., & Hanson, D. (1999). Aerodynamic measurements of patients with Parkinson disease. *Journal of Voice, 13*, 583–591.

Jiang, J. J., & Titze, I. R. (1994). Measurement of vocal fold pressure and impact stress. *Journal of Voice, 8*, 132–145.

Johns, D. E. (Ed.). (1985). *Clinical management of neurogenic communicative disorders* (2nd ed.). Austin, TX: PRO-ED.

Johnson, A. F., & Jacobson, B. H. (Eds.). (1998). *Medical speech-language pathology: A practitioner's guide.* New York: Thieme.

Johnson, T. S. (1983). Treatment of vocal abuse in children. In W. H. Perkins (Ed.), *Voice disorders: Current therapy of communication disorders.* New York: Thieme-Stratton.

Johnson, T. S. (1985). *Vocal abuse reduction program.* Austin, TX: PRO-ED.

Juarbe, C., Shemen, L., Wang, R., Anand, V., Eberle, R., Sirovatka, A., Malanaphy, K., & Klatsky, I. (1989). Tracheoesophageal puncture: For voice restoration after extended laryngopharyngectomy. *Archives of Otolaryngology: Head and Neck Surgery, 115*, 356–359.

Jung, J. H. (1989). *Genetic syndromes in communication disorders.* Austin, TX: PRO-ED.

Kaban, L. B., Conover, M., & Mulliken, J. B. (1986). Midface position after Le Fort III advancement: A long-term follow-up study. *Cleft Palate Journal, 23* (Suppl. 1), 75–77.

Kahane, J. C. (1982). Growth of the human prepubertal and pubertal larynx. *Journal of Speech and Hearing Research, 25*, 446–455.

Kahane, J. C. (1987). Connective tissue changes in the larynx and their effects of voice. *Journal of Voice, 1*, 27–30.

Kahane, J. C., & Mayo, R. (1989). The need for aggressive pursuit of healthy childhood voices. *Language Speech & Hearing Services in Schools, 20*(1), 102–107.

Kalat, J. W. (1981). *Biological psychology.* Belmont, CA: Wadsworth.

Kalb, M. B., & Carpenter, M. A. (1981). Individual speaker influence on relative intelligibility of esophageal speech and artificial larynx speech. *Journal of Speech and Hearing Disorders, 46*, 77–80.

Kaplan, E. M. (1977). The occult submucous cleft palate. *Cleft Palate Journal, 14*, 356–368.

Kaplan, S. L. (1982). Mutational falsetto. *Journal of the American Academy of Child Psychiatry, 21*, 82–85.

Karling, J., Henningsson, G., Larson, O., & Isberg, A. (1999). Comparison between two types of pharyngeal flap with regard to configuration at rest and function and speech outcome. *Cleft Palate—Craniofacial Journal, 36*, 154–165.

Karnell, M. P. (1992). Adductor and abductor spasmodic dysphonia: Related until proven otherwise. *American Journal of Speech-Language Pathology, 1*, 17–18.

Karnell, M. P. (1994). *Videoendoscopy: From velopharynx to larynx.* San Diego, CA: Singular.

Karnell, M. P., & Langmore, S. (1998). Videoendoscopy in speech and swallowing for the speech-language pathologist. In A. F. Johnson & B. H. Jacobson (Eds.), *Medical speech-language pathology: A practitioner's guide.* New York: Thieme.

Kay, N. J. (1982) Voice nodules in children: Aetiology and management. *Journal of Laryngology and Ontology, 96*, 731–736.

Kelchner, L. N., Stemple, J. C., Gerdeman, B., Le Borgne, W., & Adam, S. (1999). *Journal of Voice, 13*, 592–601.

Kemker, E. J., & Zarajczyk, D. R. (1989). Audiological management in patients with cleft palate. In K. R. Bzoch (Ed.), *Communicative disorders related to cleft lip and palate* (3rd ed.). Austin, TX: PRO-ED.

Kempster, G. B., Larson, C. R., & Kistler, M. K. (1988). Effects of electrical stimulation of cricothyroid and thyroarytenoid muscles on voice fundamental frequency. *Journal of Voice, 2*, 221–229.

Kent, R. D. (1994a). A clinical science of motor speech disorders. In J. A. Till, K. M. Yorkston, & D. R. Beukelman (Eds.), *Motor speech disorders: Advances in assessment and treatment.* Baltimore: Brookes.

Kent, R. D. (1994b). *Reference manual for communicative sciences and disorders.* Austin, TX: PRO-ED.

Kent, R. D. (1997). *The speech sciences*. San Diego, CA: Singular.

Kent, R. D., & Ball, M. J. (2000). *Voice quality measurement*. San Diego: Singular.

Kent, R. D., Kent, J. F., Duffy, J., & Weismer, G. (1998). The dysarthrias: Speech-voice profiles, related dysfunctions, and neuropathology. *Journal of Medical Speech-Language Pathology*, 6, 165–200.

Kent, R. D., Kent, J. E., & Rosenbek, J. C. (1987). Maximum performance tests of speech production. *Journal of Speech and Hearing Disorders, 52*, 367–387.

Kent, R. D., Kim, H. H., Weismer, G., Kent, J. E., Rosenbek, J. C., Brooks, B. R., & Workinger, M. (1994). Laryngeal dysfunction in neurological disease: Amyotrophic lateral sclerosis, Parkinson disease, and stroke. *Journal of Medical Speech-Language Pathology*, 2, 157–175.

Keuning, K. H. D., Wieneke, G. H., & Dejonckere, P. H. (1999). The intrajudge reliability of the perceptual rating of cleft palate speech before and after pharyngeal flap surgery: The effect of judges and speech samples. *Cleft Palate—Craniofacial Journal*, 36, 328–333.

King, J. B., Ramig, L. O., Lemke, J. H., & Horii, Y. (1994). Parkinson's disease: Longitudinal changes in acoustic parameters of phonation. *Journal of Medical Speech-Language Pathology*, 2, 29–42.

Kirchner, J. A. (1998). *Atlas on the surgical anatomy of laryngeal cancer*. San Diego, CA: Singular.

Kiritani, S. (2000). High-speech digital image recording for observing vocal fold vibration. In R. D. Kent & M. J. Ball (Eds.), *Voice quality measurement*. San Diego, CA: Singular.

Kitch, J. A., & Oates, J. (1994). The perceptual features of vocal fatigue as self-reported by a group of actors and singers. *Journal of Voice, 8*, 207–214.

Klasner, E. R., Yorkston, K. M., & Strand, E. A. (1999). Patterns of perceptual features in speakers with ALS: A preliminary study of prominence and intelligibility considerations. *Journal of Medical Speech-Language Pathology*, 7, 117–125.

Kleinsasser, O. (1986). Microlaryngoscopic and histologic appearances of polyps, nodules, cysts, Reinke's edema, and granulomas of the vocal cords. In J. A. Kirchner (Ed.), *Vocal fold histopathology: A symposium*. San Diego, CA: College-Hill.

Knox, A. W., Eccleston, V., Maurer, J. E., & Gordon, M. C. (1987). Correlates of sophisticated listener judgments of esophageal air intake noise. *Journal of Communication Disorders, 20*, 25–39.

Kolb, B., & Whishaw, I. Q. (1990). *Fundamentals of human neuropsychology* (3rd ed.). New York: Freeman.

Koller, W. C., & Busenbark, K. L. (1997). Essential tremor. In R. L. Watts & W. C. Koller (Eds.), *Movement disorders: Neurologic principles and practice*. New York: McGraw-Hill.

Kotby, D., & Carlson, E. (1993). Accent method. In J. C. Stemple (Ed.), *Voice therapy clinical studies*. St. Louis, MO: Mosby.

Kostyk, B. E., & Rochet, A. P. (1998). Laryngeal airway resistance in teachers with vocal fatigue: A preliminary report. *Journal of Voice, 12*, 287–299.

Kotby, M. N. (1995). *The accent method of voice therapy*. San Diego, CA: Singular.

Kotby, M. N., El-Sady, S. R., Basiouny, S. E., Abou-Ross, Y. A., & Hegazi, M. A. (1991). Efficacy of the accent method of voice therapy. *Journal of Voice, 5*, 316–320.

Kotby, M. N., Shiromoto, O., & Hirano, M. (1993). The accent method of voice therapy: Effect of accentuations on FO, SPL, and airflow. *Journal of Voice, 7*, 319–325.

Koufman, J. A. (1995). Evaluation of laryngeal biomechanic by fiberoptic laryngoscopy. In J. S. Rubin, R. T. Sataloff, G. S. Korovin, & W. J. Gould (Eds.), *Diagnosis and treatment of voice disorders*. New York: IGAKU-SHOIN.

Koufman, J. A., & Burke, A. J. (1996). The causes and pathogenesis of laryngeal cancer. *Visible Voice, 5*, 26–46.

Kreiborg, S., & Aduss, H. (1986). Pre- and post-surgical facial growth in patients with Crouzon's and Apert's syndromes. *Cleft Palate Journal, 23*(Suppl. 1), 78–90.

Kreiman, J., & Gerratt, B. (2000). *Measuring voice quality*. In R. D. Kent & M. J. Ball (Eds.), *Voice quality measurement*. San Diego, CA: Singular.

Kreiman, J., Gerratt, B. R., Kempster, G. B., Erman, A., & Berke, G. S. (1993). Perceptual evaluation of voice quality: Review, tutorial, and a framework for future research. *Journal of Speech and Hearing Research, 36,* 21–40.

Kreiman, J., Gerratt, B. R., Precoda, K., & Berke, G. S. (1992). Individual differences in voice quality perception. *Journal of Speech and Hearing Research, 35,* 512–520.

Kuehn, D. P., & Moon, J. B. (1998). Velopharyngeal closure force and levator veli palatini activtion levels in varying phonetic contexts. *Journal of Speech and Hearing Research, 41,* 52–62.

Kuehn, D. P., & Moon, J. B. (2000). Induced fatigue effects on velopharyngeal closure force. *Journal of Speech and Hearing Research, 43,* 486–500.

Kummer, A. W., Strife, J. L., Grau, W. H., Creaghead, N. A., & Lee, L. (1989). The effects of Le Fort I osteotomy with maxillary movement on articulation, resonance, and velopharyngeal function. *Cleft Palate Journal, 26,* 193–199.

Kurien, M., & Zachariah, N. (1999). External laryngotracheal trauma in children. *International Journal of Pediatric Otorhinolaryngology, 49,* 115–119.

Laing, A. (1992). *Speaking as a woman*. King of Prussia, PA: Creative Design Services.

Lancer, J. M., Syder, O., Jones, A. S., & LeBoutillier, A. (1988). Vocal cord nodules: A review. *Clinical Otolaryngology, 13*(1), 43–51.

Lapco, P. E., Forbes, M. M., Murry, T., & Rosen, C. A. (1999). Laryngeal botulinum toxin A for spastic dysarthria associated with cerebral palsy: A case study. *Journal of Medical Speech-Language Pathology, 7,* 63–68.

LaPointe, L. L. (1994a). Neurogenic disorders of communication. In E. D. Minifie (Ed.), *Introduction to communication sciences and disorders*. San Diego, CA: Singular.

LaPointe, L. L. (1994b). Neurogenic disorders of speech. In G. H. Shames, E. H. Wiig, & W. A. Secord (Eds.), *Human communication disorders: An introduction*. New York: Merrill.

LaPointe, L. L., Case, J. L., Duane, D. D., & Date, A. (1994). *Head positions as they affect voice in normals*. Paper presented at the International Congress of Movement Disorders, Orlando, FL.

Larson, C. R., Kempster, G. B., & Kistler, M. K. (1987). Changes in voice fundamental frequency following discharge of single motor units in cricothyroid and thyroarytenoid muscles. *Journal of Speech and Hearing Research, 30,* 552–558.

Lawson, W., Biller, H. E., & Suen, J. Y. (1989). Cancer of the larynx. In E. N. Myers & J. Y. Suen (Eds.), *Cancer of the head and neck* (2nd ed.). New York: Churchill Livingstone.

Leder, S. B., & Blom, E. D. (1998). Tracheoesophageal voice prosthesis fitting and training. In E. D. Blom, M. I. Singer, & R. C. Hamaker (Eds.), *Tracheoesophageal voice restoration following total laryngectomy*. San Diego, CA: Singular.

Leder, S. B., Spitzer, J. B., & Kirchner, J. C. (1987). Speaking fundamental frequency of postlingually profoundly deaf adult men. *Annals of Otology, Rhinology, and Laryngology, 96,* 322–324.

Lee, L. (2000a). Modification of speech breathing in a patient with chronic asthma. In J. C. Stemple (Ed.), *Voice therapy clinical studies*. San Diego, CA: Singular.

Lee, L. (2000b). Refocusing laryngeal tone. In J. C. Stemple (Ed.), *Voice therapy clinical studies* (2nd ed.). San Diego, CA: Singular.

Lee, L., Stemple, J. C., & Kizer, M. (1999). Consistency of acoustic and aerodynamic measures of voice production over 28 days under various testing conditions. *Journal of Voice, 13,* 477–483.

Leeper, H. A., Sills, P. S., & Charles, D. H. (1993). Prosthodontic management of maxillofacial and palatal defects. In K. T. Moller & C. D. Starr (Eds.), *Cleft palate: Interdisciplinary issues and treatment—for clinicians by clinicians*. Austin, TX: PRO-ED.

Leonard, R. (1999). Voice therapy: Objectives and outcomes. *Phonoscope, 2,* 217–226.

Lerman, J. W. (1991). The artificial larynx. In S. J. Salmon & K. H. Mount (Eds.), *Alaryngeal speech rehabilitation—for clinicians by clinicians*. Austin, TX: PRO-ED.

Lerman, J. W. (1999). Group therapy for laryngectomees. In S. J. Salmon (Ed.), *Alaryngeal speech rehabilitation—for clinicians by clinicians*. Austin, TX: PRO-ED.

Lewin, J. S. (1999). Tracheoesophageal communication: Beyond traditional speech treatment. In S. J. Salmon (Ed.), *Alaryngeal speech rehabilitation—for clinicians by clinicians*. Austin, TX: PRO-ED.

Lewis, K. E., Watterson, T., & Quint, T. (2000). The effect of vowels on nasalance scores. *Cleft Palate—Craniofacial Journal, 37*, 584–589.

Lieberman, P. (1977). *Speech physiology and acoustic phonetics*. New York: Macmillan.

Lieberman, P., Harris, K., Wooler, P., & Russell, J. (1971). Newborn infant cry and nonhuman primate vocalization. *Journal of Speech and Hearing Research, 14*, 718–727.

Lieu, J. E. C., Muntz, H. R., Prater, D., & Stahl, M. B. (1999). Passy-Muir valve in children with tracheotomy. *International Journal of Pediatric Otorhinolaryngology, 50*, 197–203.

Lin, E., Jiang, J., Hone, S., & Hanson, D. G. (1999). Photoglottographic measures in Parkinson disease. *Journal of Voice, 13*, 25–35.

Lim, R. Y., & Chang, H. H. (1986, February). *Malignant regeneration of a laryngeal papilloma*. Paper presented at the annual meeting of the American Academy of Otolaryngology: Head and Neck Surgery, San Antonio, TX.

Lindestad, P. A., & Hertegard, S. (1994). Spindle-shaped glottal insufficiency with and without sulcus vocalis: A retrospective study. *Annals of Otology, Rhinology, and Laryngology, 103*, 547–553.

Ling, D. (1975). Amplification for speech. In D. R. Calvert & S. R. Silverman (Eds.), *Speech and deafness*. Washington, DC: Alexander Graham Bell Association for the Deaf.

Link, D. T., Rutter, M. J., Liu, J. H., Willging, J. P., Myer, C. M., & Colton, R. T. (1999). Pediatric type 1 thyroplasty: An evolving procedure. *Annals of Otology, Rhinology, Laryngology, 108*, 1105–1110.

Linville, S. E. (2000). The aging voice. In R. D. Kent & M. J. Ball (Eds.), *Voice quality measurement*. San Diego, CA: Singular.

Linville, S. E., Skarin, B. D., & Fornatto, E. (1989). The interrelationship of measures related to vocal function, speech rate, and laryngeal appearance in elderly women. *Journal of Speech and Hearing Science, 32*, 323–330.

Logemann, J. A. (1998a). Dysphagia: Basic assessment and management issues. In A. F. Johnson & B. H. Jacobson (Eds.), *Medical speech-language pathology: A practitioner's guide*. New York: Thieme.

Logemann, J. A. (1998b). *Evaluation and treatment of swallowing disorders* (2nd ed.). Austin, TX: PRO-ED.

Long, J., Williford, H. N., Olson, M. S., & Wolfe, V. (1998). Voice problems and risk factors among aerobics instructors. *Journal of Voice, 12*, 197–207.

Long, R. E., Semb, G., & Shaw, W. C. (2000). Orthodontic treatment of the patient with complete clefts of the lip, alveolus, and palate: Lessons of the past 60 years. *Cleft Palate—Craniofacial Journal, 37*, 533.

Loney, R. W., & Bloem, T. J. (1987). Velopharyngeal dysfunction: Recommendations for use of nomenclature. *Cleft Palate Journal, 24*, 334–335.

Lopez, M. J., Kraybill, W., McElroy, T. H., & Guena, O. (1987). Voice rehabilitation practice among head and neck surgeons. *Annals of Otology, Rhinology, and Laryngology, 96*, 261–263.

Loudon, R. G., Lee, I., & Holcomb, B. J. (1988). Volumes and breathing patterns during speech in healthy and asthmatic subjects. *Journal of Speech and Hearing Research, 31*, 219–227.

Lovetri, J., Lesh, S., & Woo, P. (1999). Preliminary study on the ability of trained singers to control the intrinsic and extrinsic laryngeal musculature. *Journal of Voice, 13*, 219–226.

Lucente, F. E., & Joseph, E. M. (1999a). Nasal obstruction, congestion, and drainage. In F. E. Lucente, H. Grady, & G. Har-El (Eds.), *Essentials in otolaryngology* (4th ed.). Philadelphia: Lippincott-Williams & Wilkins.

Lucente, F. E., & Joseph, E. M. (1999b). Physical examination. In F. E. Lucente & H. Grady (Eds.), *Essentials of otolaryngology* (4th ed.). Philadelphia: Lippincott-Williams & Wilkins.

Ludlow, C. L. (1995). Management of the spasmodic dysphonias. In J. S. Rubin, R. T. Sataloff, G. S. Korovin, & W. J. Gould (Eds.), *Diagnosis and treatment of voice disorders*. New York: IGAKU-SHOIN.

Lundy, D. S., Casiano, R. R., Shatz, D., Reisberg, M., & Xue, J. W. (1998). Laryngeal injuries after short- versus long-term intubation. *Journal of Voice, 12*, 360–365.

Lundy, D. S., Lu, F. L., Casiano, R. R., & Xue, J. W. (1998). The effect of patient factors on response outcomes to Botox treatment of spasmodic dysphonia. *Journal of Voice, 12*, 460–466.

MacArthur, C. J., & Healy, G. B. (1995). Acquired voice disorders in the pediatric population. In J. S. Rubin, R. T. Sataloff, G. S. Korovin, & W. J. Gould (Eds.), *Diagnosis and treatment of voice disorders*. New York: IGAKU-SHOIN.

Mao, V. H., Abaza, M., Spiegel, J. R., Mandel, S., Hawkshaw, M., Heuer, R. J., & Sataloff, R. T. (2001). Laryngeal myasthenia gravis: Report of 40 cases. *Journal of Voice, 15*, 123–130.

Mann, E. A., McClean, M. D., Gurevich-Uvena, J., Barkmeier, J., McKenzie-Garner, P., Paffrath, J., & Patow, C. (1999). The effects of excessive vocalization on acoustic and videostroboscopic measures of vocal fold condition. *Journal of Voice, 13*, 294–302.

Manyam, B. V. (1997). Uncommon forms of tremor. In R. L. Watts & W. C. Koller (Eds.), *Movement disorders: Neurologic principles and practice*. New York: McGraw-Hill.

Maragos, N. E. (1998). The type I thyroplasty window: Implications of normal thyroid cartilage thickness. *Journal of Voice, 12*, 107–111.

Marelli, R. A., Biddinger, P. W., & Gluckman, J. L. (1992). Cytomegalovirus infection of the larynx in the acquired immunodeficiency syndrome. *Otolaryngology–Head and Neck Surgery, 106*, 296–301.

Martin, E. G. (1988). Tutorial: Drugs and vocal function. *Journal of Voice, 2*, 338–344.

Mathy, P., Yorkston, K. M., & Gutmann, M. L. (2000). ACC for individuals with amyotrophic lateral sclerosis. In D. R. Beukelman, K. M. Yorkston, & J. Reichle (Eds.), *Augmentative and alternative communication for adults with acquired neurological disorders*. Baltimore: Brookes.

Matthews, G. G. (2000). *Introduction to neuroscience*. Malden, MA: Blackwell Science.

Mattson, P. J. (1980). *Vocal abuse from cheerleading: A case study*. Unpublished master's thesis, Arizona State University, Tempe.

Mazaheri, M. (1996). Palatal lift prosthesis for the treatment of velopharyngeal incompetency and insufficiency. In S. Berkowitz (Ed.), *Cleft lip and palate with an introduction to other craniofacial anomalies: Perspectives in management* (Vol. 2). San Diego, CA: Singular.

McDermott, A., Raj, P., Glaholm, J., Pearman, K., Macnamara, M. A., & Phil, M. (2000). De novo laryngeal carcinoma in childhood. *Journal of Laryngology and Otology, 114*, 293–295.

McFarlane, S. C., & Von Berg, S. (1998). Facilitative techniques in intervention for dysphonia. *Current Opinion in Otolaryngology & Head and Neck Surgery, 6*, 161–165.

McFarlane, S. C., & Von Berg, S. (2000). Voice facilitating techniques for unilateral vocal fold paralysis. In J. C. Stemple (Ed.), *Voice therapy clinical studies* (2nd ed.). San Diego, CA: Singular.

McFarlane, S. C., & Watterson, T. L. (1990). Vocal nodules: Endoscopic study of their variations and treatment. In S. C. McFarlane (Ed.), *Seminars in speech and language, 11*(1). New York: Thieme Medical.

McHugh-Munier, C., Scherer, K. R., Lehmann, W., & Scherer, U. (1997). Coping strategies, personality, and voice quality in patients with vocal nodules and polyps. *Journal of Voice, 11*, 452–461.

McNeil, M. R. (1997). *Clinical management of sensorimotor speech disorders*. New York: Thieme.

Mecham, M. J. (1996). *Cerebral palsy* (2nd ed.). Austin, TX: PRO-ED.

Melcon, M., Hoit, J., & Hixon, T. (1989). Age and laryngeal airway resistance during vowel production. *Journal of Speech and Hearing Disorders, 54*, 282–286.

Mendoza, E., & Carballo, G. (1999). Vocal tremor and psychological stress. *Journal of Voice, 13*, 105–112.

Merson, R. M. (1999, September/October). What is the role of voice therapy in the treatment of SD? How might a medical team work together? Explain the voice therapy curve. *International Dystonia Symposium Summary*, 13–14.

Meyerhoff, W. L., & Rice, D. H. (1992). *Otolaryngology–Head and neck surgery*. Philadelphia: Saunders.

Milczuk, H. A., Smith, J. D., & Everts, E. C. (2000). Congenital laryngeal webs: Surgical management and clinical embryology. *International Journal of Pediatric Otorhinolaryngology, 52*, 1–9.

Mirra, S. S., Schneider, J. A., & Gearing, M. (1997). Neuropathology of movement disorders: An overview. In R. L. Watts & W. C. Koller (Eds.), *Movement disorders: Neurologic principles and practice*. New York: McGraw-Hill.

Mishra, S., Rosen, C. A., & Murry, T. (2000). 24 hours prior to curtain. *Journal of Voice, 14*, 92–98.

Mizuno, Y., Ikebe, S.-I., Hattori, N., Mochizuki, H., Nakagawa-Hattori, Y., & Kondo, T. (1997). Etiology of Parkinson's disease. In R. L. Watts & W. C. Koller (Eds.), *Movement disorders: Neurologic principles and practice*. New York: McGraw-Hill.

Moller, K. T., & Starr, C. D. (Eds.). (1993). *Cleft palate: Interdisciplinary issues and treatment—for clinicians by clinicians*. Austin, TX: PRO-ED.

Moon, J. B., Smith, A. E., Folkins, J. W., Lemke, J. H., & Gartlan, M. (1994). Coordination of velopharyngeal muscle activity during position of the soft palate. *Cleft Palate—Craniofacial Journal, 31*(1), 45–55.

Moore, C. A. (1992). The correspondence of vocal tract resonance with volumes obtained from magnetic resonance images. *Journal of Speech and Hearing Research, 35*, 1009–1023.

Moore, G. R. (1998). Neuropathology and pathophysiology of the multiple sclerosis lesion. In D. W. Patty & G. C. Ebers (Eds.), *Multiple sclerosis*. Philadelphia: Davis.

Moore, P., & von Leden, H. (1958). *The function of the normal larynx* [Film]. Los Angeles: Wexler Film Productions.

Moran, M. J., & Pentz, A. L. (1987). Otolaryngologists' opinions of voice therapy for vocal nodules in children. *Language, Speech and Hearing Services in Schools, 18*, 172–178.

Morrison, M., & Rammage, L. (1998). *The management of voice disorders*. San Diego, CA: Singular.

Moses, P. J. (1954). *The voice of neurosis*. New York: Grune & Stratton.

Mowrer, D. E. (1982). *Methods of modifying speech behaviors* (2nd ed.). Columbus, OH: Merrill.

Mowrer, D. E., & Case, J. L. (1982). *Clinical management of speech disorders*. Austin, TX: PRO-ED.

Murdoch, B. E. (1990). *Acquired speech and language disorders: A neuroanatomical and functional neurological approach*. London: Chapman & Hall.

Murdoch, B. E., Chenery, H. J., Bowler, S., & Ingram, J. C. L. (1989). Respiratory function in Parkinson's subjects exhibiting a perceptible speech deficit: A kinematic and spirometric analysis. *Journal of Speech and Hearing Disorders, 54*, 610–626.

Murphy, A. T. (1964). *Functional voice disorders*. Englewood Cliffs, NJ: Prentice Hall.

Murry, T., Abitbol, J., & Hersan, R. (1999). Quantitative assessment of voice quality following laser surgery for Reinke's edema. *Journal of Voice, 13*, 257–264.

Murry, T., & Woodson, G. E. (1992). Comparison of three methods for the management of vocal fold nodules. *Journal of Voice, 6*, 271–276.

Murry, T. K., & Rosen, C. A. (2000). Phonotrauma associated with crying. *Journal of Voice, 14*, 575–580.

Myers, D., & Michel, J. (1987). Vibrato and pitch transitions. *Journal of Voice, 1*(4), 168–171.

Myers, E. N., & Suen, J. Y. (Eds.). (1989). *Cancer of the head and neck* (2nd ed.). New York: Churchill Livingstone.

Narcy, P., Contencin, P., & Viala, P. (1990). Surgical treatment for laryngeal paralysis in infants and children. *Annals of Otology, Rhinology, and Laryngology, 99*, 124–128.

Nasseri, S. S., & Maragos, N. E. (2000). Combination thyroplasty and the "twisted larynx": Combined type IV and type I thyroplasty for superior laryngeal nerve weakness. *Journal of Voice, 14,* 104–111.

Neely, J. L., & Rosen, C. (2000). Vocal fold hemorrhage associated with coumadin therapy in an opera singer. *Journal of Voice, 14,* 272–277.

Nellis, J. L., Neiman, G. S., & Lehman, J. A. (1992). Comparison of nasometer and listener judgments of nasality in the assessment of velopharyngeal function after pharyngeal flap surgery. *Cleft Palate—Craniofacial Journal, 29,* 157–163.

Netsell, R., & Hixon, T. J. (1978). A noninvasive method for clinically estimating subglottal air pressure. *Journal of Speech and Hearing Disorders, 43,* 326–330.

Netsell, R., Lotz, W. K., Peters, J. E., & Schulte, L. (1994). Developmental patterns of laryngeal and respiratory function for speech production. *Journal of Voice, 8,* 123–131.

Netter, E. H. (1983). *The CIBA collection of medical illustrations:* Vol. 1. *The nervous system, Part I, anatomy and physiology.* West Caldwell, NJ: CIBA Pharmaceutical.

Newman, S. R., Butler, J., Hammond, E. H., & Gray, S. D. (2000). Preliminary report on hormone receptors in the human vocal fold. *Journal of Voice, 14,* 72–81.

Ng, M. L., Kwok, C.-L. I., & Chow, S.-F.W. (1997). Speech performance of adult Cantonese-speaking laryngectomees using different types of alaryngeal phonation. *Journal of Voice, 11,* 338–344.

Nichols, A. C. (1999). Nasalance statistics for two Mexican populations. *Cleft Palate—Craniofacial Journal, 36,* 57–63.

Niedzielska, G., & Kocki, J. (2000). Evaluation of bcl-2 gene expression in papilloma of larynx in children. *International Journal of Pediatric Otorhinolaryngology, 53,* 25–29.

Offer, D. (1980). Normal adolescent development. In H. I. Kaplan, A. M. Freedman, & B. J. Saddock (Eds.), *Comprehensive textbook of psychiatry* (3rd ed., Vol. 3). Baltimore: Williams & Wilkins.

Oguz, F., Citak, A., Unuvar, E., & Sidal, M. (2000). Airway foreign bodies in childhood. *International Journal of Pediatric Otorhinolaryngolgy, 52,* 11–16.

Olanow, C. W., Freeman, T. B., & Kordower, J. H. (1997). Transplantation strategies for Parkinson's disease. In R. L. Watts & W. C. Koller (Eds.), *Movement disorders: Neurologic principles and practice.* New York: McGraw-Hill.

Olshan, M. (2000, February). Voice lessons speaking with ALS. *ASHA Leader,* pp. 4–5.

Ong, D., & Stone, M. (1998). Three dimensional vocal tract shapes in /r/ and /l/: A study of MRI, ultrasound, electropalatography, and acoustics. *Phonoscope, 1,* 1–13.

Orlikoff, R. F. (1998). Scrambled EGG: The uses and abuses of electroglottography. *Phonoscope, 1,* 37–53.

Orlikoff, R. F., & Baken, R. J. (1993). *Clinical speech and voice measurement: Laboratory exercises and instructor's manual.* San Diego, CA: Singular.

Orlikoff, R. F., Kraus, D. H., Budnick, A. S., Pfister, D. G., & Zelefsky, M. J. (1999). Vocal function following successful chemoradiation treatment for advanced laryngeal cancer: Preliminary results. *Phonoscope, 2,* 67–77.

Orticochea, M. (1970). Results of the dynamic muscle sphincter operation in cleft palates. *British Journal of Plastic Surgery, 23,* 108–114.

Pabon, J. P. H., & Plomp, R. (1988). Automatic phonetogram recording supplemented with acoustical voice-quality parameters. *Journal of Speech and Hearing Research, 31,* 710–722.

Pannbacker, M. (1985). Common misconceptions about oral pharyngeal structure and function. *Language, Speech, and Hearing Services in Schools, 16*(1), 29–33.

Pannbacker, M. (1998). Voice treatment techniques: A review and recommendations for outcome studies. *American Journal of Speech-Language Pathology, 7,* 49–64.

Pannbacker, M., Lass, N., Middleton, G., Crutchfield, E., Trapp, D., & Scherbick, K. (1984). Current clinical practices in the assessment of velopharyngeal closure. *Cleft Palate Journal, 11,* 33–37.

Pannbacker, M., Lass, N. J., Scheuerle, J. E., & English, P. J. (1992). Survey of services and practices of cleft palate-craniofacial teams. *Cleft Palate—Craniofacial Journal, 29*, 164–167.

Pannbacker, M., Lass, N. J., & Stout, B. M. (1990). Speech-language pathologists' opinions on the management of velopharyngeal insufficiency. *Cleft Palate Journal, 27*, 68–71.

Patty, D. W., & Ebers, G. C. (Eds.). (1998). *Multiple sclerosis.* Philadelphia: Davis.

Pauloski, B. R. (1998). Acoustic and aerodynamic characteristics of tracheoesophageal voice. In E. D. Blom, M. I. Singer, & R. C. Hamaker (Eds.), *Tracheoesophageal voice restoration following total laryngectomy.* San Diego, CA: Singular.

Pauloski, B. R., Fisher, H. B., Kempster, G. B., & Blom, E. D. (1989). Statistical differentiation of tracheoesophageal speech produced under four prosthetic/occlusion speaking conditions. *Journal of Speech and Hearing Research, 32*, 591–599.

Peppard, R. (2000). Functional falsetto. In J. C. Stemple (Ed.), *Voice therapy case studies* (2nd ed.). St. Louis, MO: Mosby Yearbook.

Perry, A. (1998). Preoperative tracheoesophageal voice restoration assessment and selection criteria. In E. D. Blom, M. I. Singer, & R. C. Hamaker (Eds.), *Tracheoesophageal voice restoration following total laryngectomy.* San Diego, CA: Singular.

Perry, A., & Shaw, M. A. (2000). Evaluation of functional outcomes (speech, swallowing, and voice) in patients attending speech pathology after head and neck cancer treatment(s): Development of a multi-centre database. *Journal of Laryngology & Otology, 114*, 605–615.

Pershall, E., & Boone, D. R. (1987). Supraglottal contribution to voice quality. *Journal of Voice, 1*, 186–190.

Peterson-Falzone, S. J., & Graham, M. S. (1990). Phoneme-specific nasal emission in children with and without physical anomalies of the velopharyngeal mechanism. *Journal of Speech and Hearing Disorders, 55*, 132–139.

Peterson-Falzone, S. J., Hardin-Jones, M. A., & Karnell, M. P. (2001). *Cleft palate speech* (3rd ed.). St. Louis, MO: Mosby.

Phoenix Fire Department operations manual. (2000). Vol. 2. Phoenix, AZ: Author.

Pinho, S. R., Navas, D. M., Case, J. L., & LaPointe, L. L. (1993, November). *Vocal fry in the treatment of puberphonia.* Paper presented at the annual meeting of the American Speech-Language-Hearing Association, Los Angeles.

Poburka, B. J. (1999a). A new stroboscopy rating form. *Journal of Voice, 13*, 403–413.

Poburka, B. J. (1999b). Therapy for adults with vocal nodules: A framework for treatment. *Phonoscope, 2*, 43–49.

Poewe, W., & Granata, R. (1997). Pharmacological treatment of Parkinson's disease. In R. L. Watts & W. C. Koller (Eds.), *Movement disorders: Neurologic principles and practice.* New York: McGraw-Hill.

Pontes, P., & Behlau, M. (1993). Treatment of sulcus vocalis: Auditory, perceptual and acoustical analysis of the slicing mucosa surgical technique. *Journal of Voice, 7*, 365–376.

Portnoy, R. A., & Aronson, A. E. (1982). Diadochokinetic syllable rate and regularity in normal and in spastic and ataxic dysarthric subjects. *Journal of Speech and Hearing Disorders, 47*, 324–328.

Powell, D. M., Karanfilov, B. I., Beechler, K. B., Treole, K., Trudeau, M. D., & Forrest, L. A. (2000). Paradoxical vocal cord dysfunction in juveniles. *Archives of Otolaryngology—Head and Neck Surgery, 126*, 29–34.

Poyry, M. (1996). Dental development in 0- to 3-year-old children with cleft lip and palate. In S. Berkowitz (Ed.), *Cleft lip and palate with an introduction to other craniofacial anomalies: Perspectives in management* (Vol. 2). San Diego, CA: Singular.

Prater, M. E., & Deskin, R. W. (1998). Bronchoscopy and laryngoscopy findings as indications for tracheotomy in the burned child. *Archives of Otolaryngology—Head and Neck Surgery, 124*, 1115–1117.

Prator, R. J., & Swift, R. W. (1984). *Manual of voice therapy.* Austin, TX: PRO-ED.

Ramig, L. O. (2000). Lee Silverman voice treatment for individuals with neurological disorders: Parkinson disease. In J. C. Stemple (Ed.), *Voice therapy clinical studies* (2nd ed.). San Diego, CA: Singular.

Ramig, L. O., Bonitati, C. M., Lemke, J. H., and Horii, Y. (1994). Voice treatment for patients with Parkinson disease: Development of an approach and preliminary efficacy data. *Journal of Medical Speech-Language Pathology, 2,* 191–209.

Ramig, L. O., Countryman, S., O'Brien, C., Hoehn, M., & Thompson, L. (1996). Intensive speech treatment for patients with Parkinson disease: Short and long-term comparison of two techniques. *Neurology, 47,* 1496–1504.

Ramig, L. O., Countryman, S., Thompson, L. L., & Horii, Y. (1995). Comparison of two forms of intensive speech treatment for Parkinson Disease. *Journal of Speech and Hearing Research, 38,* 1232–1251.

Ramig, L. O., Horii, Y., & Bonitati, C. (1991). The effectiveness of speech therapy for patients with Parkinson's disease. *NCVS (National Center for Voice and Speech) June Status and Progress Report, 1,* 61–86.

Ramig, L. O., & Ringel, R. L. (1983). Effects of physiological aging on selected acoustic characteristics of voice. *Journal of Speech and Hearing Research, 26,* 22–30.

Ramig, L. O., Scherer, R. C., Klasner, E. R., Titze, I. R., & Horii, Y. (1990). Acoustic analysis of voice in amyotrophic lateral sclerosis: A longitudinal case study. *Journal of Speech and Hearing Disorders, 55,* 2–14.

Ramig, L. O., Scherer, R. C., Titze, I. R., & Ringel, S. P. (1988). Acoustic analysis of voices of patients with neurologic disease: Rationale and primary data. *Annals of Otology, Rhinology, and Laryngology, 97,* 164–171.

Ramig, L. O., & Shipp, T. (1987). Comparative measures of vocal tremor and vocal vibrato. *Journal of Voice, 1,* 162–167.

Ramig, L. O., & Verdolini, K. (1998). Treatment efficacy: Voice disorders. *Journal of Speech, Language, and Hearing Research, 41,* 101–116.

Rammage, L. O., Morrison, M., & Nichol, H. (2001). *Management of the voice and its disorders* (2nd ed.). San Diego, CA: Singular.

Raney, C., & Silverman, E. H. (1992). Attitudes toward nonspeaking individuals who use communication boards. *Journal of Speech and Hearing Research, 35,* 1269–1270.

Rantala, L., & Vilkman, E. (1999). Relationship between subjective voice complaints and acoustic parameters in female teacher' voices. *Journal of Voice, 13,* 484–495.

Rastatter, M. P., & Hyman, M. (1982). Maximum phoneme duration of /s/ and /z/ by children with vocal nodules. *Language, Speech and Hearing Services in Schools, 13,* 197–199.

Redenbaugh, M. A., & Reich, A. R. (1989). Surface EMG and related measures in normal and vocally hyperfunctional speakers. *Journal of Speech and Hearing Disorders, 54,* 68–73.

Reeves, S. D. (1999). Alaryngeal speech rehabilitation training: Past, present, and future. In S. J. Salmon (Ed.), *Alaryngeal speech rehabilitation—for clinicians by clinicians* (2nd ed.). Austin, TX: PRO-ED.

Rehm, D. (1999). *Finding my voice.* New York: Knopf.

Reich, A., & McHenry, M. (1987). Respiratory volumes in cheerleaders with a history of dysphonic episodes. *Folia Phoniatrica, 39,* 71–77.

Reich, A., McHenry, M., & Keaton, A. (1986). A survey of dysphonic episodes in high school cheerleaders. *Language, Speech, and Hearing Services in Schools, 17,* 63–71.

Reich, A. R., Mason, J. A., Frederickson, R. R., & Schlauch, R. S. (1989). Factors influencing fundamental frequency range estimates in children. *Journal of Speech and Hearing Disorders, 54,* 429–438.

Reisberg, D. J. (2000). Dental and prosthodontic care for patients with cleft or craniofacial conditions. *Cleft Palate—Craniofacial Journal, 37,* 534–537.

Rekart, D. M., & Begnal, C. E. (1989). Acoustic characteristics of reticent speech. *Journal of Voice, 3,* 324–336.

Riise, T., & Wolfson, C. (Eds.). (1997). The epideomiologic study of exogenous factors in the etiology of multiple sclerosis. *Neurology, 49* (Suppl. 2), 1–82.

Riski, J. E., Hoke, J. A., & Dolan, E. A. (1989). The role of pressure flow and endoscopic assessment in successful palatal obturator revision. *Cleft Palate Journal, 26,* 56–62.

Riski, J. E., Ruff, G. L., Georgiade, G. S., Barwick, W. J., & Edwards, P. D. (1992). Evaluation of the sphincter pharyngoplasty. *Cleft Palate—Craniofacial Journal, 29,* 254–261.

Robbins, J., Christensen, J., & Kempster, G. (1986). Characteristics of speech production after tracheoesophageal puncture: Voice onset time and vowel duration. *Journal of Speech and Hearing Research, 29,* 499–504.

Roland, T. J., Rothstein, S. G., Khushbakhat, M. R., & Perksy, M. S. (1993). Squamous cell carcinoma in HIV-positive patients under age 45. *Laryngoscope, 103,* 509–511.

Rollin, W. J. (1987). *The psychology of communication disorders in individuals and their families.* Englewood Cliffs, NJ. Prentice Hall.

Rontal, E., Rontal, M., Wald, J., & Rontal, D. (1999). Botulinum toxin injection in the treatment of vocal fold paralysis associated with multiple sclerosis: A case report. *Journal of Voice, 13,* 274–279.

Rosen, C. A., & Murry, T. (2000). Voice handicap index in singers. *Journal of Voice, 14,* 370–377.

Rosen, C. A., Murry, T., & DeMarino, D. P. (1999). Late complication of type I thyroplasty: A case report. *Journal of Voice, 13,* 417–423.

Rosen, D. C., & Sataloff, R. T. (1997). *Psychology of voice disorders.* San Diego, CA: Singular.

Rosen, D. C., & Sataloff, R. T. (1998). Psychological aspects of voice disorders. In R. T. Sataloff (Ed.), *Vocal health and pedagogy.* San Diego, CA: Singular.

Rosin, D. E., Handler, D. S., Potsic, W. P., Wetmore, R. E., & Tom, L. W. C. (1990). Vocal cord paralysis in children. *Laryngoscope, 100,* 1174–1179.

Ross, K. K. (2000, September). The emotional aspects of the dystonia patient survey. *Dystonia Dialogue,* pp. 12–13.

Roth, C. R., Poburka, B. J., & Workinger, M. S. (2000). The effect of a palatal lift prosthesis on speech intelligibility in amyotrophic lateral sclerosis: A case study. *Journal of Medical Speech-Language Pathology, 8,* 365–370.

Rothenberg, M. (1992). A multichannel electroglottograph. *Journal of Voice, 6,* 36–43.

Rothman, H. B., & Arroyo, A. A. (1987). Acoustic variability in vibrato and its perceptual significance. *Journal of Voice, 2,* 123–141.

Roy, N. (2000). Manual circumlaryngeal technique in the assessment and treatment of muscle tension dysphonia (MTD). In J. C. Stemple (Ed.), *Voice therapy clinical studies.* San Diego, CA: Singular.

Roy, N., Bless, D. M., & Heisey, D. (2000). Personality and voice disorders: A multitrait–multidisorder analysis. *Journal of Voice, 14,* 521–548.

Roy, N., Bless, D. M., Heisey, D., & Ford, C. N. (1997). Manual circumlaryngeal therapy for functional dysphonia: An evaluation of short- and long-term treatment outcomes. *Journal of Voice, 11,* 321–331.

Roy, N., & Leeper, H. A. (1993). Effects of manual laryngeal musculoskeletal tension reduction technique as a treatment for functional voice disorders: Perceptual and acoustic measures. *Journal of Voice, 7,* 242–249.

Roy, N., Ryker, K. S., & Bless, D. M. (2000). Vocal violence in actors: An investigation into its acoustic consequences and the effects of hygienic laryngeal release training. *Journal of Voice, 14,* 215–230.

Rubin, W. (1987). Dietary, chemical, stress, and hormonal influences in voice abnormalities. *Journal of Voice, 1,* 378–385.

Russell, A., Oates, J., & Greenwood, K. M. (1998). Prevalence of voice problems in teachers. *Journal of Voice, 12,* 467–479.

Safak, M. A., Gocmen, H., Korkmaz, H., & Kilic, R. (2000). Computerized tomographic alignment of Silastic implant in type 1 thyroplasty. *American Journal of Otolaryngology, 21,* 179–183.

Salmon, S. J. (1999). *Alaryngeal speech rehabilitation—for clinicians by clinicians* (2nd ed.). Austin, TX: PRO-ED.

Salvatore, A. P., Cannito, M. P., & Gutierrez, G. S. (1999). Spasmodic dysphonia: A neural net activity. *Journal of Medical Speech-Language Pathology, 7,* 169–174.

Sander, E. K. (1989). Arguments against the aggressive pursuit of voice therapy for children. *Language Speech & Hearing Services in Schools, 20*, 94–101.

Sanders, I. (1995). The microanatomy of the vocal folds. In J. S. Rubin, R. T. Sataloff, G. S. Korovin, & W. J. Gould (Eds.), *Diagnosis and treatment of voice disorders*. New York: IGAKU-SHOIN.

Sanders, I., Han, Y., Wang, J., & Biller, H. (1998). Muscle spindles are concentrated in the superior vocalis subcompartment of the human thyroarytenoid muscle. *Journal of Voice, 12*, 7–16.

Sapienza, C. M., Brown, J., Martin, D., & Davenport, P. (1999). Inspiratory pressure threshold training for glottal airway limitation in laryngeal papilloma. *Journal of Voice, 13*, 382–388.

Sapienza, C. M., & Stathopoulos, E. T. (1994). Respiratory and laryngeal measures of children and women with bilateral vocal fold nodules. *Journal of Speech and Hearing Research, 37*, 1229–1243.

Sapir, S. (1993). Vocal attrition in voice students: Survey findings. *Journal of Voice, 7*, 69–74.

Sasaki, Y., Okamura, H., & Yumoto, E. (1991). Quantitative analysis of hoarseness using a digital sound spectrograph. *Journal of Voice, 5*, 36–40.

Sataloff, R. T. (Ed.). (1987). [Special issue]. *Journal of Voice, 1*, 123–171.

Sataloff, R. T. (1988). Editorial: Respiration and singing. *Journal of Voice, 2*, 1–50.

Sataloff, R. T. (1991). *Professional voices: The science and art of clinical care*. New York: Raven.

Sataloff, R. T. (1994). Vocal tract response to toxic injury: Clinical issues. *Journal of Voice, 8*, 63–64.

Sataloff, R. T. (1998a). Endocrine dysfunction. In R. T. Sataloff (Ed.), *Vocal health and pedagogy*. San Diego, CA: Singular.

Sataloff, R. T. (1998b). Medications for traveling performers. In R. T. Sataloff (Ed.), *Vocal health and pedagogy*. San Diego, CA: Singular.

Sataloff, R. T. (1998c). *Vocal health and pedagogy*. San Diego, CA: Singular.

Sataloff, R. T. (1999). [Review of the video programs *Assessing Dysphonia: The Role of Videostroboscopy* and *Atlas of Dynamic Laryngeal Pathology*]. *Journal of Voice, 13*, 459.

Sataloff, R. T., Castell, D. O., Katz, P. O., & Sataloff, D. M. (1999). *Reflux laryngitis and related disorders*. San Diego, CA: Singular.

Sataloff, R. T., Feldman, M., Darby, K. S., Carroll, L. M., Spiegel, J. R., & Schiebel, B. R. (1988). Arytenoid dislocation. *Journal of Voice, 1*, 368–377.

Sataloff, R. T., Hawkshaw, M., & Rosen, D. C. (1998). Medications: Effects and side-effects in professional voice users. In R. T. Sataloff (Ed.), *Vocal health and pedagogy*. San Diego, CA: Singular.

Sataloff, R. T., Hawkshaw, M., & Spiegel, J. R. (1999). *Atlas of laryngology*. San Diego, CA: Singular.

Sataloff, R. T., & Sataloff, J. (1998). Hearing loss in singers and other musicians. In R. T. Sataloff (Ed.), *Vocal health and pedagogy*. San Diego, CA: Singular.

Sataloff, R. T., Spiegel, J. R., Carroll, L. M., Schiebel, B. R., Darby, K. S., & Ruinick, R. (1987). Strobovideolaryngoscopy in professional voice users: Results and clinical value. *Journal of Voice, 1*, 359–364.

Sataloff, R. T., Spiegel, J. R., Heuer, H., & Rosen, D. C. (1995). Medical management of benign voice disorders. In J. S. Rubin, R. T. Sataloff, G. S. Korovin, & W. J. Gould (Eds.), *Diagnosis and treatment of voice disorders*. New York: IGAKU-SHOIN.

Saxon, K., & Schneider, C. M. (1994). *Vocal exercise physiology*. San Diego, CA: Singular.

Schaefer, S. D., & Close, L. G. (1989). Acute management of laryngeal trauma. *Annals of Otology, Rhinology, and Laryngology, 98*, 98–104.

Scherer, R. C. (1995). Laryngeal function during phonation. In J. S. Rubin, R. T. Sataloff, G. S. Korovin, & W. J. Gould (Eds.), *Diagnosis and treatment of voice disorders*. New York: IGAKU-SHOIN.

Schmidt, P., Klingholz, E., & Martin, E. (1988). Influence of pitch, voice sound pressure, and vowel quality on the maximum phonation time. *Journal of Voice, 2*, 245–249.

Schneider, C. M., Saxon, K., & Dennehy, C. A. (1998). Exercise physiology: Perspective for vocal training. In R. T. Sataloff (Ed.), *Vocal health and pedagogy*. San Diego, CA: Singular.

Schneider, E., & Shprintzen, R. J. (1980). A survey of speech pathologists: Current trends in the diagnosis and management of velopharyngeal insufficiency. *Cleft Palate Journal, 17*, 249–253.

Schneider, P. (1993). Tracking change in dysphonia: A case study. *Journal of Voice, 7*, 179–188.

Schultz, G. M., Sulc, S., Leon, S., & Gilligan, G. (2000). Speech motor learning in Parkinson disease. *Journal of Medical Speech-Language Pathology, 8*, 243–247.

Schwan, C., Case, J. L., & LaPointe, L. L. (1996, November). *Vocal pathology in aerobic instructors*. Paper presented at the annual meeting of the American Speech-Language-Hearing Association, New Orleans.

Sedory, S. E., Hamlet, S., & Connor, N. P. (1989). Comparisons of perceptual and acoustic characteristics of tracheoesophageal and excellent esophageal speech. *Journal of Speech and Hearing Disorders, 54*, 209–214.

Seidman, M. D., Arenberg, J. G., & Shirwany, N. A. (1999). Palatal myoclonus as a cause of objective tinnitus: A report of six cases and a review of the literature. *Ear, Nose & Throat Journal, 78*, 292–297.

Seikel, J. A., King, D. W., & Drumright, D. G. (1997). *Anatomy and physiology for speech, language, and hearing* (2nd ed.). San Diego, CA: Singular.

Shanks, J. C. (1999). Consequences of total laryngectomy in daily living activities. In S. J. Salmon (Ed.), *Alaryngeal speech rehabilitation—for clinicians by clinicians* (2nd ed.). Austin, TX: PRO-ED.

Shaw, J. D., & Lancer, J. M. (1987). *A colour atlas of fiberoptic endoscopy of the upper respiratory tract*. Ipswich, England: Wolfe Medicine.

Sherrard, K. C., Marquardt, T. P., & Cannito, M. P. (2000). Phonatory and temporal aspects of spasmodic dysphonia and pseudobular dysarthria: An acoustic analysis. *Journal of Medical Speech-Language Pathology, 8*, 271–277.

Shipp, T. (1987). Vertical laryngeal position: Research findings and application for singers. *Journal of Voice, 1*, 217–219.

Shons, A. R. (1993). Surgical issues and procedures. In K. T. Moller & C. D. Starr (Eds.), *Cleft palate: Interdisciplinary issues and treatment—for clinicians by clinicians*. Austin, TX: PRO-ED.

Shprintzen, R. J. (1989). Nasopharyngoscopy. In K. R. Bzoch (Ed.), *Communicative disorders related to cleft lip and palate* (3rd ed.). Austin, TX: PRO-ED.

Shprintzen, R. J. (1997). *Genetics, syndromes, and communication disorder*. San Diego, CA: Singular.

Shulman, S. (2000). Symptom modification for abductor spasmodic dysphonia: Inhalation phonation. In J. C. Stemple (Ed.), *Voice therapy clinical studies* (2nd ed.). San Diego, CA: Singular.

Silva, A. B., Muntz, H. R., & Clary, R. (1998). Utility of conventional radiography in the diagnosis and management of pediatric airway foreign bodies. *Annals of Otology, Rhinology, and Laryngology, 107*, 834–838.

Silverman, E. H. (1989). *Communication for the speechless* (2nd ed.). Englewood Cliffs, NJ: Prentice Hall.

Simberg, S., Laine, A., Sala, E., & Ronnemaa, A.-M. (2000). Prevalence of voice disorders among future teachers. *Journal of Voice, 14*, 231–235.

Singer, M. I., Blom, E. D., & Hamaker, R. C. (1989). Voice rehabilitation following laryngectomy. In E. N. Myers & J. Y. Suen (Eds.), *Cancer of the head and neck* (2nd ed.). New York: Churchill Livingstone.

Singh, S., & Kent, R. (2000). *Singular's illustrated dictionary of speech-language pathology*. San Diego, CA: Singular.

Skolnick, M. L. (1996). Videofluoroscopic studies of the velopharyngeal portal during phonation. In S. Berkowitz (Ed.), *Cleft lip and palate* (Vol. 2). San Diego, CA: Singular.

Skolnick, M. L., McCall, G. N., & Barnes, M. (1973). The sphincteric mechanisms of velopharyngeal closure. *Cleft Palate Journal, 10*, 286–305.

Sloan, G. M. (2000). Posterior pharyngeal flap and sphincter pharyngoplasty: The state-of-the-art. *Cleft Palate—Craniofacial Journal, 37*, 112–122.

Smith, B. E., Weinberg, B., Feth, L. L., & Horii, Y. (1978). Vocal roughness and jitter characteristics of vowels produced by esophageal speakers. *Journal of Speech and Hearing Research, 21*, 240–249.

Smith, D. O., Callanan, V., Harcourt, J., & Albert, D. M. (2000). Intracordal cyst in a neonate. *International Journal of Pediatric Otorhinolaryngology, 52*, 277–281.

Smith, E., Gray, S. D., Dove, H., Kirchner, L., & Heras, H. (1997). Frequency and effects of teachers' voice problems. *Journal of Voice, 11*, 81–87.

Smith, E., Kirchner, L., Taylor, M., Hoffman, H., & Lemke, J. H. (1998). Voice problems among teachers: Differences by gender and teaching characteristics. *Journal of Voice, 12*, 328–334.

Smith, M. E., & Ramig, L. O. (1995). Neurological disorders of the larynx. In J. S. Rubin, R. T. Sataloff, G. S. Korovin, & W. J. Gould (Eds.), *Diagnosis and treatment of voice disorders*. New York: IGAKU-SHOIN.

Smith, S., & Thyme, K. (1976). Statistic research on changes in speech due to pedagogic treatment (the accent method). *Folia Phoniatria, 28*, 98–103.

Smitheran, J., & Hixon, T. J. (1981). A clinical method for estimating laryngeal airway resistance during vowel production. *Journal of Speech and Hearing Disorders, 46*, 138–146.

Solomon, N. P., & DiMattia, M. S. (2000). Effects of vocally fatiguing task and systemic hydration on phonation threshold pressure. *Journal of Voice, 14*, 341–362.

Solomon, N. P., Garlitz, S. J., & Milbrath, R. L. (2000). Respiratory and laryngeal contributions to maximum phonation duration. *Journal of Voice, 14*, 331–340.

Solomon, N. P., & Hixon, T. J. (1993). Speech breathing in Parkinson's disease. *Journal of Speech and Hearing Research, 36*, 294–310.

Solomon, N. P., McCall, G. N., Trosset, M. W., & Gray, W. C. (1989). Laryngeal configuration and constriction during two types of whispering. *Journal of Speech and Hearing Research, 32*, 161–174.

Solomon, N. P., McKee, A. S., Larson, K. J., Nawrocki, M. D., Tuite, P. J., Eriksen, S., Low, W. C., & Maxwell, R. E. (2000). Effects of pallidal stimulation on speech in three men with severe Parkinson's disease. *American Journal of Speech-Language Pathology, 9*, 241–256.

Sonninen, A., & Hurme, P. (1992). On the terminology of voice research. *Journal of Voice, 6*, 188–193.

Sowerby, D., Newcomer, J., & Schonauer, B. (1999). *Speechless: Living with spasmodic dysphonia*. Chicago: National Spasmodic Dysphonia Association.

St. Louis, K. O., & Ruscello, D. M. (1987). *Oral Speech Mechanism Screening Examination* (Rev. ed.). Austin, TX: PRO-ED.

Stal, S., & Hicks, M. J. (1998). Classic and occult submucous cleft palates: A histopathologic analysis. *Cleft Palate—Craniofacial Journal, 35*, 351–358.

Starr, C. D. (1993). Behavioral approaches to treating velopharyngeal closure and nasality. In K. T. Moller & C. D. Starr (Eds.), *Cleft palate: Interdisciplinary issues and treatment—by clinicians for clinicians*. Austin, TX: PRO-ED.

Steinberg, B., Padwa, B. L., Boyne, P., & Kaban, L. (1999). State of the art in oral and maxillofacial surgery: Treatment of maxillary hypoplasia and anterior palatal and alveolar clefts. *Cleft Palate—Craniofacial Journal, 36*, 283–291.

Stemple, J. C. (Ed.). (2000). *Voice therapy and clinical studies* (2nd ed.). San Diego, CA: Singular.

Stemple, J. C., Glaze, L. E., & Klaben, B. G. (2000). *Clinical voice pathology theory and management*. San Diego, CA: Singular.

Stewart, C. F., Allen, E. L., Tureen, P., Diamond, B. E., Blitzer, A., & Brin, M. F. (1997). Adductor spasmodic dysphonia: Standard evaluation of symptoms and severity. *Journal of Voice, 11*, 95–103.

Stone, R. E., Jr. (1983). Issues in clinical assessment of laryngeal function: Contraindications for subscribing to maximum phonation time and optimal frequency. In D. M. Bless & J. H. Abbs (Eds.), *Vocal fold physiology: Contemporary research and clinical issues*. San Diego, CA: College-Hill.

Stone, R. E., Jr., Chagnon, E., & Ossoff, R. H. (1994, November). *Understanding and treating vascular-based dysphonia*. Paper presented at the annual meeting of the American Speech-Language-Hearing Association, New Orleans.

Stone, R. E., Cleveland, T. F., & Sundberg, J. H. (1999). Formant frequencies in country western singers' speech and singing. *Journal of Voice, 13*, 161–167.

Strand, E. A., Buder, E. H., Yorkston, K. M., & Ramig, L. O. (1994). Differential phonatory characteristics of four women with amyotrophic lateral sclerosis. *Journal of Voice, 8*, 327–339.

Strassei, M. (1999). Living with a laryngectomy. In S. J. Salmon (Ed.), *Alaryngeal speech rehabilitation* (2nd ed.) Austin, TX: PRO-ED.

Subtelny, J., Li, W., Whitehead, R., & Subtelny, J. D. (1989). Cephalometric and cineradiographic study of deviant resonance in hearing-impaired speakers. *Journal of Speech and Hearing Disorders, 54*, 249–263.

Suen, J. Y., & Stern, S. J. (1995). Premalignant lesions of the larynx. In J. S. Rubin, R. T. Sataloff, G. S. Korovin, & W. J. Gould (Eds.), *Diagnosis and treatment of voice disorders*. New York: IGAKU-SHOIN.

Sun, J. D., Weatherly, R. A., Koopmann, C. F., & Carey, T. E. (2000). Mucosal swabs detect HPV in laryngeal papillomatosis patients but not in family members. *International Journal of Pediatric Otorhinolarygology, 53*, 95–103.

Sundberg, J. (1994). Perceptual aspects of singing. *Journal of Voice, 8*, 106–122.

Sundberg, J., Cleveland, T. F., Stone, R. E., & Iwarsson, J. (1999). Voice source characteristics in six premier country singers. *Journal of Voice, 13*, 168–183.

Swift, E. (2000). Treatment of an athlete with paradoxical vocal fold motion. In J. C. Stemple (Ed.), *Voice therapy clinical studies*. San Diego, CA: Singular.

Tachimura, T., Nohara, K., & Wada, T. (2000). Effect of placement of a speech appliance on levator veli palatini muscle activity during speech. *Cleft Palate—Craniofacial Journal, 37*, 478–482.

Tait, N. A., Michel, J. E., & Carpenter, M. A. (1980). Maximum duration of sustained /s/ and /z/ in children. *Journal of Speech and Hearing Disorders, 45*, 239–246.

Tardy, M. E., Jr., Toriumi, D., & Broadway, D. (1989). Facial plastic and reconstructive surgery in an aging population: A critical review. In J. C. Goldstein, H. K. Kasbima, & C. E. Koopmann, Jr. (Eds.), *Geriatric otolaryngology*. Toronto, Ontario, Canada: Decker.

Theodoros, D. G., Ward, E. C., Murdoch, B. E., Silburn, P., & Lethlean, J. (2000). The impact of pallidotomy on motor speech function in Parkinson disease. *Journal of Medical Speech-Language Pathology, 8*, 315–322.

Thomasson, M., & Sundberg, J. (1999). Consistency of phonatory breathing patterns in professional operatic singers. *Journal of Voice, 13*, 529–541.

Thompson, A. E., & Hixon, T. J. (1979). Nasal airflow during normal speech production. *Cleft Palate Journal, 16*, 412–420.

Thompson, J. W., Rosenthal, P., & Camilon, E. S., Jr. (1990). Vocal cord paralysis and superior laryngeal nerve dysfunction in Reye's syndrome. *Archives of Otolaryngology—Head and Neck Surgery, 116*, 46–48.

Thorpe, C. W., Cala, S. J., Chapman, J., & Davis, P. J. (2001). Patterns of breath support in projection of the singing voice. *Journal of Voice, 15*, 86–104.

Thumfart, W. F., Platzer, W., Gunkel, A. R., Maurer, H., & Brenner, E. (1999). *Surgical approaches in otolaryngology*. New York: Thieme.

Titze, I. R. (1990). Interpretation of the electroglottographic signal. *Journal of Voice, 4*, 1–9.

Titze, I. R. (1992). Rationale and structure of a curriculum in vocology. *Journal of Voice, 6*, 1–9.

Titze, I. R. (1994). *Principles of voice production*. Englewood Cliffs, NJ: Prentice Hall.

Titze, I. R., Luschei, E. S., & Hirano, M. (1989). Role of the thyroarytenoid muscle in regulation of fundamental frequency. *Journal of Voice, 3*, 213–224.

Tjaden, K. (2000). An acoustic study of coarticulation in dysarthric speakers with Parkinson disease. *Journal of Speech and Hearing Research, 43*, 1466–1480.

Tomblin, J. B., Morris, H. L., & Spriestersbach, D. C. (1994). *Diagnosis in speech-language pathology.* San Diego, CA: Singular.

Toohill, R. J. (1975). The psychosomatic aspects of children with vocal nodules. *Archives of Otolaryngology—Head and Neck Surgery, 101*, 591–595.

Trost-Cardamone, J. E. (1989). Coming to terms with VPI: A response to Loney and Bloem. *Cleft Palate Journal, 26*, 68–70.

Trudeau, M. D. (1998). Paradoxical vocal cord dysfunction among juveniles. *ASHA SID3 Newsletter, 8*, 11–13.

Tsui, J. (1999, September/October). *Explain the differences among Botox, NeuroBloc, and ITX: Are there differences in the degrees of success?* International Dystonia Symposium Summary, 11–12.

Tucker, H. M. (1997). Combined surgical medialization and nerve-muscle pedicle reinnervation for unilateral vocal fold paralysis: Improved functional results and prevention of long-term deterioration of voice. *Journal of Voice, 11*, 474–478.

Tucker, H. M. (1999). Long-term preservation of voice improvement following surgical medialization and reinnervation for unilateral vocal fold paralysis. *Journal of Voice, 13*, 251–256.

Tucker, H. M., & Lavertu, P. (1992). Paralysis and paresis of the vocal folds. In A. Blitzer, M. F. Brin, C. T. Sasaki, S. Fahn, & K. S. Harris (Eds.), *Neurologic disorders of the larynx.* New York: Thieme Medical.

Turvey, T. A., Vig, K. W. L., & Fonseca, R. J. (1996). *Facial clefts and craniosynostosis principles and management.* Philadelphia: Saunders.

Van Riper, C., & Irwin, J. V. (1958). *Voice and articulation.* Englewood Cliffs, NJ: Prentice Hall.

Veivers, D., & Laccourreye, O. (2000). Supracricoid partial laryngectomy for severe laryngeal stenosis. *Archives of Otolaryngology—Head and Neck Surgery, 126*, 663–664.

Velasco, M. G., Ysunza, A., Hernandez, X., & Marquez, C. (1988). Diagnosis and treatment of submucous cleft palate: A review of 108 cases. *Cleft Palate Journal, 25*, 171–173.

Verdolini, K. (1999). Critical analysis of common terminology in voice therapy: A position paper. *Phonoscope, 2*, 1–8.

Verdolini, K., Hess, M. M., Titze, I. R., Bierhals, W., & Gross, M. (1999). Investigation of vocal fold impact stress in human subjects. *Journal of Voice, 13*, 184–202.

Verdolini, K., Ramig, L. O., & Jacobson, B. (1998). Outcome measurements in voice disorders. In C. M. Frattali (Ed.), *Measuring outcomes in speech-language pathology.* New York: Thieme Medical.

Verdolini, K., Titze, I. R., & Fennell, A. (1994). Dependence of phonatory effort on hydration level. *Journal of Speech and Hearing Research, 37*, 1001–1007.

Verdolini-Marston, K., Sandage, M., & Titze, I. R. (1994). Effect of hydration treatments on laryngeal nodules and polyps and related voice measures. *Journal of Voice, 8*, 30–47.

Victoria, L., Graham, S. M., Karnell, M. P., & Hoffman, H. T. (1999). Vocal fold paralysis secondary to cardiac countershock (cardioversion). *Journal of Voice, 13*, 414–416.

Vinturri, J., Alku, P., Lauri, E.-R., Sala, E., Sihvo, M., & Vilkman, E. (2001). Objective analysis of vocal warm-up with special reference to ergonomic factors. *Journal of Voice, 15*, 36–53.

Vitek, J. L. (1997). Stereotaxic surgery and deep brain stimulation for Parkinson's disease and movement disorders. In R. L. Watts & W. C. Koller (Eds.), *Movement disorders: Neurologic principles and practice.* New York: McGraw-Hill.

Vogel, D., Carter, J. E., & Carter, P. B. (2000). *The effects of drugs on communication disorders* (2nd ed.). San Diego, CA: Singular.

Von Berg, S., Watterson, T. L., & Fudge, L. A. (1999). Behavioral management of paradoxical vocal fold movement. *Phonoscope, 2*, 143–147.

von Leden, H. (1988). Legal pitfalls in laryngology. *Journal of Voice, 2,* 330–333.

von Leden, H., Abitbol, J., Bouchayer, M., Hirano, M., & Tucker, H. (1989). Phonosurgery. *Journal of Voice, 3,* 175–182.

Walsh, P. (2000). *Physician's desk reference* (54th ed.). Montvale, NJ: Medical Economics.

Wang, E., Kompoliti, K., Jiang, J. J., & Goetz, C. G. (2000). An instrumental analysis of laryngeal responses to apomorphine stimulation in Parkinson's disease. *Journal of Medical Speech-Language Pathology, 8,* 175–186.

Warren, D. W. (1989). Aerodynamic assessment of velopharyngeal performance. In K. R. Bzoch (Ed.), *Communicative disorders related to cleft lip and palate.* Austin, TX: PRO-ED.

Warren, D. W., Hairfield, W. M., & Dalston, E. T. (1990). The relationship between nasal airway size and nasal-oral breathing in cleft lip and palate. *Cleft Palate Journal, 27,* 46–52.

Warren, D. W., Odont, D., Drake, A. F., & Jefferson, U. D. (1996). The nasal airway in breathing and speech. In S. Berkowitz (Ed.), *Cleft lip and palate with an introduction to other craniofacial anomalies: Perspectives in management* (Vol. 2). San Diego: Singular.

Warrick, P., Dromey, C., Irish, J., & Durkin, L. (2000). The treatment of essential voice tremor with botulinum toxin A: A longitudinal case report. *Journal of Voice, 14,* 410–421.

Wasz-Hockert, O., Lind, J., Vuorenkoski, V., Partenen, T., & Valanne, E. (1968). *The infant cry.* London: Heinemann.

Watanabe, H., Takemoto, S., Matsuo, H., Okuno, E., Tsuji, T., Matsuoka, M., Fukaura, J., & Matsunaga, H. (1994). Studies on vocal fold injection and changes in pitch associated with alcohol intake. *Journal of Voice, 8,* 340–346.

Watterson, T., Cox, T. L., & McFarlane, S. C. (1998). Speech intelligibility using four different electric-neck larynges. *Phonoscope, 1,* 21–26.

Watterson, T., Hansen-Magorian, H. J., & McFarlane, S. C. (1990). A demographic description of laryngeal contact ulcer patients. *Journal of Voice, 4,* 71–75.

Watterson, T., Lewis, K. E., & Deutsch, C. (1998). Nasalance and nasality in low pressure and high pressure speech. *Cleft Palate—Craniofacial Journal, 35,* 293–298.

Watterson, T., Lewis, K. E., & Homan-Foley, N. (1999). Effect of stimulus length on nasalance scores. *Cleft Palate—Craniofacial Journal, 36,* 243–247.

Watterson, T., & McFarlane, S. C. (1992). Adductor and abductor spasmodic dysphonia: Different disorders. *American Journal of Speech-Language Pathology, 1,* 19–20.

Watterson, T., McFarlane, S. C., & Menicucci, A. L. (1990). Vibratory characteristics of Teflon-injected and noninjected paralyzed vocal folds. *Journal of Speech and Hearing Disorders, 55*(1), 61–66.

Webster, D. B. (1999). *Neuroscience of communication* (2nd ed.). San Diego, CA: Singular.

Weinberg, B. (1980). *Readings in speech following total laryngectomy.* Baltimore: University Park Press.

Weinstein, G. S., Laccourreye, O., Brasnu, D., & Laccourreye, H. (2000). *Organ preservation surgery for laryngeal cancer.* San Diego, CA: Singular.

Weismann, J. L., & Curtin, H. D. (1995). The current approach to imaging the larynx. In J. S. Rubin, R. T. Sataloff, G. S. Korovin, & W. J. Gould (Eds.), *Diagnosis and treatment of voice disorders.* New York: IGAKU-SHOIN.

Welch, G. E., Sergeant, D. C., & MacCurtain, E. (1988). Some physical characteristics of the male falsetto voice. *Journal of Voice, 2*(2), 151–163.

Whurr, R., Lorch, M., Lindsay, M., Brookes, G. B., Marsden, C. D., & Jahanshahi, M. (1998). Psychological function in spasmodic dysphonia before and after treatment with botulinum toxin. *Journal of Medical Speech-Language Pathology, 6,* 81–91.

Wierzbicki, M. (1999). *Introduction to clinical psychology: Scientific foundations to clinical practice.* Boston: Allyn & Bacon.

Wilder, C. N. (1998). Speech pathology and the professional voice user. In R. T. Sataloff (Ed.), Vocal health and pedagogy. San Diego, CA: Singular.

Williams, C. E., & Stevens, K. N. (1972). Emotions and speech: Some acoustical correlations. Journal of the Acoustical Society of America, 52, 1238–1250.

Williams, J. K., Ellenbogen, R. G., & Gruss, J. S. (1999). State of the art in craniofacial surgery: Nonsyndromic craniosynostosis. Cleft Palate—Craniofacial Journal, 36, 471–485.

Wilson, D. K. (1987). Voice problems of children (3rd ed.). Baltimore: Williams & Wilkins.

Winholtz, W. S., & Ramig, L. O. (1992). Vocal tremor analysis with the Vocal Demodulator. Journal of Speech and Hearing Research, 35, 562–573.

Wirz, S. (1992). Voice disorders and their management (2nd ed.). San Diego, CA: Singular.

Witzel, M. A. (1989). Commentary. Cleft Palate Journal, 26, 199–200.

Witzel, M. A., Rich, R. H., Margar-Bacal, E., & Cox, C. (1986). Velopharyngeal insufficiency after adenoidectomy: An 8-year review. International Journal of Pediatric Otorhinolaryngology, 11, 15–20.

Wolfe, V. I., Ratusnik, D. L., Smith, F. H., & Northrop, G. (1990). Intonation and fundamental frequency in male-to-female transsexuals. Journal of Speech and Hearing Disorders, 55, 43–50.

Wolfe, V. I., & Steinfatt, T. M. (1987). Prediction of vocal severity within and across voice types. Journal of Speech and Hearing Research, 30, 230–240.

Woo, P., Colton, R., Casper, J., & Brewer, D. (1991). Diagnostic value of stroboscopic examination in hoarse patients. Journal of Voice, 5, 231–238.

Woo, P., Colton, R., & Shangold, L. (1987). Phonatory airflow analysis in patients with laryngeal disease. Annals of Otology, Rhinology, and Laryngology, 96, 549–555.

Woodson, G. (1998). Endoscopy and stroboscopy. In A. Blitzer, H. C. Pillsbury, A. F. Jahn, & W. J. Binder (Eds.), Office-based surgery in otolaryngology. New York: Thieme.

Wyke, B. (1983). Neuromuscular control systems in voice production. In D. M. Bless & J. H. Abbs (Eds.), Vocal fold physiology: Contemporary research and clinical issues. San Diego, CA: College-Hill.

Yamaguchi, H., Yotsuktira, Y., Sata, H., Watanabe, Y., Hirose, H., Kobayaskhi, N., & Bless, D. (1993). Pushing exercise program to correct glottal incompetence. Journal of Voice, 7, 250–256.

Yanagihara, N. (1967). Significance of harmonic changes and noise components of hoarseness. Journal of Speech and Hearing Research, 10, 531–541.

Yanagisawa, E., & Driscoll, B. P. (1995). Laryngeal photography and videography. In J. S. Rubin, R. T. Sataloff, G. S. Korovin, & W. J. Gould (Eds.), Diagnosis and treatment of voice disorders. New York: IGAKU-SHOIN.

Yanagisawa, E., Isaacson, G., Kmucha, S. T., & Hirokawa, R. (1989). Selection of video cameras for stroboscopic videolaryngoscopy: A comparison of fiberscopic, telescopic, and microscopic documentation. Annals of Otology, Rhinology, and Laryngology, 98, 15–20.

Yang, S., & Mu, L. (1989) A study on the mechanism of functional dysphonia. Journal of Voice, 3(4), 337–341.

Ylitalo, R., & Hammarberg, B. (2000). Voice characteristics, effects of voice therapy, and long term follow-up of contact granuloma patients. Journal of Voice, 14, 557–566.

Yorkston, K. M., Strand, E., Miller, R., Hillel, A., & Smith, K. (1993). Speech deterioration in amyotrophic lateral sclerosis: Implication for the timing of intervention. Journal of Medical Speech-Language Pathology, 1, 35–46.

Young, J. M., & McNicoll, P. (1998). Against all odds: Positive life experiences of people with advanced amyotrophic lateral sclerosis. Health and Social Work, 23, 35–40.

Younger, D. S., Lange, D. J., Lovelace, R. E., & Blitzer, A. (1992). Neuromuscular disorders of the larynx. In A. Blitzer, M. E. Brin, C. T. Sasaki, S. Fahn, & K. S. Harris (Eds.), Neurologic disorders of the larynx. New York: Thieme Medical.

Yumoto, E., Sanuki, T., & Hyodo, M. (1999). Three-dimensional endoscopic images of vocal fold paralysis by computed tomography. Archives of Otolaryngology—Head & Neck Surgery, 125, 883–890.

Zeitels, S. M., & Sataloff, R. T. (1999). Phonomicrosurgical resection of glottal papillomatosis. *Journal of Voice*, *13*, 123–127.

Zemlin, W. R. (1998). *Speech and hearing science: Anatomy and physiology* (4th ed.). Boston: Allyn & Bacon.

Zraick, R. I., LaPointe, L. L., Case, J. L., & Duane, D. D. (1993). Acoustic correlates of vocal quality in individuals with spasmodic torticollis. *Journal of Medical Speech-Language Pathology*, *1*, 261–269.

Zraick, R. I., & Liss, J. M. (2000). A comparison of equal-appearing interval scaling and direct magnitude estimation of nasal voice quality. *Journal of Speech and Hearing Research*, *43*, 979–988.

Zraick, R. I., Liss, J. M., Dorman, M. F., Case, J. L., LaPointe, L. L., & Beals, S. P. (2000). Multidimensional scaling of nasal voice quality. *Journal of Speech and Hearing Research*, *43*, 989–996.

Zraick, R. I., Nelson, J. L., Montague, J. C., & Monoson, P. K. (2000). The effect of task determination of maximum phonational frequency range. *Journal of Voice*, *14*, 154–160.

Zwirner, P., Murry, T., & Woodson, G. E. (1993). Perceptual-acoustic relationships in spasmodic dysphonia. *Journal of Voice*, *7*, 165–171.

Zwitman, D. H., & Calcaterra, T. C. (1973). The "silent cough" method for vocal hyperfunction. *Journal of Speech and Hearing Disorders*, *38*, 119–125.

Author Index

Subject Index

About the Author

Dr. James L. Case is a professor in the Department of Speech and Hearing Science at Arizona State University. He received his master's and doctoral degrees from the University of Utah. He is a member of the American Speech-Language-Hearing Association, the American Cleft Palate–Craniofacial Association, and the Arizona Speech-Language-Hearing Association. He is a Fellow in the American Speech-Language-Hearing Association and has been granted the Honors of the Association from the Arizona Speech-Language-Hearing Association. He is a member of the Southwest Craniofacial Team in Phoenix. Dr. Case was chosen as an outstanding teacher in the College of Liberal Arts and Sciences at Arizona State University. He has presented workshops on the clinical management of voice disorders in many states and in Brazil and Japan. He and his wife, Diane, have four children, all of whom are married, and 13 wonderful grandchildren.